TABLE OF CONTENTS

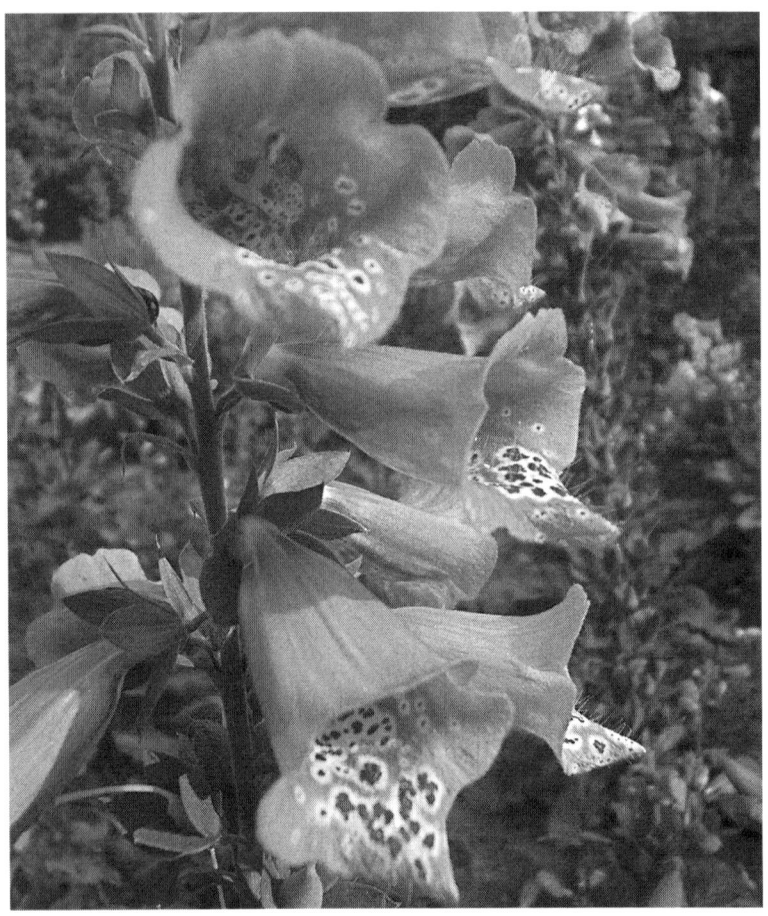

Foxglove - Early source of digitalis

This heart acts not as central king or pump, but as the circulation itself, sensitive to many things in many places. **JAMES HILLMAN**

The blood is not propelled by pressure, but rather moves with its own biological momentum and with its own intrinsic flow pattern.
RALPH MARINELLI

Only a reductionist science would need to "prove" the ridiculously obvious: that our hearts are perceptual organs, crucial to our humanness. **BUHNER**

The intellect is powerless to express thought without the aid of the heart. **THOREAU**

As a man thinketh in his heart, so is he. **PROVERBS 23:7**

ROGERS' SCHOOL OF HERBAL MEDICINE

VOLUME THREE:

CARDIOVASCULAR SYSTEM

ROBERT DALE ROGERS RH (AHG)

COVER
Top: Hawthorn berry
Middle: Lily of the Valley
Bottom Left: Candytuft flowers
Bottom Right: Scotch Broom

Copyright © Prairie Deva Press 2014 by Robert Dale Rogers.

All rights reserved.

No portion of this book, except for a brief review,
may be reproduced, or copied and transmitted,
without permission of author.

This book is for educational purposes only. The suggestions, recipes and historical information are not meant to replace a medical advisor. The author assumes no liability for unwise or unsafe usage by readers of this book.

For those interested in using herbal medicine, seek the advice of a professional.

THE CARDIOVASCULAR SYSTEM

The cardiovascular system consists physically of the heart, arteries, and veins.

Cardiovascular disease has been the number one cause of death in North America, every year since 1918.

The American Heart Association estimated that some 58 million citizens had one or more type of heart disease in 1998, with yearly costs of more than $250 billion. The numbers have increased dramatically in past fifteen years.

Liver health plays a key role in cardiovascular health and herbs for that important organ are covered in that book. Kidney health also plays a role in hypertension, and this will also be covered in another volume.

The respiration system plays a role in cardiovascular health, as our diaphragm and breathing also help propel blood. Muscle tension, of course, makes our muscles and heart work harder, suggesting that Tai Chi, Yoga and Qi Gong all help promote heart health, as does the capacity, metaphysically speaking, to love and receive love.

The heart produces a number of hormones, acting more like an endocrine gland than a mechanical pump. It is an organ of feeling and is more than a muscle that pumps blood.

Blood courses through the arteries like two cyclonic vortexes, one clock-wise and the other counter. The heart does not "pump" the blood but influences speed and volume through judicious production of hormones.

In fact, we have three brains, including the gut brain and heart brain. The heart may be the most important endocrine gland in the body, producing a hormone that effects the limbic system or the ancient or emotional brain.

Work by neurocardiologists has discovered that nearly two-thirds of the cells in our heart are neural, not muscle cells as previously thought. The ganglia of these nerves are linked to every major organ in the body. Nearly half of these neural cells help translate information coming from various parts of the body and respond appropriately.

The other half carry on a discussion with our brain in a manner we still don't fully understand.

There are 40,000 sensory neurons relaying information from the heart to the brain, leading some researchers to call it the "little brain".

The heart communicates via nervous system, hormones, blood pressure waves and electro-magnetic fields. In fact, the heart emits more electrical activity than the brain, up to sixty times greater in amplitude, and an electro-magnetic field 5000 times stronger than brain.

The neurons within the heart enable it to learn, remember and make decisions that are independent of the brain's cerebral cortex.

For greater insight into this and related emotional and spiritual connection, I highly recommend *The Secret Teachings of Plants* by Stephen Harrod Buhner.

A few definitions are in order:

Arteriosclerosis- This comes from the Greek, meaning " hardening of the arteries", suggesting loss of arterial elasticity, and associated thickening.

Atherosclerosis- This is a form of above that involves the buildup of plaque and fats on the interior lining of the blood vessel.

Arrhythmia- This is a loss of rhythm or irregular heart beat of the heart. Disturbances of the sinoatrial node are believed to cause this electrical impulse disturbance.

Tachycardia- This is a quickening and speeding up of the heart beat, sometimes arrhythmic, and at times simply accelerated.

Myocarditis, pericarditis and endocarditis are swollen, inflammatory conditions of the heart muscle, sheath surrounding the heart and heart muscle lining respectively.

Congestive Heart Failure (CHF) is the result of the inability to nourish, cleanse and strengthen the heart. Advanced forms create fluid buildup in the lungs, liver, and ankles, creating conditions such as pulmonary edema.

Hyperlipidemia- This is a condition of high serum levels of cholesterol and triglycerides in the bloodstream.

LDL- low density lipoproteins

HDL- high density lipoproteins

Triglycerides- saturated fatty acids- related to high blood sugar

In herbal medicine, cardiotonics do not always contain cardiac glycosides and yet have benefit to the heart and blood vessels.

Ginkgo leaf (*Ginkgo biloba)* is a peripheral vasodilator and vascular tonic. It is covered under the volume on Brain.

Cardioactive herbs are utilized whenever there is a picture of congestive heart failure (CHF). This introductory course does not provide enough scope to include anything addressing mild CHF, most often associated with aging.

Cardioactive herbs contain cardiac glycosides that create positive inotropic activity, increasing heart contractibility, frequency, volume of blood and stimulate cardiac function.

Circulatory stimulants include Cayenne (*Capsicum annuum*) and Rosemary (*Rosmarinus officinalis*).

Rosemary and Stinging Nettle are especially useful in cases of low blood pressure.

Linden, Garlic and Mistletoe (*Viscum album*) all assist in lowering blood pressure. Combining Garlic and fish oils (omega 3 fatty acids) speeds up the benefit.

Prickly Ash (*Zanthoxylum americanum),* Gingko (*G. biloba*) and Ginger (*Zingiber officinale*) are peripheral vasodilators.

Ginger has been found to contain gingerol, which mildly increases the heart's force of contraction by stimulating beta adrenergic activity.

Prickly Ash is considered a diffusive, meaning that it causes a diffusing sensation through the nerves, and is thus considered a nervous stimulant as well. Many herbs do not fit into tidy categories, and Prickly Ash is one of these.

Cardiac palpitations can be related to a number of related conditions.

In the case of nervous involvement, Valerian (Nervous system), Motherwort, and Linden Flowers should be considered.

Although these herbs also possess mild anti-spasmodic activity, the use of Crampbark (*Viburnum opulus*) could be considered in cases of hypertension with stress, headache, bronchitis, indigestion, and premenstrual syndrome. See Reproductive system.

Varicose veins, poor venous tone and congestion , leading to hemorrhoids, phlebitis and thrombophlebitis can be helped by herbs such as Horse Chestnut (*Aesculus hippocastanum*), Witch Hazel (*Hamamelis virginiana*), and Stoneroot (*Collinsonia canadensis*).

It should be noted that Witch Hazel tincture is used for internal use, and the distilled water or hydrosol for external use.

Rutin, a bioflavonoid derived from Buckwheat or the white inner peel of citrus fruit also helps to strengthen fragile capillaries and tone vascular tissue. This is generally taken as a supplement with meals for a period of time.

Shepherd's Purse (*Capsella bursa pastoris*) is an important hemostatic herb that helps reduce internal bleeding. It is frequently used by herbalists for menstrual and birthing issues, and will be discussed further under Reproduction.

Both Alfalfa and Stinging Nettle are rich in vitamin K, which plays a role in blood clotting, as well as bone formation. Both of these herbs will be covered in other volumes.

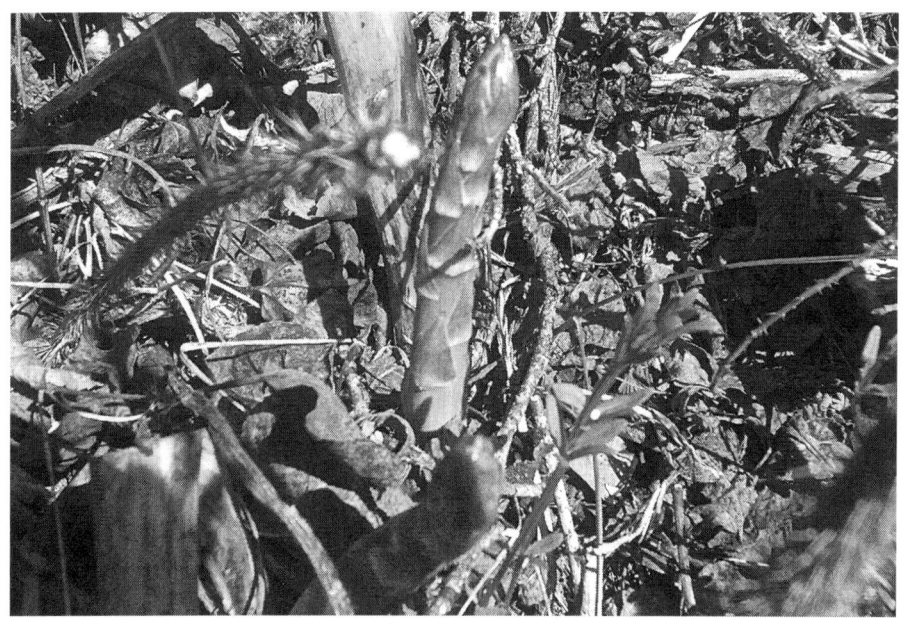

Asparagus shoot

ASPARAGUS
(*Asparagus officinalis* L.)
PARTS USED- spear, seeds, root

RIDDLE

"What killed a queen to love inclined,
What on a beggar oft we find,
Show, to ourselves if aptly joined,
A plant which we in bundles bind."

ANSWER: Asp-a rag-us

Asparagus, enjoyed in the food, brings lusty desires to men.

MATTHIOLUS

"No herbe is sooner converted into good blood than Asparagus".

LANGHAM

Aspagago was added to the Latin language from the Greek, as a synonym for "foremost, tender, choice". The root word **SPARGAO**, according to Jonathan Roberts, "has lustful, tumescent connotations, and it is easy to see how the connection was made."

Asparagus is derived from a Greek word signifying "the tearer", in allusion to the spikes of some species. Or it may be originally from the Persian **SPURGAS**, meaning a shoot; and hence the Greek **ASPHARAGOS** meaning to shoot or sprout, or **ASPARASSO**, to rip or tear. Another possibility is "as long as one's throat", as diners swallowed the spears whole. I do myself!

Swallow Grass derives from this allegory, or may be a dialect variation of asparagus. Sparrow may come from the Greek **SPORGILOS** sparrow or **PSAR** for starling.

The ancient Greeks believed asparagus grew from a ram's horn sunk in the ground. Later, the English, filled trenches with cattle horns, to improve on cultivation. There are only 20 varieties of asparagus considered edible out of the 300 known.

Ancient Egyptian tomb drawings from 4000 BC suggest the use of asparagus for urinary and nematocidal application.

Asparagus is one of those spring vegetables that I look for with great anticipation. When the spears start popping from the perennial root, they can grow up to ten inches in a single day!

The female spear is slimmer, while the superior male is shorter and stockier. It has long been found that modern cultivars, like Saxon, Franklin, and Lucullus, are all male.

They are a pre-historic vegetable, dating back to the age of reptiles, when horsetail and ferns were the dominant plants. Wild Asparagus is one of the oldest known plants, believed grown in the salt marshes of Asia Minor, thousands of years before recorded history.

Asparagus has distinct male spears that are skinny, and the plump female that matures into an inedible fern with green, and later orange berries.

The Greeks said the roots were the most beneficial, containing the strongest qualities. Hippocrates recommended it for overweight patients with blemished skin. Dioscorides recommended chewing the root for aching teeth.

Galen considered Asparagus root one of the 4 opening roots, a remedy that stimulates both kidney and liver function.

The Greeks and Romans boiled it so quickly that the phrase- "faster than asparagus is cooked" came to mean quickly or in a jiffy.

Liebig, or some other early scientist, said asparagin helped develop form in the human brain.

Its phallic symbolism is unmistakable, and yet its reputation as a sex food is not without foundation, being rich in vitamin E, and other constituents.

The Greeks used asparagus for bridal garlands and for weaving baskets in the harvest festival, Thesmophoria. They dedicated the vegetable to Aphrodite, the goddess of love, and Perigune, the goddess of the cornfield, who hid to escape her wicked father.

The Perfumed Garden, a book of aphrodisiac foods from the Arab tradition in the 14th century says this about asparagus, or Halioun, as it was known:

"He who boils Halioun and then fries them in fat, and then pours upon them the yolks of eggs with pounded condiments, and eats every day of this dish, will grow very strong for the coitus and find a stimulant for amourous desires."

This was important in harem situations, where the coveted position of favourite wife was not the prettiest or best in bed, but the woman with greatest number of sons. Every mother-in-law prodded the sheik to grant her daughter's wish for more, to which he could never plead exhaustion.

Culpepper picked up on this and wrote, "the decoction of the roots boiled in wine and being taken fasting several mornings together, stirreth up bodily lust in man or woman."

The shoot is slightly warming, with a bitter and pungent flavour. It helps to reduce phlegm and mucous, sooth constipation, and other mucous membranes.

In Italy, the root is decocted as a diuretic and sedative; as well as in cardiac disorders. A wine was traditionally made from asparagus in Britain.

In both China and India, the vegetable has been used for a wide range of ailments from toothaches, cancer, parasites, rheumatism, and constipation.

Sparrow Grass is a common Chinese name for the herb.

The seeds are used to treat parasitic diseases and the roots for fatigue (yin tonic).

In Japan, Asparagus root, or Tenmondo, as it is known in Kampo medicine, is used to nourish the kidneys. It is considered a gentle diuretic that is appropriate for diabetics.

In Mexico, it is considered a heart tonic, while the Spanish minced either the buds of the fruit, or the long branches and decocted it in bits of chicken broth for urine retention.

In various formulas, the root is used to relieve fevers, and dry respiratory symptoms like dry mouth, unproductive coughs, and phlegm difficult to expel.

The spears and extracts have been used for cleaning the face and drying acne and sores.

When Alexander the Great invaded Bactria he was smitten by the legendary Princess Roxana, reputed to have the most beautiful complexion in the world. She loved to roam the salt marshes, picking her favourite food, asparagus. Today, the topical application of the plant powder has a drying effect on acne.

Even the berries can be used. Dutch physicians boiled the berries, and had barren women eat them with vinegar, oil, and sugar to become fertile. The berry seeds can be roasted and ground as a coffee substitute.

My dearly departed friend and mentor, Jean Chancelet from Joussard, grew lots of asparagus in his lakeshore garden.

Every spring he would rejuvenate his kidneys and liver, with steamed asparagus and dandelion bud/garlic salads. It was said to be President Jefferson's favorite vegetable.

Sauer, in his Compendius Herbal, mentions collecting asparagus in flower and after drying in shade, added a bag to a barrel of poor wine to enhance the flavour and odour.

Asparagus juice sprayed on tomato plants will protect them from nematodes, including rootknot, sting, stubby root and meadow nematodes. Tomatoes protect against asparagus beetles due to their solanine content, making the two good companion plants. Asparagus and parsley also enjoy each other's company.

The Cherokee infused the introduced plant for rickets; while the Iroquois decocted the root with other plants as a foot soak for rheumatism, or with tree barks before meals as a blood cleanser.

MEDICINAL

CONSTITUENTS- stalk- asparagine, asparagose, chelidonic acid, arginine (1.8%), histidine, tryptophan, tyrosine, succinic acid, sarsapogenin, blumenol, ferulic acid, asparenyn, asparenyol, methyl esters of asparagusic acid, coniferin, steroid saponins, folacin (18 ppm), rutin, flavonoids, filicins A and B, filicinosides C and D, pentosans (70,000 ppm), phenylalanine, lutein, hyperoside, isoquercitin. Recently identified antioxidants include racemofuran, asparagamine A, and racemosol.
Viamins A, B, C, K and E, and minerals including, potassium and zinc (12-124 ppm), vanadium (0.3-2 ppm), strontium (19-200 ppm), zirconium (2.4 ppm), and boron (104 ppm); PUFA (up to 12,387 ppm), and lysine (18,710 ppm). It has a potassium/sodium ratio of 15:1.
root- nine steroidal glycosides (asparagosides), coniferin glycoside, bitter glycosides such as officinalisin I and II, inulin flavonoids, bitter steroid saponins including sarsasapogenin, asparagin, arginin, smilagenin, diosgenin (0.27-0.46%) tyrosine, and aspartic saponin I. Aspartic acid (sulphur containing), esters 3-mercapto-butyric acid, alpha-aminodimethyl-gamma-butyrothetin, 3-methylthio-isobutyric acid, diisobutyric acid disulphide, berstein and chelidonic acids, methyl mercaptan, asparagose, asparagusic acid, choline, purine, inulin, mannan.
seed- alanine (1.8%)

Asparagus shoots contain vitamin E and folic acid, both good for the heart.

Folic acid acts as a floodgate, controlling the amount of homocysteine allowed in the bloodstream.

When folate drops, the other levels rise, causing damage to the tender arteries supplying blood to the heart and brain.

Enlarged heart associated with edema and congestive heart failure may be relieved by the use of this plant in the diet.

Folic acid is needed by pregnant women to prevent neural tube (spinal cord) birth defects in their babies.

Folate is a protectant against cancer. Studies have revealed that low levels of folate in blood are directly related to developing colon cancer. Folic acid is useful, as well, in those prone to iron-deficient anemia.

Glutathione is a small amino acid grouping and powerful anti-oxidant that helps mop up free radicals. According to the NCI, asparagus is the richest food source of glutathione, an important anti-oxidant also found in Sea Buckthorn fruit, and Milk Thistle seed. It contains rich sources of selenium, another important anti-oxidant.

Asparagus contains histones, protein compounds believed to act as cell growth normalizers on cancer cell division. This may partially explain the reversal of various cancers, involving cooked asparagus juice.

Asparagine is a strong, persistent diuretic that will give some individuals a violet odour to their increased urine flow. The peculiar smell of asparagus urine is due to the sulphur compound S-methylprop-2-enethioate, a metabolite of asparagusic acid. Mitchell SC & Waring RH, *Phytochemistry* 2014 97 5-10. The presence of two adjacent sulphur atoms leads to chemical reactivity, including the ability to substitute for alpha lipoic acid in an alpha keto-acid oxidation system.

It relates to aspartic acid, or asparagin, an amino acid that some people lack the enzyme to break down. It is a harmless phenomenon.

According to Darcy Williamson, there are two camps regarding the unique smell. Some scientists believe that about half the population have a gene that breaks down the sulphur compounds into smelly odors. Others think it is in the olfactory nerves and that only half of us have the gene that enables detection of odor that is there.

William LeSassier called it a nutritive diuretic as it strengthens the kidneys rather than forcing them to work harder.

It relieves swollen ankles caused by edema of cardiac origin. In Germany, the root, but not the stalk, is approved for use as a diuretic for helping prevent kidney stones and treat urinary tract inflammation.

Asparagus juice can be very helpful in some cases of acne, by alkalizing an overly acidic body aggravated by sugar and fats. Eczemas, especially weeping types, respond favorably. It is useful in lifestyle related hyperuricemia, but may not help those who have inherited the tendency. The cooked shoots dissolve uric and oxalic acid that can aggravate arthritic and gouty conditions.

Michael Moore suggested, "The fresh root tincture seems to be a useful preventative in times of stress and dehydration (as in training or heat) for the anabolic mesomorph with a history of passing uric acid-cysteine stones; use 60-90 drops up to four times daily in a glass of water."

Keep in mind that asparagus contains purines that in large amounts, over time, can be aggravating to gouty conditions, cystitis and rheumatism. Discretion is advised.

Recent work by Ting Sun et al, *J Ag Food Chem* 2007 55:1 found rhamnosidase activity can change rutin in asparagus juice to quercitin-3-glucoside, an even more potent anti-oxidant.

Work by Dae Sik Jang et al, *J Ag Food Chem* 2004 52 found new compounds in asparagus stalks that exhibit significant COX-2 inhibition. Regulation of the COX pathway is associated with anti-inflammatory and cancer chemo-preventative activity.

The cladophylls and bottom stems significantly reduced systolic and diastolic pressure, fasting glucose and total cholesterol in a trial of 28 volunteers. Nishimura M et al, *Journal Traditional Complementary Medicine* 2013 3:4 250-5.

A compound in stems inhibits ACE activity in the kidney, preventing hypertension and protecting kidney function. Sanae M & Yasuo A, *J Ag Food Chem* 2013 61:23 5520-5.

Enzyme treated asparagus extracts show cytoprotection of neuronal cells, and attenuate effects of cognitive impairment in SAMP8 mice. Sakurai T et al, *Nat Prod Commun* 2014 9:1. Another mouse study fouond a strong anti-anxiety effect from water extracts of stems. Cheng L et al, *Evid Based Complement Altern Med* 2013 Nov 20.

Asparagus contains SMM, or S-methylmethionine, which is found in cabbage and malt barley. This substance helps sooth gastric and duodenal ulcers, and may be of value in Crohn's disease of the ileum, as well as irritable bowel syndrome. The inulin and other starches help grow *Bifidus* bacteria in the colon.

Asparagus juice can be purchased commercially, and is a great aid in those desiring a weight loss regime. Take two tablespoons of the fresh juice morning and evening for two weeks.

The root is chopped into small cubes and dried for later use in gout and uric acid related joint inflammation.

The root tea is a gentle but effective laxative, when an irritating cathartic would be ill advised; such as the elderly or during pregnancy. By promoting secretions, it relieves dry intestinal conditions. Dry coughs with little phlegm, and heat, such as croup and chronic bronchitis, may also benefit from the addition of asparagus root to a herbal formula especially when accompanied by excess urination of low specific gravity.

Asparagus root is an aphrodisiac, and helps increase breast milk flow in new mothers.

Althein (asparagin) occurs in crystals, and is found in the root of marshmallow and licorice. One grain three times daily was used traditionally for relieving dropsy from disease of a dilated heart. Syrup of asparagus is used medically in France, for rheumatism.

Asparagus contains rutin, an important bioflavonoid that keeps blood vessels healthy, and strengthens varicose veins. Rutin helps antidote radiation and x-rays to some degree.

The herb is highly recommended in rheumatism and congestive heart failure associated with pulmonary edema; as well as of some benefit in mild diabetes.

Asparagus root moistens dry and irritated eyes, especially related to kidney or liver dehydration. Asparagin and resins in asparagus combine to gently sedate the heart, calm palpitations and nervous excitement.

The plant contains anti-viral agents. Aquino R et al, *Journal of Chemotherapy* 1991 3:5.

In studies by Shimoyamada et al, anti-fungal activity was detected in the bottom cut thrown away as factory waste.

The activity was specific to *Candida* and *Cryptococcus* species, *Trichophyton rubra* (0.5 ug/ml), *Microsporum gypseum* 0.5 ug/ml and *Epidermophyton floccosum* (1.0 ug/ml). The saponin is identical to collettinside III from *Dioscorea collettii*. *J of Science Food and Agric* 1996 72:4.

According to Bensky and Gamble, the root tea has antibiotic effect on 3 strains of *Streptococcus* and *Staphylococcus aureus* skin infections.

Shao-Yu et al, presented a paper at the *Ninth International Asparagus Symposium* in July 1997, showing asparagus spears contain two saponins (oligofurostanosides) that effectively inhibit the growth of human leukemia cells. *Cancer Letters* 1996 104:1.

Previous work by Sasaki et al, showed fibres isolated from the vegetable had mutagen absorbing or cancer preventing properties. *Chemistry Abstracts* 1986 104.

Scientists have identified steroidal glycosides in asparagus roots. Smilagenin, one of many steroidal saponins, is used in the partial synthesis of cortisone and other steroids.

Asparagusic acid has been shown, in clinical studies, to be nematocidal. Asparagine is an amino succinic acid, vital to biological energy yielding cycles.

The inedible bottom part is often discarded as waste. Wang J et al, *J Sci Food Agric* 93:6 1492-1498, found saponins in these old stems suppress cancer cell lines of breast, colon and pancreas through modulation of Rho GTPase signaling pathway.

The young shoots and leaves both up-regulate alcohol dehydrogenase and aldehyde dehydrogenase, protecting the liver from toxic insult. Kim et al, *J Food Sci* 74:7. This suggests a use for leaf parts that are usually discarded.

White, or blanched asparagus activates TRAIL apoptosis in human colon cancer cell lines. Bousserouel S et al, *Int J Oncol* 2013 43:2 394-404.

The seeds have some use in powdered form for calming stomach upset, as well as remedies for neuritis and rheumatism.

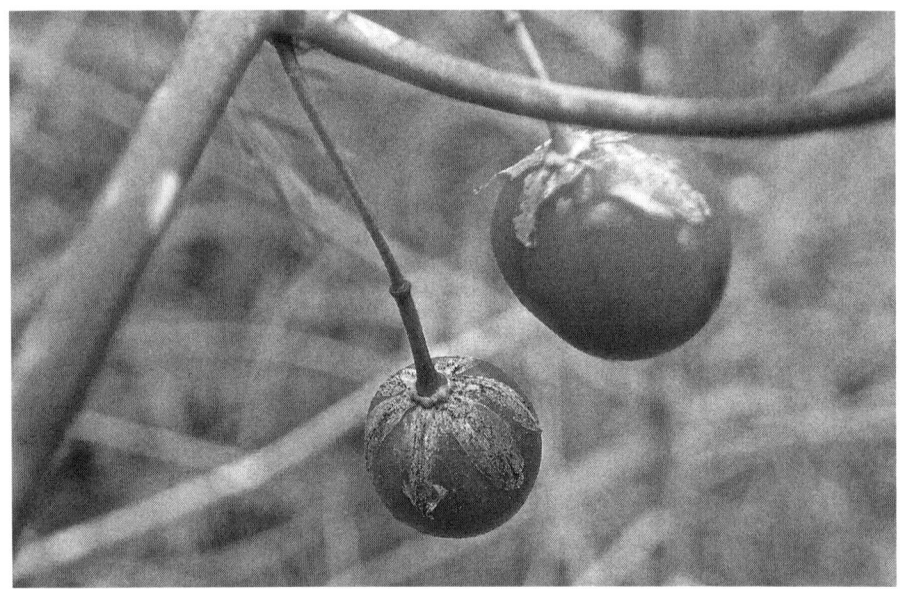
Asparagus berries

The seeds are used to relieve toothaches, stimulate hair growth, and to treat cancer.

The berries have been reportedly used as contraceptives. Barnes et al, *Lloydia* 1978; Brondegaard *Planta Medica* 1973 23:2. I would advise caution with this information.

Methyl mercaptan can be irritating in cystitis, and may aggravate the bladder during an acute infection. Asparagus stalks are relatively high in purines that can aggravate gout; but the root is fine. Asparagus root preparations are not to be used by individuals with cardiac edema or inflammatory kidney disease, according to German Commission E monographs. In some women, kidney stimulation during the last trimester of pregnancy could be undesirable. Individuals with gout or acute joint rheumatism, those individuals of a nervous, easily irritated temperament, or suffering diarrhea may find asparagus aggravates their condition. Asparagoside A is a sapogenin used to manufacture compounds of the pregnane series of pharmaceuticals.

HOMEOPATHY

Common Garden Asparagus (*A. officinalis*) has a marked and immediate action on urinary secretion. It is useful in cases of heart palpitation with oppression in the chest, intermittent pulse, and pain in the left shoulder and heart, associated with bladder disturbances. Complaints from suppression of perspiration.

The urination may be frequent with fine stitches in orifice of the urethra, and a burning sensation. It can be used for cystitis, associated with mucous, pus and stones or small gravel.

It is also indicated for rheumatic pain in the back, especially near the shoulder and limbs.

The head may feel heavy, with profuse, thin fluids from the nose, or aching forehead in the morning. The throat feels rough, with coughing of copious, tenacious mucous.

It can antidote both Aconite (Monkshood) and Apis, so choose appropriately.

DOSE- Sixth potency. The mother tincture is prepared from the fresh root in fall. Proving by Buchner with four provers and tincture of shoots in 1840; clinical observations by Hering, Twentyman and Vithoulkas in *Materia Medica Viva*.

ESSENTIAL OIL

The dry roots of asparagus (*A. officinalis*) have been steam distilled and yield 0.0108% of dark, brown oil with an intensely acidic odour. The specific gravity is 0.8777, and contains palmitic acid.

The above ground asparagus contains asparagusic acid (1,2-dithiolane-4-carboxylic acid), dihydroasparagusic acid (3,3'dimercaptoisobutyric acid), and S-acetyldihydroasparagusic acid. All three act as growth inhibitors.

Oil has been isolated from the small pale rose flowers of the related *A. sprengeri*. The odour is intense and narcotic, resembling fatty aldehydes.

HYDROSOLS

The distilled water of asparagus should be used especially, by those who are inclined toward gravel, stones and lumbago. This purges the gravel and stones, as well as the scummy matter on which the stones form. This iscuretic possesses a first rate capacity for opening obstructions, and provokes the urine briskly. It controls dripping urine and jaundice, and fortifies against the cold evil or cold piss. It also loosens up the liver and spleen and in addition to the above ailments, when taken in 4-5 loth (two to 2.5 ounce) doses each morning and evening.   **SAUER**

Asparagus root, stalk and herb are all distilled into a water that is good for drying the urine out so quickly it smells like the water. It is for pain in the limbs and bladder, gout in the gut, opening stoppages of the liver and spleen, painful urination, pain in the head and yellow jaundice. Brunschwig, Book of Distillation 1530.

FLOWER ESSENCES

Asparagus flower essence helps eliminate hidden fears and negative thoughts, especially when picked up from the lower astral planes.
                                                            PEGASUS

Asparagus flower essence promotes peace of mind, a loving nature, a good memory and calm spirit.   **DARCY WILLIAMSON**

PERSONALITY TRAITS

My mother always told me you could assess someone's sexual abilities by the way they ate asparagus; and you can certainly assess their class bracket in this country. I remember being deeply anxious when a friend brought their latest flame to dinner and he ate his asparagus precisely with a knife and fork, leaving the tips!

After much experimentation I have found my mother to be totally accurate.   **WRIGHT**

MYTHS AND LEGENDS

The Greek myth of Perigune begins with Perigune's father, Sinus, who lived on the island of Corinth and personified the north wind. Sinus was a bandit, and he acquired the name Pitokamptes, or Pine Bender, for his ability to bend the tops of pine trees down to the ground with his bare hands. Sinus typically asked travelers to help him, and when they did, he quickly released his hold and sent the unwitting victims catapulting to their deaths. The Greek hero Theseus put an end to that by releasing his hold first. After killing Sinus, he noticed the daughter Perigune hiding behind an asparagus bush, terribly frightened. She was talking to the asparagus, and promising the plant that if it hid her safely, she would never harm it. The use of asparagus in her myth likely reflected its phallic symbolism.

Perigune emerged from behind the asparagus and immediately fell in love with Theseus. Soon she bore him a son, Melanippus, who became the ancestor of the Ioxids, who venerated asparagus.

TAMRA ANDREWS

RECIPES

ROOT JUICE- Two tablespoons up to 4 times daily.

STEM JUICE- Three tablespoons 3x daily. The stems are steamed and then juiced.

DECOCTION- Simmer one teaspoon of dry root to one cup of water for 45 minutes. Drink between meals.

It should not be used in loss of appetite or diarrhea, or if there are aches and pains from influenza.

ROOT TINCTURE- 2-5 ml. The fresh root is prepared at 1:2; the dry at 1:5, both with 50% alcohol.

ROOT POWDER- 10-50 grams twice daily.

TO GROW- Plant asparagus in a sunny area, with light, well-mulched sandy soil. Trenches of well-aged manure are ideal, with plants set one foot apart. Do not cut for first two years. You can start from seed, but first year roots are inexpensive.

In the 1800's it was recommended that salt be added to the soil. Obviously, asparagus is a salt marsh plant and can tolerate some salinity. In the 1950s when herbicides replaced salt for weed control, the *Fusarium* fungus became a problem. Studies by Cole et al, 1992 have shown that chlorine increases resistance to *Fusarium*.

NOTE- Animal studies suggest asparagus shoots reduce milk production.

ROCK GARDEN BROOM
(*Cytisus pilosa* L.)
PURPLE BROOM
(*C. purpureus* Scop. *var. procumbens*)
GOLDEN BROOM
(*C. ratisbonensis* Schaeff.)
SCOTCH BROOM
GREEN BROOM
(*C. scoparius* [L.] Link.)
(*Spartium scoparium* L.)
(*Sarothamnus scoparius* Koch.)
SHRUB BROOM
(*C. nigricans* L.)
PARTS USED- aerial parts

Sweep the house with blossomed brooms in May
You are sure to sweep the head of the house away.
The broom, yellow and bright, as bullion unalloyed her blossoms.
COWPER

O, the Broom, the bonnie, bonnie Broom,
The Broom o' the Cowden knowes,
Fain would I be in my ain country,
Herdin' my father's yowes. **TRADITIONAL SCOTTISH SONG**

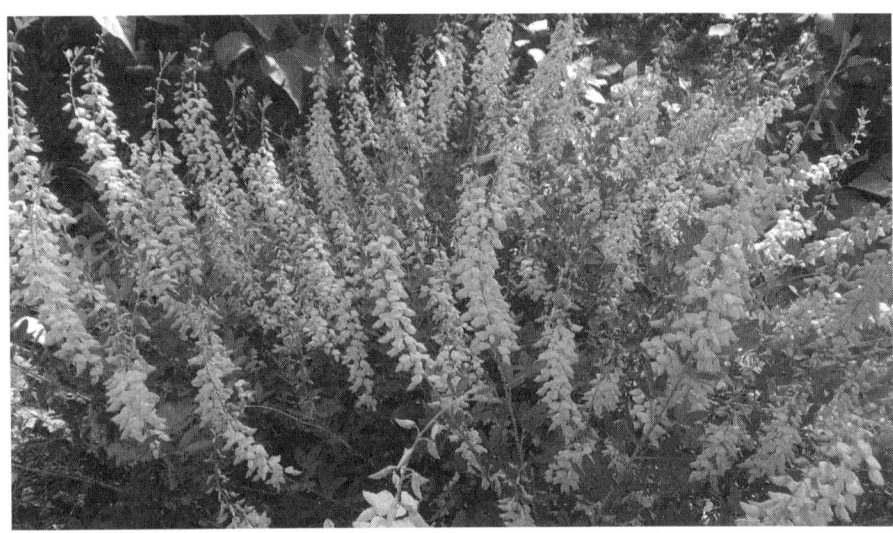

Shrub Broom

14

Broom is named for its former use to sweep floors in Scotland. Broom is derived in turn from the Anglo Saxon **BROM**, meaning foliage. Shrubs used to make brooms were called **BESOMS**.

In Holland, a ship with a besom tied to the top of the mast was advertising for a new owner. This led to the saying of a woman seeking a new husband, "she hangs out the broom".

Cytisus is from the Greek name for a shrubby clover **KUTISOS**, and in turn the Greek island of Cythera.

Pilosa means covered with long, soft hairs; purpureus means purple or violet, referring to the flower colour.

Broom is not remarkably hardy on the prairies, and yet a fine specimen can be found at the Devonian Gardens, southwest of Edmonton, a zone 3 climate. On the coast of British Columbia, grows the related Scotch Broom (*C. scoparius/Sarthamnus scoparius*). It is practically cursed as a noxious weed, after its introduction to Vancouver Island by Captain Walter Grant in 1850.

He picked up some seeds from the British consul in Hawaii, and although only three germinated near Sooke, they soon colonized most of southern Vancouver Island.

Gerard, the 17th century English herbalist wrote, "that worthy Prince of famous memorie Henrie 8, King of England, was woont to drinke the distilled water of Broome floures against surfets and diseases thereof arising". Spanish gypsies used the aromatic flowers as a perfumed cologne.

In those days, Broom was used instead of Hops, as bitter agent in making beer.

Gerard recommended the young flower buds be salted and vinegared like capers.

Various kings, and generals throughout Europe, have used Broom as a helmet crest or rallying symbol for troops in the field. Richard II of England portrayed it in his Great Seal, and its facsimile decorates his tomb. It is associated with Mars.

Broom extracts may be used externally for skin protection against oxidative damage. Gonzalez N et al, *J Photochem Photobiol B* 2013 Aug 5: 125.

Brooms, hardy to the harsh prairie climate, are in no danger of escaping and becoming too plentiful.

Although small, in comparison to their coastal cousins, our Brooms possess the same medicinal qualities.

The dried herb has been smoked by a number of people who claim that just one cigarette produces several hours of euphoria and calm. Sparteine resembles nicotine in some ways, but I doubt very much that the effects are that strong.

In Peru, broom is added to fermenting chichi, a corn beer, to improve inebriation. I can attest to that!

Other hardy species include *C. nigricans*, and *C. decumbens*.

MEDICINAL

CONSTITUENTS- flowering tops- various aklaloids including sparteine, and cytisine, various flavonoid glycosides, including scoparin, vitexin, luteolin, and quercitin, the isoflavonoid beta sitosterol, tyramines, bitters, epinene (epinephrine), dopamine, tannins and essential oils.

Broom flowering tops are used for those individuals with low blood pressure and a weakened heart condition.

The herb is a useful in cardiac edema, relying upon both its diuretic and peripheral vaso-constrictive properties.

It combines well with both Hawthorn and Lily of the Valley in the treatment of cardiovascular conditions, but due to its hypertensive action, is not recommended for those suffering high blood pressure.

Dr. Rudoph Weiss, in Herbal Medicine, refutes this.

"It is sometimes stated that broom will elevate blood pressure and is therefore indicated in cases of hypotension. This is not the case. The drug is able to get rid of the extra-systoles that are not uncommon with this condition and therefore give subjective relief. Low blood pressure as such is not among its indications".

Weiss felt that Broom acts on the conductivity of the heart. The active constituents "slow down the pathologically accelerated stimuli arising in the atrium, reduce increased irritability in the conduction system and regulate the action of the heart, evidently improving venous return at the same time. Atrial and ventricular fibrillation disappear. Extra systoles also respond to long term treatment." He believed the action similar to quinine and quinidine, but much gentler and less dangerous.

"Like quinine, broom stimulates uterine contractions, which gives it styptic properties. Broom is therefore used in obstetrics much in the same way as quinine."

Broom can be useful in excessive menstruation, especially in women nearing the menopausal transition. It combines hemostatic effect with its astringent venous decongesting action.

Although contraindicated in pregnancy due to its uterine stimulating properties, this same activity gives good response in stalled labor, postpartum bleeding and slow uterine involution.

Work by Raschak, *Arzneimittel-Forschung* 1974 24:5 showed sparteine can slow the heart, inhibit arrhythmia and extra systoles by damping overstimulation of the system responsible for conducting nerve impulses through the heart.

Work by Thies, *Pharm in Unserer Zeit* 1986 6 found sparteine to work in this manner.

Other investigation by Steinegger and Hansel, *Lehrbuch der Pharmakognosie* 1972 found scoparoside (a glycoside) largely responsible for the herb's diuretic effects.

The plant tips are best collected in early spring when alkaloids are still high, and the yellow flowers are rich in flavonoids.

Sparteine is responsible for the cardiotonic effect, while scoparin possesses the diuretic effect. Tyramine acts as an indirect sympathicomimetic, vasoconstrictor and hypotensive.

As such, it falls into what Traditional Chinese Medicine would term Heart Yang deficiency, with scanty urine, water retention and cardiac insufficiency.

As Peter Holmes notes: "Again, from the clinical point of view, it's interesting to note that Broom top is the inverse of Valerian root- a bitter cooling remedy for heart weakness, as opposed to a pungent warming one. This simply indicates using Broom for those tending to hot conditions rather than cold ones".

Broom is indicated in long-term treatment, as it is largely non-toxic. In fact, its best work appears to be over the long term, making it of special use in treating extra-systolic activity and post infectious myocarditis with arrhythmia.

It is not recommended for acute or chronic angina or tachycardia, but for those individuals suffering mild cardiac insufficiency with water retention and occasional skipped heartbeat. It improves venous bloos return.

Sparteine inhibits sodium and potassium transport across the cell membrane, and in cardiac cells this mimics the activity of drugs such as quinidine and procainamide.

It undergoes oxidative metabolism via the P-450 cytochrome activity of the liver and should not be combined with beta-blockers, and other cardiac drugs.

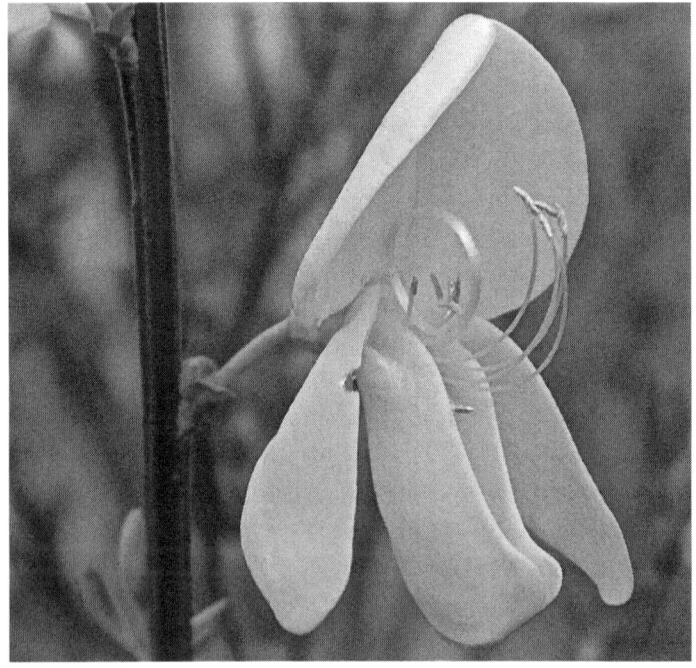

Scotch Broom

18

Although sparteine exhibits quinidine like effects, cytosine is nicotine-like in action with ganglion stimulating activity greater than ganglion blocking.

Initially, it causes excitement and then paralysis of the autonomic nervous system. Plants grown in shade contain less sparteine.

Cytisine, also found in *Baptisia, Lupinus, Aconitum* and *Genista* species, docks to the acetylcholine receptors of the central nervous system, the ganglia, and neuro-muscular endplate. This effect is similar to nicotine and causes strychnine-like spasms, hallucinations and unconscious-ness. During World War I, the leaves of various plants containing cytosine were used as a tobacco substitute. These cigarettes caused the same nausea to non-smokers as a real tobacco, while those already addicted did not notice any discomfort. In fact, toxicity symptoms are parallel to nicotine poisoning.

Cytisine protects cortical neurons, in part, by inhibiting the level of GluN2B-containing NMDA receptors and regulating Bcl-2 family. *Neurotoxicity* 2013 34 219-25.

HOMEOPATHY

Broom (*Spartium Scoparium*) is indicated in heart disturbance and fear, stabbing pains in the heart and palpitations at night that make the patient get up and walk about. The condition is aggravated by lying on the left side.

Excited and quarrelsome feeling, nervous excitement and hysteria. Anxiety, melancholy, depression, no drive or ambition, sadness and palpitations.

Dreams of glorifying and idealizing oneself, and of dead people.

DOSE-Mother tincture to 2x and 30C. The mother tincture is prepared from the fresh flowers *of Cytisus scoparius*. Hinsdale attempted first proving on three students in 1918. Proving by Schier with two females and four males with tincture, 2x, 10x in 1896; proving by Mezger with 27 provers with tincture, 2x and 4x in 1951-2.

HYDROSOL

Broom water is good against the stone, yellow jaundice, provokes urine, and helps the bladder and kidneys, as well as joints.

BRUNSCHWIG

FLOWER ESSENCES

Scotch Broom flower essence helps promote positive and optimistic feelings about the world and future events; helping promote sun-like forces of caring, encouragement and purpose.

When imbalanced, a person may feel weighed down and depressed, or overcome with pessimism and despair, especially regarding one's personal relationship to world events. Scotch Broom helps alleviated these feelings. **FLOWER ESSENCE SOCIETY**

Purple Broom flower essence is for those individuals frustrated with their spiritual development or lack thereof. It helps those persons who feel constrained by the dogma of religious institutions.

It can benefit the transition from feeling unworthy in God's presence, to experiencing one's own God within. **PRAIRIE DEVA**

SPIRITUAL PROPERTIES

Broom (Cytisus) appears in various forms, but all show the same unusual feature. The small, delicate leaves grow on hard angular shoots or stems. Those at the base of the stem each have three lobes and are attached with a stalk, while those at the top of the stem are simple leaves with no stalk.

This difference in the form of leaves between one end of the shoot and the other seems to indicate that the leaves and the stems originally came from two species that through crossing were reborn in the broom. Thus the qualities of broom are renewal and rebirth, as evidenced by the bright yellow flowers that grow from the previous year's growth. The broom's roots fix nitrogen, feeding and renewing the soil it grows in, and although the broom burns readily in fire, it soon grows back again, being reborn from its ashes like the mythical Phoenix.

BOUCHARDON

I use broom flowers to increase my awareness of the environment. Scotch broom is a mild psychotropic drug. It is not nearly as strong as the commonly misused drugs, but it has the effect of allowing one to be more aware of the world. It is as though one can see with the third eye, as odd as that may sound. I think that this is an important thing to do at this time, as humans attempt to rediscover a benevolent interaction with nature.

Plants do affect us. Understanding the deeper messages coming to us through interactions with plants is important for our survival.

MITCHELL

Broom is a symbol for astral travel, a process described in the language of the shaman and the Druid as Otherworld journeying, whereby a person's spirit leaves the body and travels independently of earthly reality. This links broom with Morpheus, the Greek god of dreams, and with his equivalents from other belief systems. Otherworld experience can be linked to broom's narcotic properties, although intoxication is not in any way essential to astral travel nor to exploring related aspects of the mind outside general experience. Narcotics can open this door, but the effect can be illusory. However, with both great healing potential and narcotic effect, broom has long, firm-rooted associations with healers and magicians, with wise women and shamans. **GIFFORD**

PERSONALITY TRAITS

Broom is helpful each time we have to make a new beginning after a period of change. Life is always challenging us to change, whether in the major steps described below, or in taking the most banal of day to day decisions. Broom helps us to integrate the challenges we are presented with. **BOUCHARDON**

The Broom person is often large, and can retain much abdominal fluid. General fluid secretion and excretion will be unbalanced, and there will be a danger of uric acid related problems.

Today's Broom may have these symptoms originating from either the spleen, or the blood related processes the spleen manages. Anemia in varying degrees may be present, and may be intermittently present together with disordered iron absorption and metabolism. In acupuncture terminology, this is a "wet (damp)-spleen" person.

Emotionally, Broom can be loud and brash, but sometimes, quite the opposite. There can be self-effacing and self-critical depressed periods.

The negative chronic Broom can strut about, acting and declaiming. They can be headstrong, verging on manic behaviour in extreme cases; the depression that follows can be typical too. As well as the tender spleen and consequent blood quality problems, there can be adrenal incompetence and massive fluid secretion-excretion imbalances. Volatile, unpredictable, geniuses, mad professors and even mentally unstable; are all valid comments on their natures. Creatures of extremes of feeling, these may cause massive surges in blood pressure.

Severe cardiac symptoms may eventually present. The heart grows tired of these surges in blood pressure, and failing kidneys put an even more uneven load on the major circulation. The spleen may become grossly enlarged, and very tender even to the touch.

The Positive Broom heart is beating strongly and without extra or dis-rhythmic pulses.

Spleen begins to reduce in size, and more stable diuretic hormone production and distribution is the improvement in adrenal glands and through kidneys. Fluid excretion is better managed. Emotionally, this person is subject still to extremes.

Although treatment with Broom and other herbs will reduce the peaks and raise the valleys of these emotional zigzaggers, giving them (and you!) a relatively calmer ride through life, their tendencies are always exaggerated emotional and physical responses to stimuli. Adrenaline pumps, the heart flutters, and strong secondary pulses may be found. Those around them often spend much of their nervous energy trying to placate and stabilize them in order to avoid another up and another down. **HALL**

Broom is a wonderful Witch's name. Of course, we jokingly refer to secretive Witches as being "in the broom closet", and we have many old customs and uses for the magical broom in circle and out.

Broom is a good name for people of either sex, and is just as applicable to a youthful person as it is to a crone. Broom is a name which suggests fertility, cleansing, honor, protection and freedom.
MCFARLAND

RECIPES

TINCTURE- 10-15 drops three times daily in warm water before meals. The fresh flowering tops are prepared in a 1:5 tincture at 25% alcohol.

INFUSION- 2-4 grams of flowering tops in 180 mls of water three times daily. Dosage is tablespoon three to four times daily. Do not use the tops before flowering, or the seeds.

POWDER- 5-15 grains.

CAUTION- Do not use Broom in pregnancy, high blood pressure, or for those taking MAO inhibitors, the latter due to the tyramine content of both twigs and flowers. Its activity may well interfere with a pacemaker. No kidding!

Sparteine is a marker of the metabolic activity of CYP2D6. About 6-9% of Caucasians are poor metabolizers so interaction with drugs is likely.

BUCKWHEAT

(*Fagopyrum esculentum* Moench)
(*F. sagittatum* Gilib.)
(*Polygonum fagopyrum* L.)
TARTARY BUCKWHEAT
(*F. tataricum* [L] Gaertn.)
(*P. tataricum*)
WILD BUCKWHEAT
BLACK BINDWEED
(*P. convolvulus* L.)
(*Fallopia convolvulus* [L.] Á. Löve)
(*Bilderdykia convolvulus*)
(*Tiniaria convolvulus*)
PARTS USED- seeds, flowers, leaves, hulls, pollen.

Soba is deep. The more you know, the more there is to know.

HIROMI ARAI

Kasha on the spoon, baby will walk soon. **RUSSIAN SAYING**

When the husk gets separated from the kernel, almost all men run after the husk and pay their respects to that. It is only the husk of Christianity that is so bruited and wide spread in this world; the kernel is still the very least and rarest of all things. There is not a single church founded on it. To obey the higher law is generally considered the last manifestation of littleness. **THOREAU**

A field of Buckwheat...is a magnet in the days when birds are wandering. They love to linger many days in the stubble; and when bird music is rare, their occasional songs are precious to the ear.

FRANK BOLLES

Shchi and kasha, that's our real food. **RUSSIAN SAYING**

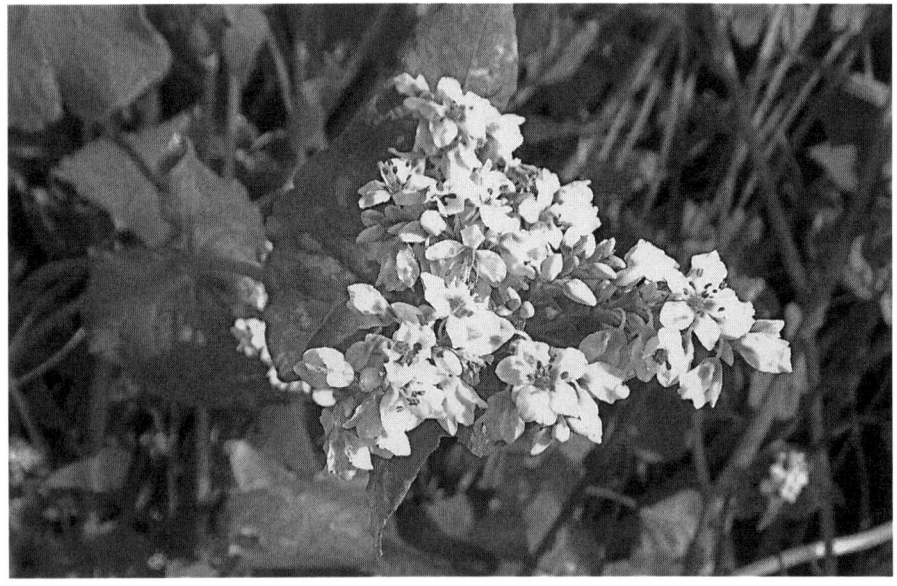

Buckwheat in full flower

Buckwheat may be a corruption of **BOEK-WEIT** from the Dutch. In German, it is known as **BUCHWEIZEN**, or Beech-wheat. In turn this is from a translation of the Latin **FAGOPYRUM**; **PHEGOS** meaning, beech, and **PYROS**, meaning wheat.

Or, maybe from the Scandinavian word for beech **BOC**, because the shape and colour of the grain resembles beech nut. Or, it is from the Scottish word "Buck", meaning the beech tree; and **WHOET**, meaning wheat.

My personal favourite is the old German **BUKWETEN**, meaning "goat's wheat", alluding to perceived inferiority to true wheat. Esculentum means edible.

Convolvulus is from Latin **CUM** or **CON**, for common bindweed, and **VOLVERE**, to roll, referring to the twining vine.

Polygonum means many knees or many seeds, both of which are true.

Buckwheat is native to central Asia, but widely grown throughout the world. It is believed to have originated from the wild perennial *F. cymosum*, then cultivated in China for over one thousand years.

It was introduced into Europe about 1440 AD. It's French name, **BLE SARRASIN**, alludes to Middle Eastern origins.

On the prairies, it is grown for it's nutty cereal, as a green manure crop, and nectar for bees. Worldwide, over two million hectares are under cultivation with two-thirds in northern Russia. Estimated value of our largely exported crop is $5.5 million annually.

Canadian farmers planted 50,000 acres in 1998, 30,000 of those in Manitoba. Average yield is about 20 bushels per acre, with $8-9 per bushel at present time.

Rutin content, plant height and herbage yield are highest in rows 50 cm apart, at sowing rate of 80 kilograms per hectare. Rutin content of buckwheat appears related to solar radiation, with long summer days producing the richest buckwheat flour.

Work by Lee et al, *Prep Biochem Biotech* has found hairy root culture can be used to produce rutin in large amounts. More about that later.

When used for choking out weeds, including persistent Canada thistle, or as a turned over green manure, higher rates would be used.

Buckwheat honey is a rich, dark and aromatic treat that goes great on buckwheat pancakes or waffles.

One acre of buckwheat will allow bees to produce up to 150 pounds of honey per season.

The groats, raw or roasted, are known as kasha, and used in many traditional European dishes like cabbage rolls. Kasha is from the medieval Russian, meaning "meal, feast or porridge" in reference to any grain, whereas in North America it means roasted or cooked

25

buckwheat. Russian expressions such as "you can't make kasha with him", means you won't get anywhere with him.

Another saying "he's got kasha in his head", means he's mixed up, and "you can't spoil kasha with butter" means you can't have too much of a good thing.

Do not use the term kasha for buckwheat in Japan. Kasha is a ghoul, in that country, that feeds off human bodies left unguarded before cremation, a type of cannibalistic spirit.

Of all the grains, or more correctly, a fruit seed, buckwheat has the longest transit time, and is therefore most filling and stabilizing of blood sugars. It must be remembered that sunlight rapidly deteriorates buckwheat. It must be stored in the dark.

In parts of Germany, it is used in beer making, and at one time to make gin.

Blini is a Russian buckwheat pancake, and in France the galette is a crepe from flour. In India, the flour is called kutu or kootu, and used in pakoras, chapattis and even liquors.

Buckwheat grits cooked in buttermilk with hot sugar syrup are a Dutch favorite.

Studies in Brazil have confirmed buckwheat flour does not contain toxic prolamines that affect celiac and other gluten-sensitive patients. It should, however, be used with caution by those with skin eruptions, as it may aggravate. Likewise, it is not recommended for nervous, and emotionally unstable individuals with high fevers, thirst and high blood pressure.

The Hindu of India eat buckwheat on fasting days; while in Japan, it is made into soba noodles. The grain is steamed, dried and eaten when boiled, or made into Manju, a small cake or bread. Recently, Japan's oldest woman died at age 114. She was vegetarian who ate soba and played the guitar until the ripe age of 107.

Eating soba noodles on New Year's Eve ensures good luck with money for the year.

The dried seeds are infused to make a nutty beverage.

Japanese goldsmiths use the dough to gather gold dust in their shops.

Buckwheat noodles and a hearty black polenta (Polenta nera), are made from buckwheat flour in northern Italy.

Koto is a recent, and first, black seed-coat buckwheat released as a new variety in Canada. It is desired for its increased size and plumpness, and starch content by the Japanese market.

Kade Research from Morden, Manitoba is a major player in the development of new type and varieties of buckwheat. They have successfully crossed the frost-resistant tartary buckwheat with common buckwheat, and other related species from China. Clayton Campbell, who formed the company, went to Asia to collect native buckwheat samples. There, he met a Japanese plant breeder who had found a new self-pollinating species in the mountains of China. He gave Campbell a few seeds, and the rest is history.

The new cross is frost tolerant, and gives 30-40% increased yield. The new cross shows a 50% freeze-off at -7° C, significantly extending the season.

Buckwheat requires fairly high levels of phosphorus in the soil to set seed and mature.

A study conducted by Takahashi et al, at the Yokohama City University School of Medicine, found buckwheat allergies and sensitivity are not rare in school children. They suggest buckwheat be withdrawn from school lunch meals to avoid anaphylactic type reactions, similar to the peanut allergy in this country.

A round worm vermifuge product has been prepared from the plant in Japan.

The young leaves make an acceptable potherb, and the thicker stems can be added to cattle feed.

As a green crop, it is best ploughed back under at full blossom; very useful for choking out weeds on organic soils.

The seeds are a rich source of lysine, compared with other cereal grains; making it a valuable food for domestic animals, and if plowed under, a green manure for poorer soils.

In studies conducted by Sure (1955), buckwheat flour at an 8% level is one of the best sources of high biological-value protein in the plant kingdom.

Work conducted for the Kissei Pharmaceutical Company found a 20% protein level of buckwheat increases muscle mass, elevates carcass protein and water, and reduces body fat in animals.

Buckwheat sprouts grow up to five inches long and are rich in B vitamins such as choline and inositol. They take up to ten days to mature and are ready when 90% of the hulls have fallen off. Make sure you use the seed, as both the groat and kasha cannot sprout. Buckwheat and tartary buckwheat sprouts are rich in anthocyanins.

Eight day sprouts possess the highest anti-oxidant, anti-cholesterol and triglyceride content. Ten day-old sprouts contain the highest rutin and GABA. Lin et al, *J Ag Food Chem* 2008 56:4.

The high lysine content of seeds may compensate for limited supply in other cereals, leading to a superior mixed-blend for livestock feed, and cereal products.

The Iroquois made use of buckwheat after its introduction to the New World. They made a decoction of the plant that was given when " the baby is sick because of the mother's adultery". I don't know if the Cree of Alberta used it medicinally, but they named it **KISEPAMICOWIN**.

Buckwheat is associated with the feminine, and planet Venus.

A few grains are added to incense burned to attract money, and are symbolically kept in kitchen to guard against poverty. In magic, buckwheat is ground into flour, and sprinkled around the house to keep away evil, or to form a magic circle on the floor.

Buckwheat hulls are used in Japan, and elsewhere as stuffing for pillows. It is the perfect material to offer support to the neck and head, and at the same time offer maximum cooling effect.

Sleeping on a pillow of buckwheat hulls is said to not only produce a more restful night's sleep but will give you more visual and prophetic dreams. I did not notice.

The hulls used are larger seed varieties easily grown on the prairies.

An article in *Allergy* 2001 56 found several children using the pillows developed nighttime wheezing and coughs, suggesting the possibility of buckwheat sensitization.

Buckwheat is used as a late-season honey crop. It has a long blooming period, especially in late summer, when other sources of nectar are limited. Nectar flow requires adequate moisture, clear still days, and cool nights. Under these conditions, an acre of buckwheat may yield up to 150 pounds of honey.

It is not uncommon for beehives to produce ten pounds of honey per day while foraging buckwheat. The plant yields more nectar in morning, so beekeepers should avoid afternoon visits, and grumpy bees.

Fagopyrin is a pigment closely related to hypericin in St. John's wort, but less phototoxic. Nonetheless, it can cause problems in some livestock.

The flowers yield a brown dye, the stems a blue colour with mordants.

In China, the ashes of buckwheat are combined with lime, and applied to virulent sores, unhealthy granulations, and centipede bites.

Buckwheat is a hyper-accumulator of lead and cadmium, even on soils with moderate amounts.

Fagopyrin is not activated by ultraviolet light but to a different part of sunlight spectrum.

Individuals who are sensitive to fagopyrism complain of feeling numb, fuzzy, buzzing impression when they scratch the skin.

Their hands feel painfully cold when exposed for very short period of time to cold objects or water. Eyes become sensitive to light and skin may swell, itch and remain abnormal for days.

The seeds of tartary buckwheat are gathered and used like common buckwheat. The plant is still grown for food in the mountains of southwest China, northern India, and Nepal. Up to 30 years ago, it was cultivated in parts of Slovenia.

Although the yield is less, the leaf rutin content is greater by 45-80%, thereby producing a greater yield of rutin per acre.

The seeds contain 11% protein, and are more suited to poultry feed than the angular buckwheat seed.

Work by Fabjan et al, *J Agric Food Chem* 2003 51 found rutin levels in tartary seeds in the range of 0.8-1.7% compared to buckwheat seeds at 0.01%.

Liu et al, *J Ag Food Chem* 2008 56:1 found rutin in Tartary Buckwheat five times higher than in the cultivated crop.

Tartary Buckwheat contains an anti-breast cancer protein. Guo et al, J *Ag Food Chem* 55:17.

Sinapic acid rutinoside shows activity against feline calicivirus, strain F9, a noro virus surrogate. Katayama S et al, *J Agric Food Chem* 2013 61:40.

Wild buckwheat (*Polygonum convolvulus*) closely resembles the field bindweeds. It is an introduced annual to cultivated fields, with vine-like stems, and small green flowers.

The seeds are available in large quantities from seed-cleaning plants, and could be utilized by farm animals. Harrold et al, *Journal of Animal Science* 1980 showed wild buckwheat possesses a 52.5% crude protein digestibility and a 2.206 kcal digestible energy per gram of dried matter. The amino acid composition is not much different than buckwheat; and the high lysine content of achenes may be of use in completing protein of other grains.

The seeds were tested for potential toxicity by Wilsdorf et al, in Berlin. They found *P. convolvulus* seed fed at 5 and 20% rations showed incipient impairment of liver metabolism in rats after 38 days. Do not feed it to your pet rat!

MEDICINAL

CONSTITUENTS-*F. esculentum* plant- rutinoside or quercitin-3-rutinoside (1-6%), dianthrone fagopyrin, proto-fagopyrin, oxalic acid, hyperin, a piperidine alkaloid, quercitrin, quercetin, isovitexin and vitexin. Rutin is a practically odourless, yellow to mat green crystalline powder extracted from buckwheat.
seeds- metalloproteinase, amylose and amylopectin, 0.01% rutin, D-chiro-inositol, molybdenum.
immature seed- aspartic proteinase
flowers- rutin (20mg/100 grams), and naphthadianthrones mainly fagopyrin and frototfagopyrin.

F. tataricum- rutin (4-5% of dry leaf wt), 3',4',5,7-tetra-0-methyl-rutin, quercitin (2% of seed weight), kaempferol and kaempferol-3-0-rutinoside, and rutin-7-0-galactoside.
seed- 11% protein, high lysine, up to 1.7% rutin; quercetrin, quercitin.
P. convolvulus- proazulenes, rutoside, kaempferol, querctin and quercitoside, hyperoside, frangula-emodin, caffeic, chlorogenic and 4-hydroxycinnamic acid.
root- coumarin and derivatives.

Buckwheat has over 90% of the food value of non-fat milk solids, is gluten-free, and has nearly twice the lysine of wheat.

The name rutin is derived from the herb rue, which was the cheapest and most readily available source during the two World Wars. Rue contains rutinoside, also found in the Rutaceae family, which includes citrus fruits.

Yields for both Tartary and cultivated buckwheat yield about 15-25 kilograms of rutin per hectare from a single harvest. Seed setting (at approximately 50 days after sowing) gives the highest rutin yield. It has been noted that rutin content is closely connected with flowering, that later flowering cultivars produce a higher content of rutin.

Darker seed strains are preferred, by the Japanese, due to the perception of increased flavonoid and rutin content. Canadian researchers have bred strains, like Koto, for this desirable quality.

The top of buckwheat serves as the raw material for rutin, which is used in treating various circulatory disturbances like hemorrhoids, varicose veins and ulcers, combining well with horsetail. Rutinoside is used for retinitis, and rheumatic fever associated conditions.

Rutin has anti-oxidant properties, which give it potential as a food preservative. This anti-oxidant quality in buckwheat extracts has been examined by Yokozawa et al, *J Agric Food Chem* 2002 50 and found to inhibit the progression of kidney failure.

Rutin is anti-tumour, anti-mutagenic, anti-carcinogenic, a smooth muscle relaxant and estrogen receptor binder. It antidotes x-rays and other forms of radiation.

Buckwheat inhibits leukemia cell proliferation and growth by inducing cellular maturity. Wu et al, *J Med Food* 2011 114:1-2.

Rutin is broken down by healthy intestinal bacteria, to aglycone quercetin, and then to the anti-oxidant phenol 3,4-dihydroxyphenylacetic acid.

Work by Kim et al, *Int Immunopharm* 2003 3:1 suggests buckwheat possesses anti-allergic action due to inhibition of histamine release and cytokine gene expression in mast cells. Except those with allergic response, of course.

The buckwheat hulls contain anti-oxidant compounds, as described by Watanabe et al, in 1997 research conducted in Japan. They found 4.3 mg/100 grams of rutin in the hulls; and four other anti-oxidant compounds.

Kim et al, *J Agric Food Chem* 2003 51:6 found buckwheat hulls possess significant anti-oxidative and protein glycation inhibitory activity. The latter term refers to a role in anti-aging and diabetic complications.

The flavonols in flour possess even more powerful anti-oxidant properties, Quettier et al, *J of Ethnopharmacology* 2000 72:1-2.

Work by Hinneburg et al, *Pharmazie* 61:3 suggests buckwheat is better anti-oxidant than isolated rutin.

An application of the flour, made into a paste, can be applied to bring back the milk flow of nursing mothers.

Studies conducted by Wojcicki et al, in Poland 1995, found rabbits fed a high fat diet and buckwheat extract, had reduced atherosclerotic plaque formation on aorta.

The same study showed reductions in serum levels of insulin, increased testosterone, as well as decreased free radicals and lower cholesterol and triglycerides in the liver. Straight rutin, however, did not show the same effect.

Choi et al, *Phytomed* June 29 2007 found buckwheat germinated for 48 hours, increased rutin content by ten times and showed potent protection of fatty liver formation in an 8 week rat study.

In a three month study reported in *Phytotherapy Research* (1996) buck-wheat showed a 26.7% regression of diabetic retinopathy, as well as decreased total cholesterol, increased HDL cholesterol, and decreased blood serum levels of glycosylated hemoglobin.

A specific treatment for hemorrhage of the retina is to combine buckwheat with linden flowers.

Metalloproteinase is an enzyme in the seed similar to that in animal and bacterial origin. In studies by Belozersky et al, in Moscow, it was found to hydrolyse three peptide bonds formed by the amino groups of Lue15, Tyr16, and Phe25 in the oxidized B-chain of insulin. Amylose, a starch, and amylopectin a water-soluble fibre are absorbed very slowly, and helping improve glucose tolerance in type 2 diabetics. The slow absorption helps keep blood sugar from swaying and causing damage to kidneys and eyes.

Buckwheat cookies given to 62 female daycare workers in a double-blind, cross-over study found lower levels of inflammation and cholesterol. Weislander, Tohuku et al, *J Exp Med* 2011 225 2.

Fagopyritol, a constituent isolated from buckwheat, is effective in lowering the symptoms of type II diabetes.

Another constituent of buckwheat is D-chiro-inositol, a stereoisomer of myo-inositol. It is a component of a phospho-glycan endogenous to the human body that appears to be involved in the post-receptor insulin-mediated signaling pathway. The compound D-pinitol found in pine needles, lentils and other plants is similar in action, and may be converted to D-chiro-inositol *in vivo*.

One study found a 14-fold increase in mean serum concentration of D-chiro-inositol after giving D-pinitol to diabetic patients at 20 mg per kg of weight per day for four weeks.

Women with polycystic ovary syndrome show insulin resistance that may be due in part to a deficiency of D-chiro-inositol or defect in tissue availability or utilization. Baillargeon et al, *Diabetes Care* 2006 29:2; Nestler et al, *N Engl J Med* 1999 340:17.

Forty-four obese women with PCOS received 1200 mg of D-chiro-inositol or placebo for 8 weeks. More women in the first group ovulated and serum testosterone levels and insulin resistance improved as well. Rice et al, *Hum Reprod* 2005 20:2.

A human study by He et al, 1995, in China, found buckwheat taken at rate of 100 grams per day, lowered total serum cholesterol, and created higher ratios of high-density lipoproteins, that show protection against coronary heart disease.

Another human study at Johns Hopkins found people who consumed the most buckwheat had the lowest blood pressure.

Rutin normalizes an increased permeability of the capillarieswhich manifests as increased lymphatic circulation, increased protein discharge and tendency towards edema. It appears that rutin exerts an inhibitory effect on an enzyme, hyaluronic acid. For circulatory problems, rutin is best combined with vitamin C, such as rosehips or lemon juice.

Rutin is valuable to those suffering high blood pressure, as it strengthens and increases the efficiency of smaller blood vessels (the arterioles and venules).

When pressure is high, these small vessels are prone to breakage. It is useful, therefore, in temporal arteritis, and in visible pulsations of the carotid artery.

Rutin is virucidal for pseudo-rabies, and exhibits weak activity against vesicular stomatitis virus. Beladi et al, 1977.

And don't forget that buckwheat is excellent for those suffering celiac disease. Being free of gluten, it can be enjoyed in a variety of meals.

Buckwheat sprouts are rich in protein, amino acids, minerals and rutin; in fact 27 times higher than the seeds. They are easy to make, and use as a fresh vegetable (see below).

Buckwheat sprouts help lower hypertension and protect arterial endothelial cells from oxidation. Kim et al, *Phytother Res* Jan 2009.

Restless leg syndrome is the inability to keep the legs still, or associated with an itching, burning or prickly feeling that may be early manifestation of chronic venous insufficiency. Buckwheat, like blueberry leaves, can help capillary permeability. Faba beans, which increase dopamine production, also help reduce this sydrome.

Purple patches on the skin, due to capillary hemorrhage, are resolved.

Buckwheat herb tea has been found to relieve leg edema in those patients with chronic venous insufficiency. A single-centre, randomized, double-blind, placebo-controlled clinical trial of 77 patients in Germany, confirmed both the efficacy and safety of this treatment. Ihme et al, *Eur J Clin Pharm* 1995 50.

Pyorrhea, an infectious disease of the gums, is often related to bioflavonoid deficiency- and improved by rutin and vitamin C supplementation.

Rutin is a useful anti-histamine. Excessive histamine dilates small blood vessels that create leakage and inflammation.

Rutin and its metabolites inhibit bone loss both by slowing down bone resorption and increasing osteoblastic activity. Horcajada-Molteni et al, *J Bone Miner Res* 2000 15:11.

Rutin appears to be one of the best remedies for Ménière's Disease. Work by Moser et al, *J Larynogoogy and Otology* 1984 98 found in double-blind study that rutin, or hydroxy-ethyl rutosides reduce hearing loss and vertigo attacks.

Water extracts of the entire plant show activity against mycobacterium.

A trypsin inhibitor from the seed has been cloned and expanded into *E. coli*. The resultant organism inhibited proliferation of IM 9 human lymphoblastoid cells. Zhang et al, *Acta Biochim Biophys Sinica* 2007 39:9.

Leung et al, *J Peptide Sci* 2007 13:11 found an anti-fungal peptide in seed inhibits HIV and the L1210 leukemia cancer cells at a low concentration of 4.0 uM.

Polysaccharides, isolated from buckwheat, show potential for therapy in leukemia, based on differentiation. Wu & Lee et al, *J Food Med* 13:3.

Buckwheat honey has anti-oxidant content equal to the ascorbic acid related anti-oxidant content of tomatoes. Researchers at University of Illinois noted honey varies widely in colour, water, sugar, ash, nitrogen and metal content, and buckwheat honey has less water and more anti-oxidants.

P-hydroxybenzoic and p-coumaric acid are main components, and 3-methylbutanoic acid is main volatile.

Buckwheat honey was found as effective or better than dextromethorphan in a trial of cough relief on 105 children aged 2-18 years.

Buckwheat honey has been found to increase serum anti-oxidant capacity in human. *Journal Agric Food Chem* 2003 51.

Buckwheat honey is a traditional ingredient of Jewish honey wine, and gingerbread in France.

The immature seed contains appreciable amounts of aspartic proteinase, with milk clotting ability, and other areas of biotech interest.

The hull has been extract with 70% ethanol and then fractionated in work by Kim et al, *J Med Food* 2007 10:2.

Various fractions show significant effect against MCF breast cancer cell lines at 89-93%, human gastric carcinoma at 82% and sarcoma 180 cell lines.

All of the above led to the pharmaceutical journal, *Pharmazeutische Zeitung*, selecting Buckwheat as Medicinal Plant of the Year in 1999.

Tartary buckwheat is commonly used in India for various abdominal complaints.

Extracts of tartary buckwheat show activity against gram positive and negative bacteria.

Because it produces a high proportion of leaves and contains 45-80% more rutin than other buckwheat, it produces the greatest yield of rutin per acre.

Research on buckwheat and tartary buckwheat found leaf powder harvested from 42 day old plants exhibits the overall highest levels of GABA, rutin and anthocyanins; up to ten times higher than other plants. Suzucki et al, *J Ag Food Chem* 2009 57:1.

Tartary buckwheat contains an anti-tumor protein. Work by Guo et al, *J Ag Food Chem* 2007 55:17 found leaves and flowers at full bloom possess the highest anti-oxidant activity. The plant is often dried and powdered as a food colorant.

The herb regulates vascular tone. Ushida et al, *J Nutr Biochem* 2008 19:10.

Tartary Buckwheat sprouts contain vitexin, also found in passionflower. Work by Abbasi et al, suggests vitexin may modulate cholinergic receptors involved in memory. *Chin J Physiol* 2013 56:3.

The related Wild Buckwheat *(F. cymosum)*, **JIN CH'AIO MAI** rhizome is used in Traditional Chinese Medicine to treat lung problems and tumours.

Chan et al, *Life Sciences* 2003 72:16 found plant extracts inhibit cancer cells from lung, liver, colon, leukocytes and bone; whereas prostate, cervix, ovary and brain cancer cells were not affected. Ironically, cancer cells from the breast, MCF-7, were stimulated by the extract. Synergistic activity between the extract and daunomycin was noted in human lung cancer cell line H460. This chemotherapy drug is often used in acute leukemia.

HOMEOPATHY

Fagopyrum (Buckwheat) has an action mainly on the skin and itching.

If there is relief from bathing in cold water, and is made worse by scratching, touching or sunlight, then it is worth a trial. Like Urtica (nettles) and Bovista (puffball), the skin is hot, swollen, irritated, especially around the knees and elbows.

There may be itching around the eyes or ears, with a hot head that is better from bending backwards. The patient may be irritable or depressed, with an inability to study and poor memory.

One symptom that can lead to Fagopyrum is pain in the eyeballs, as if they were being squeezed out. The stomach may be acidic, with hot reflux, but ironically relieved by coffee. Persistent morning nausea, and drooling may also accompany this condition.

There may be pain around the heart, and throbbing in all the arteries that is made better by lying on one's back. The female may suffer an itchy vulva with yellowish discharge, and some burning pain in the right ovary. The neck muscles may be stiff and have a bruised sensation.

DOSE- Third and 12th potency. Mother tincture is prepared from the whole fresh plant when just mature. Proving by Hitchcock with nine provers at 1st, 3rd, 10th, 15th, and 16th dilutions in 1872-3.

LEAF AND SEED OIL

The leaf fat acids of buckwheat contain 16% palmitic, 26% oleic, 17% linoleic, and 30% linolenic; with one percent each of stearic and the saturated C20, C26, and C28 acids.

The seeds of wild buckwheat (*P. convolvulus*) contain 2.9% oil; composed of 5.6% myristic, 10.9% palmitic, 3.7% stearic, 41.5% oleic, 34.4% linoleic and 2.5% linolenic acids.

ESSENTIAL OIL

Fagopyrum tataricum leaves are steam-distilled, and yield 0.36% of an essential oil composed of bornyl acetate (17.3%), alpha-terpineol (15.8%), alpha-thujene (14%) and alpha-pinene (8.76%).

POLLEN

A peptide from buckwheat pollen stimulates production of human lymphocytes.

Research conducted by Liu et al at Beijing Hospital, reported in August 1998 showed conclusively the immune-stimulating effect of buckwheat pollen. This leads to the possibility of developing a novel immuno-modulator.

DOCTRINE OF SIGNATURES

Decreasing capillary fragility by the use of rutin results in a decreased incidence of vascular complications such as retinal hemorrhage, apoplexy and coronary occlusion. Interestingly, there is a botanical signature for cardiac use. The membranous wings of the seed or achene form a heart-like shape with smooth edges.   **VERMEULEN**

FLOWER ESSENCES

Buckwheat flower essence is for integrating past lessons into current life. Understanding today, in terms of past patterns of experience, feeling and behaviour can help break any current day gridlock.

WHOLE ENERGY

Wild Buckwheat essence is used when you compare yourself to other and set yourself apart from them. When we focus on the differences between us in relationships we isolate ourselves. Wild Buckwheat helps us to find and focus on what we have in common, and helps us to blend and harmonize with others. **DESERT ALCHEMY**

SPIRITUAL PROPERTIES

To attract abundance into your life, burn some of the crushed hulls with your favorite incense. For protection, sprinkle a small handful of the ground seeds around the outside of your home.

Add Buckwheat flour to your holiday baking to bring good luck, love and prosperity to your family and friends. **SUSAN GREGG**

RECIPES

TINCTURE- FRESH PLANT- The fresh plant and seed make a crimson red tincture, with a slightly acid reaction. Use 1:4 at 50% alcohol.

FLOUR- In the case of buckwheat, the lighter buckwheat flour is actually healthier than the whole flour that adds the ground hull. This results in a darker colour flour but actually dilutes the nutrient content- the hulls adding virtually no nutrients.

BUCKWHEAT POULTICE- To help re-establish milk flow in nursing mothers, combine buckwheat flour and buttermilk into poultice. Warm it, but do not boil or make too hot. Apply warm, over entire breast, renewing every four hours. It may take 3-4 days, but usually 24 hours is sufficient.

COOKING BUCKWHEAT- You can buy both roasted and unroasted cereal. After washing and draining buckwheat, put it in a hot skillet and toss for 5 minutes. This expands and strengthens the outer skin, so it stays intact and does not mush.

For the roasted form that is cracked, add an egg white in before adding it to the pan. The albumen will keep it firm. Un-cracked kasha does not need this.

Transfer buckwheat to pot and add two cups water for each cup. Always begin with boiling water, which will seal the outer surface and hold its shape. Simmer, covered for 15 minutes or until done.

BUCKWHEAT SPROUTS- Wash the seeds to remove dust and unripe seeds, then germinate in dark for three days at approximately 25° C. Once they are 2-3 cm long they must be sprayed for one minute every three hours. After 3-4 days the sprouts are 12-15 cm long with light yellow cotyledons and bright white hypocotyls; very similar to soy sprouts.

RUTIN- 100 mg 2-3 times daily. Do not use rutin with vitamin C, even though rutin protects ascorbic acid from oxidation. Rutin slows the rate at which the vitamin is absorbed by cells.

CAUTION- Rutin may interfere with action of quinolone antibiotics. It may theoretically interact with nitrosamines found in cured and smoked meat, to form carcinogenic compounds. Fagopyrismus, or buckwheat poisoning, is an erythema on un-pigmented skin, accompanied by nervous symptoms. It is a widely known condition in livestock, especially pigs. It is due to heavy consumption of buckwheat and exposure to sunlight. The disease is cured, by moving the animals to shade.

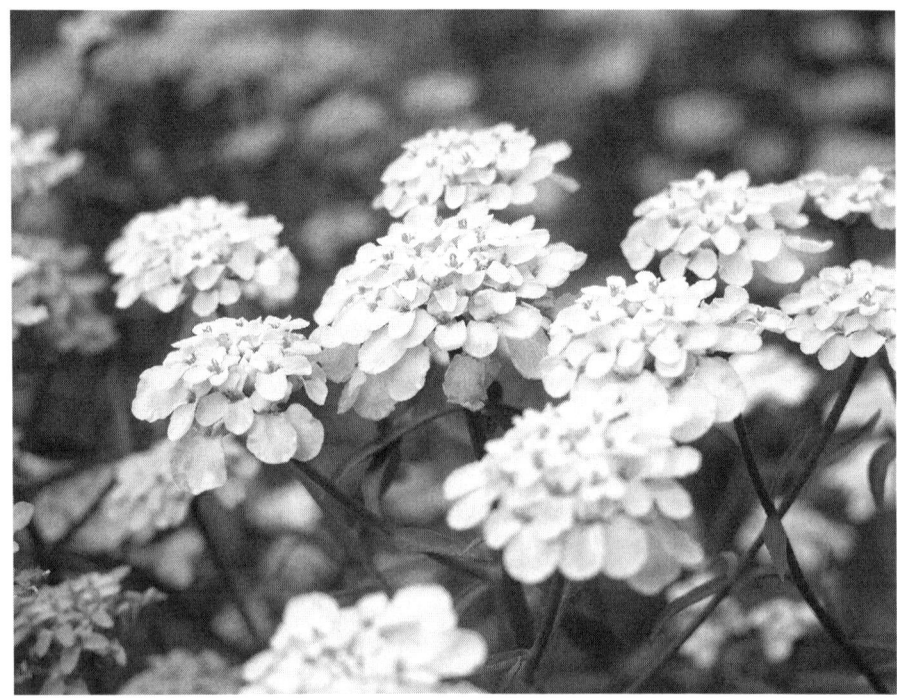

Candytuft flower

BITTER CANDYTUFT
WILD CANDYTUFT
CLOWN'S MUSTARD
(*Iberis amara* L.)
(*I. coronaria* D. Don)
FAIRY CANDYTUFT
(*I. umbellata* L.)
PERENNIAL CANDYTUFT
(*I. sempervirens* L.)
ROCK CANDYTUFT
(*I. saxatilis* L.)
PARTS USED- seeds, leaves

Iberis is the ancient name for Spain, where these flowers are prolific. The ancient Greeks said the European peninsula was named after **IBER**, an unspecified animal. Umbellata is named for the umbels of flower stalks or spokes, like the wooden struts of an ancient roman umbrella. Sempervirens means "always alive", in reference to the evergreen foliage. Amara means bitter.

Bitter or Rocket Candytuft is an introduced annual from Europe, that prefers dry, loamy soil rich in calcium. Candytuft comes from old English name for Crete. It was called Cretan Cress, when Lord Edward Zouche brought it back to England in Elizabethan times.

Many of the hybrids are grown in rock gardens, edgings, and borders. They range in colour from pink to lilac, to purple to white. Bitter Candytuft has fragrant blossoms, the Fairy Candytuft no fragrance at all.

Perennial Candytuft is an evergreen perennial or dwarf shrub that is covered in bright white flowers in early June.

It is an attractive addition to a rock garden or perennial border. It can be propagated from seed, or stem and root cuttings.

Cultivars recommended for the Prairies include Snowflake and Purity.

Rock Candytuft is another beautiful specimen with numerous, white showy blossoms.

Iberis amara is the medicinal species, used primarily in homeopathic medicine.

41

The plants can be started from seed, and reach flowering stage in about two months.

According to Grieve, all parts of the plant were used by american herbalists; leaves, stem, root and seeds. It was used for gout, rheumatism, and related ailments.

As a simple (by itself) it was used to allay excited action of the heart, especially when enlarged.

It was considered useful in asthma, bronchitis and dropsy.

MEDICINAL

CONSTITUENTS- *I. amara*- flowers various flavonoid glycosides including kaempferol-3-glycoside-7-rhamnoside, kaempferol-7-rhamnoside, quercitin-3-glycoside-rhamnoside.
leaves–minor flavonoids.
whole plant- cucurbitacin E and I; and (R)-3-methylsulfinylpropylamine, and 3-methylthiopropylamine, vitamin C.
seeds- flavonoids, 6-0-sinapoyl sucrose.

Wild Candytuft is a bitter-tasting tonic that aids digestion and relieves gas and bloating. It was traditionally taken for gout, rheumatism, arthritis, and dropsy.

According to Dr. King, "medicinally, it appears to control nervous and vascular excitement, and has been found efficient in enlargement of the heart, and some affections of the air tubes."

Ellingwood in 1915 wrote: "The most direct action of this remedy is upon an enlarged heart, where there is functional weakness. It lessens the force of the heart's action, controlling violence and irritability. It overcomes the dyspnoea of these cases, the vertigo and general sense of weakness, with other reflex symptoms. In bronchitis, asthma, dyspnoea, and in jaundice or dropsy, all of cardiac origin, it is said to be one of our best agents, in some cases acting magically."

This is interesting as the plant contains no cardenolides, but glucosinolates, suggesting it may have action on over-active thyroid.

Dr. Bastyr recommended Iberis for sea legs, wobbly legs, and vertigo.

Iberogast is a mixture of fresh plant extract from Bitter Candytuft (*Iberis amara*) and eight other herbal extracts, including angelica, chamomile, milk thistle, lemon balm, peppermint, celandine, and licorice. It has been widely used in Europe for the treatment of dyspeptic diseases and colonic disorders.

In studies conducted by Okpaanyi et al, 1983 Iberogast and its constituents were screened against acetylcholine-induced contractions of the guinea pig ileum *in vitro*.

In a recent study by Reichling and Saller, the fresh plant extract, both *in vitro* and *in vivo*, exhibited tonifying effect on the smooth muscles of the stomach and small intestine.

In rats, it showed anti-ulcer activity similar to cimetidine.

Stomach acid and leukotrine concentrations were reduced, but prostaglandin E2 content, reduced by indomethacin, was increased.

In patients with irritable bowel a clear difference was found between herbal extract and placebo, in a multi-centre, prospective, double-blind, randomized parallel group comparison. The fresh bitter Candytuft (*I. amara*) extract increased the basal resting tone and contraction of atonic and slightly contracted gut segments.

In the following year, the same researcher found that a water/alcohol extraction of the whole fresh plant showed anti-inflammatory activity against the carragenan-induced rat paw edema.

Iberogast has been the subject of 15 clinical studies with more than 80% of patients suffering non-ulcer dyspepsia, irritable bowel syndrome, gastro-esophageal reflux and drug-induced dyspepsia obtaining relief.

Two are worthy of note, both by Madisch and colleagues. The first is a multi-center, PC, DB trial of Iberogast or placebo on 60 patients with dyspepsia for four weeks. Significant improvement was noted.

The second involved 120 patients assigned to one of four groups and after eight weeks, 43.3% of patients taking Iberogast showed improvement compared to 3.3% on placebo. *Z Gastroenterol* 2001 39:7; *Digestion* 2004 69:1.

Perennial Candytuft (*I. sempervirens*) seeds and leaves have been examined and reveal activity against both gram positive and negative bacteria.

The expressed juice of Fairy Candytuft (*I. umbellata*) seedlings is active against both forms of bacteria.

The seeds of *I. amara* have strong fungi-toxic effects. In one study the seed was shown to retain its potency against fungi for nine months at room temperature.

Cucurbitacins, found in most Iberis species, are cytotoxic and anti-tumour, and possess anti-gibberellin activity.

HOMEOPATHY

Bitter Candytuft is of most value in treating arrhythmia and cardiac insufficiency.

In the foreground are the heart symptoms, with palpitations after the slightest movement, with no intrinsic cause, or palpitations with vertigo and anxiety, heaviness and pressure in the praecordium with shooting pains, and particularly a nocturnal aggravation.

At night there may be a visible throbbing of the heart, cessation of heartbeat, or fibrillation with a small, irregular pulse.

Iberis shows weakness of memory, swimming in the head with inability to fix attention, vertigo upon rising, congestion of the head with tinnitus, headache and hearing impairment with reddened eyes and optical illusions of light.

Patient is nervous or irritable upon rising in morning, dreams of home and disturbing sleep.

The right shoulder may have drawing pains with a sensation of heaviness in the left arm, and trembling in the lower limbs after movement.

The congestive heart condition may be ameliorated by increased mucous secretions and hawking up the mucous from the larynx and trachea.

There may be a sensation in the larynx as if bound up with a string, and suffocating, with shortness of breath, air hunger, and inhibited respiration.

The abdominal organs may be involved, with eructations, digestive weakness, abdominal distensions, sensations of pressure and pain in the liver region. There may also be soft, clay coloured stools, indicating biliary dysfunction.

Symptoms are worse from lying down on the left side, or in a warm room. Symptoms better from belching or expelling gas, open air.

DOSE- Tincture and 1st potency. For cardiac neurosis use 1X to 3X, and for bradycardia use 5-30th potency.

The mother tincture is made from the dried ripe seeds of the flower head. First proving by Hale with two males and one female with tincture, 1x and 4x dilutions in 1872. Jehn proved with four females and nine males at 2x, 2x, and 6x in 1955.

FLOWER ESSENCES

Iberis Candytuft has been used externally for bruises. It is useful for those who bruise easily and with chemotherapy patients whose blood may be adversely affected by the treatment. "Through self harmony, I renew by healing".

It encourages regeneration and self-healing by activating the light inherent in each cell. It enhances a balanced mineral pattern within the cell, allowing the tissues to be bathed with nutrients. **PETIT FLEUR**

SPIRITUAL PROPERTIES

Candytuft is known as the symbol of indifference. This was attributed to the plant in parts of the world where it is a small evergreen shrub.

There it bears its blossoms throughout the year. When a gardener collects the seeds, he must dive below the flowers which cover them. In bearing fruit, it does not fade, but preserves its leaves and flowers even in decay.

The seasons appear to pass by this plant without affecting it. It was experts of flower lore in the East who first, noting its disregard for the season, made the Candytuft the symbol of indifference.

CLAIRE POWELL

Candytuft flowers represent equanimity, with immutable peace and calm. **MOTHER**

PERSONALITY TRAITS

Through clinical cases, Mangialavori deems Iberis a very common remedy for modern life. He has found the remedy to be often useful in men who, in order to appear young, frantically try to reverse the process of aging by wearing clothing appropriate for much younger men and pushing themselves to feats of physical prowess, even while not really enjoying it. **VERMEULEN**

RECIPES

POWDERED SEEDS- 1-5 grains. In overdoses or too large ones, it can produce giddiness, vertigo, vomiting, nausea and diarrhea.

TINCTURE- Five drops twice daily for various conditions. Make at 1:4 at 50% alcohol from whole blooming fresh plant, with clear seed formation.

CANOLA
RAPE
(*Brassica napus subsp. oleifera*)
(*B. rapa subsp. oleifera*)
(*B. campestris subsp. rapifera*)
PARTS USED- flowers, seed, leaf

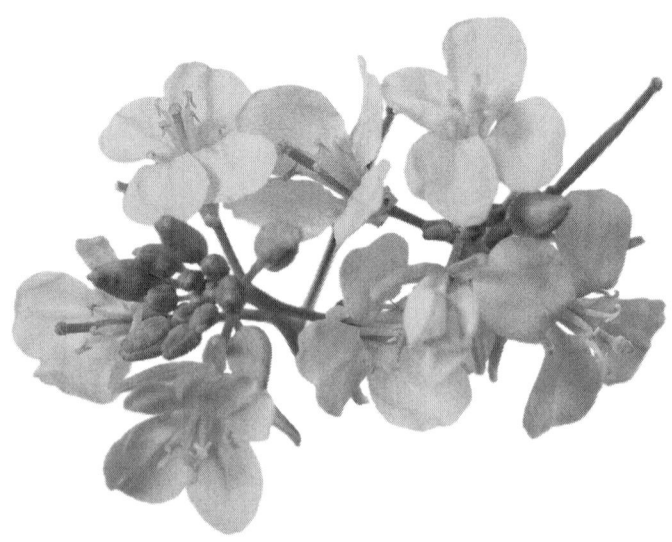

Rapeseed blossoms

Rape is derived from the Latin **RAPA** or **RAPUM** meaning turnip. Canola was name invented to market the new hybrid with low erucic acid oil about fifty years ago.

Yellow seas of canola are familiar on the prairie landscape. It is thought rapeseed was native to the Himalayas, but has adapted well to the prairies.

Canola is a very important economic plant, with Alberta exporting over $400 million of seed a year.

Through extensive research and development, a superior vegetable oil has been born (see below). The term canola was coined and trademarked for varieties of rape with two undesirable constituents, erucic acid and glucosinolate in seed and meal.

All the low glucosinolate rapeseed grown in the world today can be traced back to a single batch of Bronowski (*B. rapa*) seed, developed in Poland before WW II. Seeds from Argentina (*B. napus*) are being investigated and bred for northern climates. This variety has 30% higher yields and better disease resistance, but has a longer growing season. Argentine varieties used to, before GMO, account for 90% of canola planted on the prairies.

Gary Stringam, a canola breeder at the U of Alberta has reduced the maturity date of Argentine species to within four days of Polish canola. Ten years ago, the gap was nearly two weeks. AAFC researchers are developing a yellow-seeded species, as this trait increases seed oil and meal protein content.

The Saskatoon Research Centre is attempting to re-establish *B. rapa* as an early maturing canola for northern Saskatchewan and Alberta.

Other scientists are developing species high in oleic acid and low in linolenic acid as well as canola without glucosinolates.

Recent work by Mykytyn at the Ukrainian Agrarian Academy of Sciences, found that water extracts of uva ursi, or bearberry (*Arctostaphylos uva-ursi*) inhibit the myrosinase enzyme in rape meal, and may be a low-cost, low-tech way to improve meal feed safety.

Dr. Anne Johnson-Flanagan, at the University of Alberta, has been working on improving the freezing tolerance in oilseeds for the past seven years. She has tried two breeding techniques, one turning a winter canola into a spring variety. The other transformation is to move a cold-tolerant gene from winter into spring canola.

Double-haploid breeding has resulted, in the lab, of one particular line with a freezing tolerance in excess of -18° C. The research continues, as a work in progress.

Pollen tube growth in canola flowers is so fast that some tubes reach ovules within six hours of a pollen grain hitting the stigma. Within 2-3 hours of pollen hitting the stigma, sugar water is absorbed and swelling begins.

In Saudi Arabia, rape seeds have long been valued as an aphrodisiac. This may be due, in part to the seeds having estrogenic activity.

The black to reddish-brown canola seeds can be toasted as a tasty condiment over salads and grains. They have a mild taste, similar to radish seed, with peanut-like flavour.

The greens can be cooked like any potherb. In both India and China, the roots and leaves are considered stomachic, while a poultice of fresh leaves is applied to abscesses; and the seed tea given in cases of colic.

In Sweden, *B. campestris* seed has long been used as food for hens and pigeons, and a high quality food and lamp oil. The spring greens are eaten steamed, the older leaves in cabbage soup. The plant was used as a diuretic, and for scurvy and breathlessness.

In a test, bees fed canola pollen lived 65% versus sunflower pollen in their diet.

Lutein is a naturally-occurring carotenoid in various human tissue and has in particular an affinity for the human retina. It plays a role in preventing diabetic retinopathy, macular degeneration and other disease of the eye.

At the present time, the largest commercial source of lutein for the health market is from marigold. Given the preponderance of rape blossoms on the prairie, a little more research into the viability of using the flowers for human supplementation seems obvious.

Kull and Pfander at U of Berne in Switzerland, isolated lutein from rape petals.

Canola lends itself to creating genetically engineered plants. Monsanto, the biotech giant, purchased a patent from Calgene on genetically engineered brassica plants, including canola.

SemBioSys Genetics, a Calgary-based company created a variety of canola that contains hirudin, a substance only found in leeches, for preventing blood clots. They accomplished this by placing a protein from the salivary glands of leeches into canola. It currently costs $30/ gram on the world market to produce.

The blood anticoagulant is produced in transgenic seeds as an oleoresin fusion. The fusion protein accumulates on oil bodies and can be released in vitro from washed oil body preparations using an endoprotease. The fusion protein itself is inactive, but on release of the hirudin domain high specific activity hirudin is produced and partitions into the water phase. It never made it to market. They then switched to safflower to create insulin, and this also was never commercialized. See below.

Unfortunately, a whole brassica patent, like the one issued back in the 1980s, allows giants like Monsanto to dictate and control the global biotech industry, and squeeze the smaller, innovative companies.

Not all transgenic work with canola has been this successful, however.

Researchers at Monsanto/Calgene, took a gene from the California bay tree to produce a laurate canola containing an oil rich (38-42%) in lauric acid. This is traditionally obtained from coconut and palm oil, and widely used in shampoos, soaps and detergents.

The project, initiated in 1997, has been shelved, despite an over-production of seed.

Not only that, but as little as 1% of laurate created in commodity canola through cross-contamination, would be a disaster. Certified seed contracts call for a half-mile isolation zone, but some grower contracts require only a 100 yard buffer strip.

Cross-pollination between Monsanto's herbicide tolerant canola and conventional canola has occurred in the Sexsmith area. Whether this could migrate to "weedy" brassicas is unknown. In Britain, Monsanto finally admitted in the summer of 1999 that their GM crops can cross-breed with native plants, after GM canola found near Cambridge bred with wild turnips.

And in August 1999, a farmer from Bruno, Saskatchewan filed a civil suit against Monsanto, alleging their genetically-engineered canola has polluted and contaminated his land. Almost 80% of the 5.6 million acres of canola planted in the summer of '99 in Western Canada was herbicide resistant.

The whole matter may resolve itself economically.

A new Agriculture Canada study, conducted over two years, indicates that modified canola has bigger yields in only 60% of test fields. These results may turn the tide, considering it costs 30% more to grow the genetically modified canola.

In spring of 2001, about one thousand farmers across the prairies were forced to reseed after Quest canola, a GMO seed produced under a Monsanto license, was found contaminated with trace amounts of another herbicide resistant variety.

Lack of control over genetically modified food is a federal responsibility that is not being addressed in a timely or consistent manner. To say the least.

Monsanto scientists have created GMO canola that produces bio-degradable plastic. The yield is still too low for commercial production, and the company, in their 1998 annual report, have ended their manufacturing and research on biodegradable plastic.

Researchers believe, however, that one day, plants will be efficient producers of oils, plastics, and animal feed, all in one crop.

Dr. Suresh Narine, chair of rheology at U of Alberta, is forging ahead in manufacturing bio-plastics from flax and canola oil. The concept of green technology filling consumers demand for plastic is a good one, and may prove to be a huge industry. Time will tell.

A GM rapeseed developed by Monsanto produces oil rich in beta-carotene. They did this by using a gene from soil bacterium to increase the levels of vitamin A already present in the plant.

Fytokem, an innovative Saskatchewan nutraceutical firm, developed a phytosterol extract from canola, a tyrosinase and elastase inhibitor.

Canola oil is an excellent skin moisturizer, and may be useful for trans-dermal barrier transport systems.

Canola seedlings at day 3 to 5 have been shown to be very effective biocatalysts for the hydrolysis of fats and oils containing common and unusual fatty acids.

Work done by Jachmanian and Mukherjee at the Federal Centre for Cereal, Potato and Lipid Research in Munster, Germany found lipase from the germinating seedlings significantly increased the amount of hydrolysis in mustard, borage, and flaxseed triacylglycerols in a cheap and easy to obtain manner. *Journal of Agriculture and Food Chemistry* 1995 43.

The removal of phenolic compounds from canola meal, and their possible use as natural antioxidants would achieve two objectives.

The phenolics make the seed cake undesirable due to a bitter taste, astringency, and the inhibition of iron absorption in gastrointestinal lumen.

Work by Wanasundara et al, at Memorial University in Newfoundland has identified an anti-oxidant- 1-O-beta-D-glucopyranosyl sinapate that can be extracted.

The rapeseed press cakes contain glucosinolates that are goitergenic.

A technique to destroy these unwanted compounds has been reported through the use of the fungus *Geotrichum candidum* and its action of microbial fermentation.

Burcon NutraScience in British Columbia have developed the world's first commercial canola protein for animals.

Puratein, a canola protein isolate, has virtually undetectable levels of glycosinolates, phytates or phenolics. Studies show its nutritional effectiveness and functionality rival meat, eggs and milk protein.

And unlike processes involving soy, this patented production process uses only salt, water and meal; producing a flavorless, odorless, off-white product with excellent functionality. This has been achieved by taking advantage of the hydrophobic nature of the canola protein molecules.

A rat study for 13 weeks showed the product safe, with slight thyroid/parathyroid weight gain. Mejia et al, *Food Chem Tox* 2009 August 6.

There is incredible potential for this product, once regulatory hurdles are overcome. For more information check out www.burcon.ca.

Press cake meal possesses anti-oxidant and anti-microbial activity. Vinyl syringol, a decarboxylation product of sinapic acid, is a phenolic compound effective against formation of the pro-inflammatory mediator, prostaglandin E_2. This may have application for functional foods. Vuorela et al, *J Ag Food Chem* 2005 53.

It affects cell permeability tested with metoprolol. Sinapic acid may have an impact on drugs and other components actively transported across cell membranes.

A new cholesterol-lowering product from Sweden, Hjartans Lust Cheese, recently gained a health claim status.

A new fodder rape, OO, may have some potential on the prairies.

The seeds of *B. campestris* var. *sarason* were extracted with ethanol, in an experiment by Samir et al, at U of Rajasthan, India. They found it significantly reduced the incidence of tumours on mice skin induced by anthracene as compared to control group. *Phytotherapy Research* 1999 13:3.

Feeding canola oil to dairy cows may result in healthier milk to consumers, according to a two-month study conducted near Pickardville, Alberta. In studies with goats, adding canola oil to the diet improves the level of healthier fatty acids and reduced those linked to cholesterol.

Dr. Zahir Mir at Lethbridge Research Centre wrote, "this study confirms that we can improve the fatty acid profile of milk with dietary supplements."

It helps by increasing the milk levels of conjugated linoleic acids (CLAs). "They stimulate the immune system, protect against heart disease, and may have a role in cancer prevention." CLA levels in the study were directly proportional to increase in canola.

In Indonesia, rapeseed roots are used to treat coughs and ticklish throats.

MEDICINAL

CONSTITUENTS- petals- 80 different carotenoids, including a variety of luteoxanthins, violaxanthins, taraxanthin , a 1:1 mixture of flavoxanthin and chrysanthe-maxanthin, and various (Z)-isomers of lutein.
seed- Canola has been bred to contain less than 2% erucic acid. Sinapic acid is the predominant phenolic acid; minor acids being p-hydroxybenzoic, vanillic, gentisic, protocatechuic, syringic, p-coumaric, ferulic and caffeic. Traces of chlorogenic acid are found in the free phenolic fraction of meal. Vitamin K1 (140-200 mcg/100 grams.

A new vegetable oil, made from canola and soy oil, has been processed so that 80% of the oil is present in diglyceride form, rather than triglyceride. The oil is metabolized differently so instead of being stored as fat, it is burned as energy. This new product, called Enova, has been marketed in Japan for several years as a joint venture of ADM and the Kao Corporation, and is now the number one cooking oil in the country.

The FDA has declared the product GRAS as a cooking oil and margarine type spread. This has great potential for improving market share for canola oil into the health market.

Canola hulls, extracted with 70% acetone, exhibit anti-oxidant activity. Amarowicz et al, *J Ag Food Chem* 2000 48:7.

In Traditional Chinese Medicine, rapeseed is used to break up blood coagulations, strengthen the loins and legs, and heal rheumatism.

Rapeseed contains four potent ACE (angiotensin-converting enzyme) inhibiting peptides that lower blood pressure in animal experiments. Marczak et al, *Peptides* 2003 24.

Work by de Mar Yust et al, *Food Chem* 2004 87 treated rapeseed protein hydrolysates with food grade endoprotease and alcalase, and found two compounds with anti-HIV protease inhibition.

Pollen from *B. napus* contains flavonoids that show efficacy in benign prostatic hypertrophy, and inhibition of PSA levels. Han et al, *J Phytomed* 14:5.

A newly identified ceramide from the pollen shows significant cytotoxicity against Tca8113 human squamous carcinoma cell lines. Pei et al, *Fitoterapia* 2010 81:5.

Canola oil can be applied externally to the head to promote hair growth.

To cure acute pain in nipples and skin swelling of unknown origin, boil rape in water and crush it to make a juice. Drink a small glass of warm juice three times daily.

HOMEOPATHY

Red Seed (*B. napus*) is indicated in dropsical swellings, scorbutic mouth, voracious appetite associated with swelling and distention of the abdomen.

It is also indicated in cases of drooping nails, and gangrene.

Aversion to being approached, irritability with trifles, wants to be quiet and desire for rest. Feeling of impending doom, of being in wrong place, dreams of ascending hills, descending escalators and snow.

Desire for cold water, cold sweat during sleep. Sensation as if floating in air, weight at base of sternum as if heart were heavy, neck weak as if too long and unsupported.

DOSE- The mother tincture is prepared from the ripe seeds. Original proving with 7 provers by Jeremy Sherr at 6c and 30c in 1991. Reproving with 30c ten years later.

ESSENTIAL OIL

Using headspace analysis in field and then gas chromatography and mass spectrometry, the volatile components of canola flowers have been determined.

The major constituents are the monoterpenes limonene, sabinene, beta-mycrene, alpha farnesene and cis-3-hexen-l-ol acetate (green leaf volatile). Minor constituents include monoterpenes, sesquiterpenes, short chain aldehydes and ketones and organic suphides.

Alpha farnesene, one of the major volatiles, has been shown in studies to be the major scent to which worker bees respond.

An essential oil is produced from seedcakes, before they are fed to cattle. For canola, it is necessary to introduce an enzyme in order to decompose the precursor of the essential oil.

White mustard seed is often used for this purpose. After steam-distillation and removal of the hydrosol, the essential oil is obtained.

It is almost colorless, mobile and very pungent, with an odour reminiscent of horseradish.

It is considered toxic, although information on lethal dosage or toxicity levels has not been published.

SEED OIL

RAPESEED- eruric acid (30-60%), oleic acid (9-25%), linoleic (11-25%), alpha linolenic (5-12%) and palmitic acid (0-5%), vitamin K2.

CANOLA- oleic acid (48-60%), linoleic acid (18-30%) alpha linolenic acid (6-15%) and palmitic acid (3-6%), negligible amounts of erucic acid.

It is not as if high erucic acid oils are not desirable, they are just not edible. They have excellent lubricating properties, and special attributes for manufacturing nylons, paints and coatings that do not shrink or swell with changes of moisture.

High Erucic Acid Rapeseed (HEAR) oil is used as a synthetic rubber base, and illuminate for colour processing in magazines. World use is estimated at 80,000 tonnes per year.

The oil possesses excellent electrical insulation properties with good strength.

Erucamide is a chemical produced from erucic acid used to make bread wraps, garbage and sandwich bags. Erucamide lubricates the extruding machine during the manufacture of thin, plastic films, and after processing, migrates to the surface of the films and keeps them from clinging together. Erucic acid is used as a plasticizer in PVC cling film. Over 200 patented applications have been catalogued for C22 acids and their derivatives.

Biodegradable polyesters from rapeseed oil are being investigated in both North America and Europe. The production of 1,3-propanediol from glycerol obtained from rapeseed oil, is based on development of genetically modified microorganisms, using fermenters and membrane bioreactors.

One area of interest is the fermentation of low-grade glycerol by *Clostridium buytricum*. New biodegradable polyester based urethanes are one example of this application.

Research at the U of Alberta, led by Dr. Suresh Narine, is looking at turning canola oil into monomers for plastics, lubricants, and cosmetics.

International Lubricants in Seattle, Washington, markets automatic transmission fluid supplement (ATF) and a metal cutting oil based of derivatives of rapeseed oil. The transmission fluid supplement decreased wear by more than 50% compared to factory-filled fluid. And it produced 24% fewer acids that break down ATF fluid.

Recently, a firm patented and introduced a low calorie chocolate substitute that contains over 50% behenic acid, a derivative of eruric acid.

I find disturbing it disturbing that erucic acid is added to peanut butter to keep it from separating, without being identified on the label.

Other compounds such as brassylic and pelargonic acid have application for plasticizers, perfumes, flavors, coatings, paints, cosmetics and lubricants.

High erucic acid diet gained a brief spotlight in the movie Lorzeno's Oil. One symptom of adrenoleukodystrophy, a genetic disorder, is the difficulty of the body to deal with very long chain fatty acids, resulting in damage to the myelin sheaths that protect nerve cells. The defective gene is from the mother and only passed on to sons. Even as the film was being produced, however, the benefit of erucic acid for ALD was being disproved. Rapeseed oil is toxic, as illustrated by the 1981 poisoning and death of 600 Spaniards from commercial cooking oil made with "denatured" industrial rapeseed oil.

Mobil Oil has been marketing a biodegradable, non-toxic hydraulic fluid that is 97% rapeseed oil since 1991.

Industrial bake-on paint uses rapeseed oil due to its flexibility and impact resistance. About one-third of the billion gallons of paint used annually in the United States is of this type, used for automobiles, household appliances and machinery.

Nylon 13.13 can be made from erucic acid. It absorbs only 0.75% moisture compared to 10.5% for nylon 6, a typical commercial nylon. Polymers such as Nylon 13.13 could serve as high voltage insulators, fuel tanks in automobiles, and lightweight parts for aerospace and marine applications.

In Europe, a fuel derived from rape (rape methyl ester) is gaining in popularity as a replacement for diesel. It produces almost no sulphur and far less CO_2.

This biodiesel produces 80% less CO_2, 90% less unburned hydrocarbons, and cancer causing pollutants. It is ten times less toxic than table salt and biodegrades. It also ignites at 125° C, compared to 55° C for regular diesel.

Milligan BioTech, in Foam Lake, Saskatchewan makes canola-based fuel additives.

Duane Johnson, an alternative crop specialist at Colorado State University has developed motor oil from canola that cuts automobile pollution by 40%.

Used canola oil can be recycled into greases and chain oils; and consumers would not have to pay to dispose of the used canola oil, as they do the petro oil. One interesting use of canola oil is as a chainsaw lubricant inoculated with medicinal and gourmet mushrooms spores. As poplar or spruce are harvested, inoculation of high value added products begins.

If canola motor oil replaced just 5% of the petroleum oil used today, the US market would be roughly 50 million gallons.

Of course, the American Petroleum Institute won't certify it, as it is a huge threat to their economic lifeline. Automobile manufacturers require that only API certified oil is used in their engines, or warranties are void.

Even still, Wisconsin and Michigan state governments are in negotiations to use canola oil in their state-owned vehicles. Officials in New Zealand are considering its use.

Work by Metz, *Plant Physiology* 2000 122:3 introduced a single cDNA from Jojoba into high erucic acid rapeseed. This resulted in a portion of seed oil changing from triglycerides to waxes.

Canola oil is most valuable for health in its organic, and cold-pressed form. It contains significant amounts of vitamin K. This little understood vitamin plays a key role in bone and blood health, including clotting factors.

Canola oil is an excellent source and provides 100% of the RDA when present in the diet at greater than 15% of caloric content. Both light and heat destroy this valuable component.

Compared to other vegetable oils, canola is slightly better at lowering LDL, or bad cholesterol. It has less saturated fat than olive oil and is one of the better sources of omega 3 fatty acids. It has one of the best ratios of omega 6 to omega 3 fatty acids. While both are needed for good health, they only work effectively when present in the proper ratio. Omega 6 competes with omega 3, so that if you have too many in your diet, your body will not absorb the latter.

The ideal ration of omega 6 to 3 is less than 4 to 1, with up to 10 to 1 acceptable. Canola has a ratio of 2 to 1, versus olive with a ratio of 16 to 1 and corn oil 60 to 1.

Recent work by Vogel, 2000 found that olive oil, unless accompanied by anti-oxidant vegetables or vitamins, impeded artery function as much as a fast food meal, such as Egg McMuffin. Canola oil, on the other hand, had little or no negative effect on arterial function.

Transgenic work on canola has produced a highly enriched GLA, or gamma linolenic acid, from the seed oil. Borage seed oil contains about 23% GLA, whereas this enriched oil is 36%. Work by Wainwright et al, *Lipids* 2003 38:2, suggest it may be a suitable alternative source of GLA.

Clinical trials have shown the new, improved canola use in humans decreases both total and LDL cholesterol levels. The balance of fatty acids in canola, with relatively high levels of linolenic acid and a relatively low linoleic to linolenic acid ratio, may lower risk of clot formation, or thrombogenesis.

It is thought linolenic acid in canola oil is converted to the long chain omega 3 fatty acids in humans, such as DHA and EPA.

A recent study on mice and their unborn pups suggests that canola oil replacing corn oil lowers the cancer risk to both. This is likely due to the omega 6 fatty acids that comprise 50% of corn oil and only 20% of canola. Elaine Hardman and colleagues found CEBP alpha, a transcription factor involving breast cancer differentiation, and Egr1, a tumor suppressing gene, were up-regulated in those fed corn oil and less active in those fed canola.

Work by Kuwahara et al, *J Ag Food Chem* 2004:52 identified canolol (4-vinyl-2, 6-dimethoxyphenol) in canola oil. They found canolol prevents apoptosis in mammalian cells induced by oxidative stress. It proved toxic to cultured human colon cancer cell lines, suggesting a potential new nutraceutical.

Nexera canola, developed through traditional breeding methods, produces oil with over 70% monosaturated fatty acids, and may play a key role in providing healthy alternative to trans fatty acids prevalent in partially hydrogenated vegetable oils. Natreon canola oil is now being produced in North America, after development by Dow AgroSciences.

Australian cardiologists have shown that dietary canola helps prevent cardiac arrhythmias in laboratory experiments. Work by Fuhrman et al, *J Ag Food Chem* 2007:55 found a mixture of canola oil coating DAG, reduced atherogenic risk factors in mice studies.

The oil is used as an extracted phytosterol for skin moisturizers, and a trans-dermal barrier transport agent.

In Traditional Chinese Medicine, rapeseed oil (120 grams) is taken internally to correct intestinal intussusception (the slipping of one part of the intestine into another).

Work by Najine et al, *Can J of Botany* 1995 73 showed increasing sodium chloride content in water induced a decrease in linolenic and hexadecatrienoic acid; and an increase in linoleic and palmitic acids.

LEAF OIL

Rape leaves contain mainly palmitic acid (16%), tetradeconic acid (0.5-0.7%), hexadeca 7,10,13-trienoic (17%), and unsaturated C18 acid. The presence of so much C16 acid, and the absence of erucic acid is noteworthy.

HYDROSOL

Rape leaf is distilled and the water is used internally for gravel in the limbs and bladder, according to Brunschwig, Book of Distillation.

POLLEN

The pollen of canola contains steroidal lactones. These brassinosteroids, as they are known, when used as a leaf spray on wheat seedlings, causes the third and fourth leaf to increase, root growth increases, the soluble protein and soluble reducing sugars increase.

Honeybees have been found to live up to 65% longer on canola pollen diets that that from sunflower.

Canola honey begins to harden within weeks of collection.

FLOWER ESSENCE

Rape flower essence helps bring back drive and momentum in daily obligations. **MIRIANA**

PERSONALITY TRAITS

Canola was an Irish goddess. One night, following an argument with a lover, she left their bed and wandered into the night. She heard some beautiful music, so she sat down and soon fell asleep in the open air.

In the morning, Canola discovered the music had been made by the wind, blowing through rotted sinews clinging to a whale skeleton on the shore. Inspired by the sight and the magical sound, she built the first harp.

CAYENNE
(*Capsicum annuum*)
PARTS USED- fruit

Cayenne is a popular condiment that adds heat and zest to meals. It is tropical in origin and has a wide variation in size, shape and heat value associated with the fruit.

Work by Gagliano et al, *PLoS One* 2012 7:5 suggests that cayenne possesses some unique ways of communicating with other plants.

Capsaicin powder and oil is used in bear spray, and insect repellant, helping protect crops and trees from rodents.

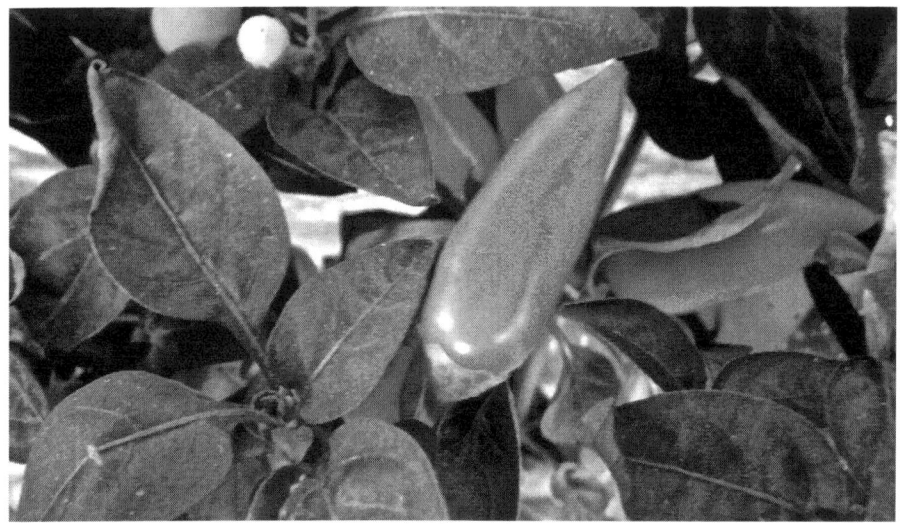
Cayenne

MEDICINAL

CONSTITUENTS- fruit- pectin, gums, capsaicin (0.1-0.2%), vanillyl amides, flavanoids, solanin, steroidal saponins, sapogenins, carotenoids, lecithin, various minerals including calcium carbonate, magnesium, potassium phosphate and iron.

Matthew Wood writes that Samuel Thomson introduced red pepper into American Herbalism over two hundred years ago.

It is a circulatory diffusive, meaning that it help distribute blood equally throughout the body. Matthew explains. "Due to weaknesses in the system, there could also be disparities between different circuits of the vasculature. For example, overeating might cause an excess blood supply to the digestive organs, smoking to the lungs, drug abuse or drinking to the liver, constipation to the large intestine, or there might be stagnation around the heart itself, or in the surface, the capillaries. When this inequality occurs a burden is placed upon the heart."

Matthew points to an unequal pulse, with one artery flaccid and the other sharp as a knife blade; or the heartbeat is not synchronized from one arm to the other. Stagnation of capillaries on the cheeks is another indicator.

The use of cayenne, helps the practitioner determine the true heart condition and recommend specific heart remedies.

One of my early teachers, Dr. John Christopher, was a real advocate of cayenne pepper. "It equalizes the blood stream from the top of the head to the bottom of the feet".

I have used cayenne pepper externally on open, gushing wounds; staunching the blood flow very quickly. Sprinkle the powder in socks and mitts to keep them warm in winter.

It can be used successfully for internal hemorrhage of the digestive system, healing gastric ulcers and improving poor stomach tone. It does not create the burning sensation one may anticipate. It does however, warm up cold digestive conditions such as Spleen Yang deficiency, representing itself as diarrhea, abdominal pain, pale complexion and atonic dyspepsia and constipation.

It helps promote sweating, and useful in rheumatic conditions, colds and flu, and repressed low-grade and intermittent fevers. Cayenne may be added to warm water gargles for sore throats, laryngitis, pharyngitis and tonsillitis.

For acute or chronic bronchitis, add to specific respiratory herbs.

Both Thomson and Christopher used cayenne internally in acute heart attacks.

When added to herbal formulas for long-term assistance of the cardiovascular system, it should not be used as more than 15% of the combination.

Externally, capsaicin is used to relieve arthritic pain in the form of a cream, liniment or oil.

Not only does cayenne act as a warming, stimulating irritant, but over time it dulls nerve pain signals, giving more permanent benefit in chronic pain. Substance P (for pain) receptors are depleted, giving symptomatic relief. Several over-the-counter topical creams are widely available, including an 8% patch.

Post-surgical pain in cancer patients may be helped, as well as pruritis and psoriasis in some cases.

If using your own liniments or oils observe extreme caution, as leaving on too long may cause blisters or dermatitis.

Capsaicin has been found to induce cell cycle arrest and apoptosis in human KB cancer cell lines. Lin CH et al, *BMC Complement Altern Med* 2013 13:46.

In vivo tests suggest it may be of benefit in cholangiocarcinoma. Wutka A et al, *PLoS One* 2014 9:4.

It may be of benefit in preventing or treating colo-rectal cancer due to up-regulation of NAG-1 gene expression and apoptosis. Lee, Seong-Ho et al, *Carcinogenesis* 2010 31:4.

In vitro studies suggest it may be cytotoxic against multi-drug resistant lymphoma, oral tumor cell lines and perhaps inhibit leukemia cell growth.

It may have potential to use in combination with 5-FU in treatment of gastric carcinoma. Meral O et al, *Tumour Biol* 2014 March 30.

One caution to note. Chemotherapeutic potential of capsaicin may be affected by impaired NK cell function. Maybe. Kim HS et al, *Carcinogenesis* 2014 April 17.

A systematic review of clinical trials suggest it may be effective in treating low back pain.

Cayenne is often added to weight loss formulas. Baek Jangmi et al, *Nutr Res Pract* 2013 7:2. It is full of carotenoids that possess analgesic, anti-oxidant and anti-inflammatory properties. Hernandez-Ortega M et al, *J Biomed Biotech* 2012.

Cayenne inhibits aromatase, suggesting use with nettle root in hormone sensitive cancers. Luqman S et al, *J Med Food* 2011 14:11.

HOMEOPATHY

Reproachful and angry about faults of other, offended at trifles, fault-finding.

Makes jokes and witty remarks, merry and content and yet slightest thing makes him angry. Dreams of being betrayed by partner or of flying.

Desire for coffee, but causes nausea. Sleepless from emotion or homesickness.

Frequently indicated for phlegmatic or melancholic types, those dreading open air.

Phytophobia, flatulence from vegetables. Coughs with bursting headache, chest or bladder. Joints painful and stiff upon beginning to move.

DOSE- Third to sixth potency. Proving by Hahnemann on 7 provers, clinical observations by Hering and Mangialavori.

FLOWER ESSENCE

Cayenne flower essence provides a catalytic spark to the soul who may be stagnating in its growth cycle.   **FLOWER ESSENCE SOCIETY**

SPIRITUAL PROPERTIES

There is a transference of the heating ability of cayenne onto the spiritual level…Because of this heating effect, the heart opens more. This is under the direction of will, so an individual may choose to use such a heart opening in ways that are appropriate to them.

The inner lesson of cayenne is to provoke choice. In fact, this is the karmic less of cayenne. Choice on the level of the heart is extremely difficult for most individuals. When you have this loving feeling, you have the opportunity to share it with many individuals or with only one person.

The development of all psychic gifts is greatly accelerated. The fourth chakra is especially opened.

The pericardium meridian is accelerated greatly and the bladder and governing vessel meridians are enhanced. The heavy metal and petrochemical miasms are eased. Adding cayenne to the water or spraying it in the air, transfers some of the cayenne's healing qualities, so that extra growth of rootlet hairs again takes place. This often pushes the plant through this difficult stage.   **GURUDAS**

RECIPES

TINCTURE- 5-10 drops in water. In formulas, no more than 10% of finished product. Make with crushed, dried fruit at 1:5 and 40% alcohol.

CAUTIONS- Cayenne may interfere with theophylline and exaggerate coughing reflex associated with drug. There is one case of erythematous dermatitis in infants breast feeding from mothers who ingested cayenne pepper flavored meals. It may aggravate peptic ulcers, and kidneys in some individuals. Asthmatics may be more sensitive to capsaicin. One study in Mexico City suggests that chili pepper consumers are at a 5.5 fold greater risk of gastric cancer than non-consumers.

GARDEN CHERVIL
(***Anthriscus cerefolium*** [L] Hoffm.**)**
(***A. longirostris***)
(***Scandix cerefolium***)
(***A. cerefolium*** var. *cerefolium*)
WILD CHERVIL
COW PARSLEY
(***A. sylvestris*** Hoffm.**)**
PARTS USED- leaf

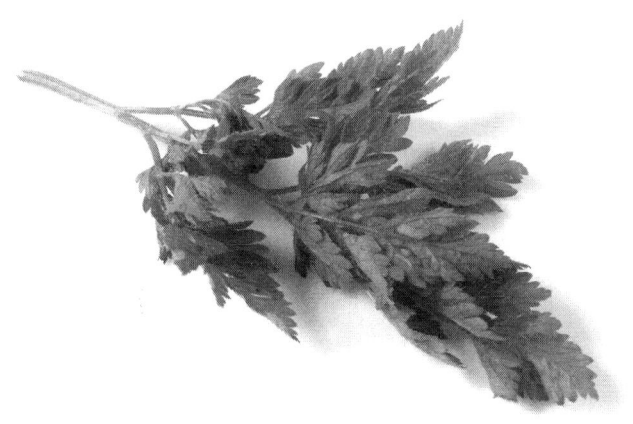

Chervil (*Anthriscus cerefolium*)

Chibolles and Chervelles and ripe chiries manye.**PIERS PLOWMAN**

See, banks and brakes now leaved how thick!
Laced they are again with fretty Chervil.   **G M HOPKINS**

Anthriscus is from Greek **ANTHRISKOS**, meaning little flower. Cerefolium was believed derived from Latin meaning "waxy or cherry-leaved", and in turn from the Greek, Chairephyllon, meaning "pleasing leaf". Chervil may derive from the Anglo-Saxon, **CERFILLE**.

Cere forms the root of cerebral, cerebrum and cerebellum, from **KER**, meaning the top of the head. Some authors allude to its powerful brain stimulation. Ceres is the Roman goddess of sowing and harvesting, and name given to our new cat.

However, garden chervil does not have waxy leaves, but soft, crisp leaves similar in appearance and texture to parsley. Cerefolium is a mis-translation of the Greek **CHAIREPHYLLON**, meaning "healthy leaf", or "leaf of rejoicing the heart". But we appear stuck with this species name, and nobody is in rush to change it.

Do not confuse this plant with the plant sweet cicely (*Myrrhis odorata*), which is called sweet chervil in many herb books. Both are rich in anise-scented anethole, and look somewhat similar, but the former herb is perennial and this is an annual.

Pliny considered the herb a tonic and aphrodisiac useful for older men. An older writer said that "the roots are very good for old people that are dull and without courage; they gladden and comfort the spirits, and do increase their lusty strength."

It was cultivated by ancient Syrians. The herb is sometimes called Gourmet or French Parsley, since it has a more delicate flavour. The Dutch add **WARMUS** to hotchpots and other culinary delights.

In medieval Europe, it was known as rich man's parsley, probably due to its more refined taste and scent.

Hildegard, the 12th century Abbess, wrote: "Chervil is of a dry nature and grows from neither strong air nor the strong moisture of the earth, but arises in weak breezes, before the fertile heat of summer... It is beneficial as a medicine, and heals broken wounds of the bowels. Pound chervil, and pour the expressed juice in wine."

Garden Chervil has a strong aromatic presence, reminiscent of anise or licorice, with a hint of tarragon. It is a hardy annual that flowers from late spring to summer, and prefers light, fertile soil that does not dry out.

It does not care for direct sun, preferring shade at some part of day.

It makes a nice addition, when finely chopped, to soup and salads. Chervil is one of the four *FINES HERBES* of French Cuisine and used to flavour potato salad.

The others, for those curious, are chives, parsley and tarragon. For soups, add the minced leaves at the last moment, to retain their flavour. I like a small amount on raw oysters, in French vinaigrettes, tabouli, and of course, in a Bechamel or Béarnaise sauce.

The herb has a unifying quality that helps blend other flavors together.

Chervil was considered one of the Celt's nine sacred herbs, the others being, mugwort, plantain, watercress, chamomile, nettle, crabapple, fennel, and the unidentified Atterlothe.

Pliny recommended chervil "to comfort the cold stomach of the aged". The boiled roots were eaten as a preventative during the plague. Apicius, a Roman gourmet, included green chervil sauce in his two thousand year-old cook book, *De Re Coquinaria*.

An ancient Arabian liqueur, called **RIG EL GHURAB**, is chervil and cherry-flavored.

In medieval times, the herb was used to thin blood clots, and dissipate the congestion of severe bruising.

It was used in treating kidney stones, as diuretic, and treatment of pleurisy. The leaves were used for the pain of rheumatism. In Ayurvedic terms, the herb helps to calm both kapha and pitta, when out of balance.

Culpepper said "it is a certain remedy to dissolve congealed or clotted blood in the body, or that which is clotted by bruises, falls, etc… the juice or distilled water thereof being drunk, and the bruised leaves laid to the place, being taken in either meat or drink, it is good to provoke urine, or expel the stone in the kidneys, to send down women's courses and to help the pleurisy and prickling of the sides."

In 1565, Evelyn wrote, "the tender tops of Cherville should never be wanting in our sallets, being exceeding wholesome and chearing the spirits." Gerard mentions Chervil "bringeth down the menses".

Sauer mentions a combination of two parts chervil with one part each of *Sanicula* species and *Pyrola rotundifolia* for blood clots congealed in body.

The herbalist Juliette de Bairacli Levy recommends it for "poor memory and mental depression".

Chervil is believed to cure hiccups. As a milk or mask, it helps cleanse the skin, prevent wrinkles and retain suppleness.

Today, in Europe, chervil tea or soup is taken on Holy Thursday as a symbol of Christ's resurrection and new life.

Used as a companion plant with radish, it is said to improve the growth and sharpen the flavour of the roots.

The fresh plant can be used to wash the scalp to clear dandruff and other scalp crustations.

Holistic veterinarians use chervil as an appetizer for animals that are poor feeders; and like carrots, help improve eyesight.

Commercially, the herb is used to flavour soups, baked goods, ice cream and non-alcoholic drinks.

Bakirci, *Nahrung* 1999 43:5 found *Anthriscus* stimulated acid production in dairy culture production of *Streptococcus thermophilus* and *Lactobacillus bulgaricus.*

Germination of the stick-like seeds in light takes up to ten days. Do not cover with soil, but also do not allow the young seedlings to dry out.

If you scatter the seeds in a small area, and cover with cheesecloth, you can then remove it when seeds have rooted. Direct sunlight can be too much for delicate chervil, so look for a somewhat shaded area, at least for part of the day.

The plant is an annual, but will self-sow readily if allowed. It prefers the cool weather of spring and fall, and will go to seed quickly in heat of summer unless continually topped. It thrives when daytime temperatures are 40-50° F, and becomes very bushy, but quickly flowers in hot weather. Brussels Winter is one cultivar that will not bolt as quickly.

Although it tolerates pH 5-8, the range of 7-8 is more optimal. The seeds have a short shelf-life and should be planted anew each year, the best being fresh seed from previous fall. Harvest can begin at 90 days when planted outdoors, and from 40-60 days in greenhouse after sowing. It does not like transplanting and will quickly bolt if grown in starter pots.

The plant does not dry well, and is best used medicinally as a fresh plant tincture, or a frozen juice. If dried, it should be under 90° F in order to retain any green colour.

The dried plant can add subtle notes to potpourri.

Work at ARC, Vegreville showed curled chervil susceptible to infection by aster yellows disease.

Ernest Small, in his excellent book, *Culinary Herbs*, mentions that binomials such as *Cerefolium cerefolium* are no longer usable in botanical classification.

Such a name is known as a tautonym, meaning the genus and species are the same. He notes, with interest, however that trinomial combinations are acceptable. Strange indeed the world of taxonomy!

Wild Chervil, or Cow Parsley is a naturalized biennial/perennial from Eurasia.

It is reputedly unlucky and must not be picked, with country names such as mother die and break your mother's heart.

This probably originated from its similar appearance to deadly Poison Hemlock.

The plant was made into a lotion by the Lesotho of Africa, or as a refreshing bath when feeling tired or sick. For chest colds, the seeds are chewed with honey.

The plant has been used traditionally, in Russia, as both a childbirth remedy and abortifacient. In Europe, the plant powder is used to heal wounds.

In Scotland, the young plant and flowering tips were used for dyeing Harris Tweed. The dried stalks made weaving bobbins.

It is considered problematic in some pastureland from Newfoundland to Ontario as well as BC. It has not naturalized to the Canadian prairies, but a small controlled plot would do no harm.

In fact, work by Bockholt & Schnittke, *Wirtschaftseigene-Futter* 1996 42:6 found Wild Chervil and twelve other mineral nutritive "weeds" might actually improve the mineral supply to cattle when preserved as hay or silage.

The roots, as well as young leaves, are edible and used in soups, casseroles, potato or bean dishes. This is spite of the fact large amounts are considered narcotic.

The leaves can be used as a parsley substitute, and to flavour alcoholic beverages.

The yellow flowers are used as a dye.

The highest content of deoxypodophyllotoxin is found in root and aerial parts in spring of second year. Anthracin, the main root lignan, is strongly insecticidal. In one study, it caused the death of 80% of mosquito larvae at only 5 ppm.

MEDICINAL

CONSTITUENTS- *A. cerefolium* leaf- rich in protein (23%), calcium (1346 mg/100 g), iron (31.95), magnesium (130), potassium (4,740), zinc (8.8), B6, A, C, B complex, E, K, and P; apiin.
A. sylvestris root- anthricin (deoxypodophyllotoxin 0.39% dried wt), isoanthricin, anthriscinol methyl ether, (Z)-2-angelolyloxymethyl-butenoic acid, falcarindiol, angelolyl podophyllotoxin, morelensin, burseherin, elemicin, nemerosin.
aerial parts- stigmasterol, 0-cresol, p-cresol, p-cymene, eugenol, anthricin, beta sitosterol, n-paraffins, n-alcohols, fatty acids, esters.
ground part- deoxypodophyllotoxin, (-)-deoxypodorhizone, nemerosin, falcarindiol.
seed- four lignans including deoxypodo-phyllotoxin, morelensin, (-)-deoxypodo-rhizone and (-)-hinonkin; a phenylpropanoid, two phenylpropanoid esters and falcarindiol.
flower only- luteolin, apigenin, caffeic acid.

Chervil is a simple, safe and reliable blood-thinner or anti-coagulant. It may be used in cases of varicose veins, or in serious cases of embolism and thrombosis. Over time, the herb will help lower blood pressure.

Unlike medical coumarins that work quickly, but can have dangerous side effects in overdose, chervil will work slowly but only thin the blood to its normal consistency, and no more.

It therefore can be very useful in treating strokes and embolism.

Women suffering irregular periods are helped by the herb, and over time the herb will normalize the cycle.

When taken over long-term, chervil will help prevent varicosities, hemorrhoids and risk of embolic complications.

The herb is used for various nodular conditions, including gouty nodes, various breast lumps and cysts. Related to this is stagnant phlegm in the lungs, for which chervil combines well with gumweed and mullein.

It is an efficient cholagogue, taken as a fresh juice, up to one half cup twice daily between meals. It will increase bile production, and increase appetite.

John Heinerman suggests that plant root and leaf help fight infection and reduce inflammation of the spleen.

A cooled, strained infusion in an eye-cup helps relieve sore, inflamed eyes. In France, for example, the herb is used for severe inflammation of the eyes, including, conjunctivitis, detached retina, cataracts and opthalmitis; combined with eyebright for even better results. The freshly crushed herb quickly relieves hemorrhoid pain and inflammation.

The herb has been used traditionally in Europe for fever, gout, jaundice and chronic skin conditions, including eczema.

Dr. Leon Binet, former Dean of Medicine in Paris created a formula for the above conditions, including glaucoma. See recipes below.

Water extracts of the aerial parts of Wild Chervil show antioxidant and anti-lipo-peroxidant quality. Fejes et al, *J of Ethnopharmacology* 2000 69:3. The herb extracts were more active than roots.

Deoxypodophyllotoxin is a phenyl tetralin-type lignan with anti-tumour activity. It shows activity against human cervix carcinoma cell lines in G2/m phase prior to apoptosis. Yong et al, *Bioorg Med Chem Lett* 2009 19:15. See flax below.

Uden et al, *J Nat Products* 60:4 found 0.39% of this compound in root and when suspended with *Linum flavum* under artificial conditions, the final yield was close to 83%.

Rotaviruses are responsible for many cases of infantile diarrhea. Song et al, *Korean J of Pharmacology* 1998 29:2 found wild chervil the third most inhibitory herb, *in vitro*. Goldthread was most inhibitory, followed by astragalus root, and then chervil of the 50 herbs tested.

Wild chervil root is used in Korean herbal medicine as an anti-tussive and diuretic. In China, the root is known as **QIAN HU**, or **E SHEN**.

Wild chervil root is cytotoxic against human tumour cell lines K562 and Colo 205. Lim et al, *Archives of Pharmacol Res* 1999 22:2. They first reported occurrence of angeloyl podophyllotoxin in nature.

Deoxypodophyllotoxin inhibits migration and MMP-2/9 activity in TNFalpha stimulated human aorta smooth muscle. Suh et al, *Vascul Pharmacol* 2009 51:1. This suggests anti-inflammatory activity and possible prevention of atherosclerosis.

The presence of a lignan with a 2,7'-cyclolignan skeleton is of particular interest to cancer research.

Ikeda et al, *Chem Pharm Bulletin* 1998 46:5 found root, seed and ground parts of herb highly inhibitory against MK-1, HeLa and B16F10 cancer cell lines, *in vitro*.

Bae Ki Wuan, found anti-angiogenic activity, and inhibition of A549 human lung cancer cells from wild chervil extracts. *Korean J of Pharmacognosy* 2000 21:3.

Anthricin (deoxypodophyllotoxin) inhibits mTOR, suggesting a combination of an autophagy inhibitor and anthricin may be a new strategy for treatment of breast cancer cells. Jung CH et al, *Evid Based Complement Altern Med* 2013 May 29.

Peudedanin, found in carrots and Meum, exhibits anti-neoplastic activity.

Cow parsley roots are extremely abortifacient; and in fact, the whole plant is to be avoided during pregnancy.

Recent work suggests terpenoids in the plant prevent ovum implantation, inhibit ovarian growth and disrupt the estrus cycle.

ESSENTIAL OILS

Chervil essential oil from the aerial parts is composed mainly of methyl chavicol (83.1%), 1-allyl-2, 4-dimethoxy-benzene (15.15%), undecane (1.75%), and beta pinene (<0.01%).

The leaf yields 0.3% and seed 0.9%. Scent is cross between tarragon and parsley.

Cow parsley flower essential oil contains 12 components, the leaf has 19.

The flower and leaf essential oil is mainly eugenol methyl ether, undecane and estragol (methyl chavicol); as well as minor amounts of p-cymene, and pentacylic terpenes.

Eugenol is highest (67%) before flowering, methyl chavicol (69%) highest during flower, and undecane (19%) after flowering.

Fresh leaf oil contain up to 39% beta phellandrene, 17% beta myrcene, 6% sabinene, 5.4% Z-beta ocimene, and 4% benzene acetaldehyde.

The root essential oil is composed of alpha pinene (4.6%) beta mycrene, delta limonene, 1-alpha fenchyl alcohol and acetate, benzaldehyde, and 17% Z-beta-ocimene.

SEED OIL

The seeds of Wild Chervil contain 12% fatty acids, composed of petroselic acid, petroselidic acid, linoleic acid, stearic acid, and hydroxy-stearic acid.

HYDROSOL

The distilled water of Chervil, taken every morning and evening in doses of four or five tablespoons, is very good for dissipating blood congealed in the body resulting from apoplexy, hard falls or severe blows. It will also heal internal injuries.

Additionally, it forces out urine and gravel, breaks up kidney stones, and is good for lumbago and pleurisy. **SAUER**

Chervil water distilled about the end of May, helps ruptures, breaks the stone, dissolves congealed blood, strengthens the heart and stomach.
CULPEPPER

FLOWER ESSENCES

Chervil flower essence activates the brow and crown charkas and the poa. It is good for the newborn, and where there may be confusion as to spiritual identity or disorientation. It enhances the ability to astral and soul project, and the desire to meditate is stimulated. It is also used to cleanse quartz crystals.   **PEGASUS**

Wild Chervil flower essence helps develop self-perception. After reclamation of contradictions, there is a feeling of inner peace.

MIRIANA

PERSONALITY TRAITS

Although chervil resembles a delicate parsley with somewhat lacy, fernlike foliage, the spirit of its flavor betrays an aristocratic subtlety. Is it any wonder that a synonym for chervil is French parsley?

TUCKER/DEBAGGIO

RECIPES

BLOOTCLOTS- Take two parts chervil, one part each of black snakeroot (*Sanicula marylandica*), and pyrola (*P. rotundifolia*), and combine as a tincture or tea.

TINCTURE- Fresh plant tincture only. Twenty drops four times daily in acute cases. For maintenance 10 drops twice daily in water before meals. Make fresh tincture at 1:4 and 40% alcohol. Only the fresh product has any meaningful activity.

DR. BINET'S EYE FORMULA- Combine one tsp of fresh chervil, parsley, roman chamomile and lavender flowers to one pint boiling water and steep off heat for one half hour. Stain and use cooled in an eyecup three times daily.

COMPLEXION MILK- Simmer one half-litre milk with a cup of fresh chervil leaves for ten minutes. Strain and refrigerate. Then slowly simmer one cup of brandy with one cup of fresh leaves.

Remove from heat, and let cool overnight. Strain and bottle. Store this at room temperature. Each morning splash chervil milk on face and rinse with spring water. Every evening, splash on the brandy. Oh go ahead, and take a swig as well!

CAUTION: Wild Chervil inhibits CYP2C9 and CYP3A4, suggesting inhibition of liver enzyme clearance.

COMMON FLAX
(***Linum usitatissimum*** L.)
LEWIS' WILD FLAX
WILD BLUE FLAX
WESTERN BLUE FLAX
(***L. lewisii*** Pursh.)
(***L. perenne ssp. lewisii*** [Pursh] Eat/ & J. Wright)
MEADOW WILD FLAX
(***L. pratense*** [Nort.] Small)
YELLOW FLAX
(***L. rigidum*** Pursh.)
PURGING FLAX
MOUNTAIN FLAX
FAIRY FLAX
(***L. catharticum*** L.)
WHITE FLAX
(***L. album*** Boiss.)
PARTS USED- flowers, stems, seeds

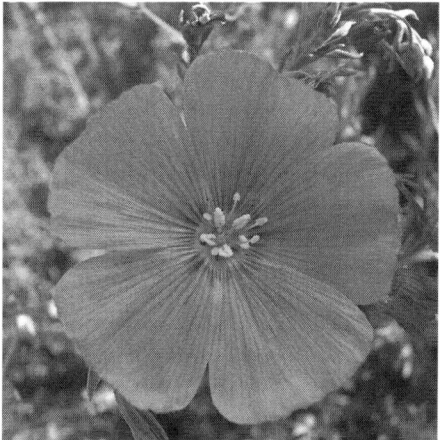

Flax flower

Oh! The goodly Flax-flower!
It groweth on the hill;
And be the breeze awake or sleep,
It never standeth still!
It seemeth all astir with life,
As if it loved to thrive,
As if it had a merry heart
Within its stem alive!   **MARY HOWITT**

And a few plots of Flax in the hollows gleamed blue with delicate flowers- childlike eyes that seemed blinking in the glare.   **KNAB**

Blue were her eyes as the fairy-flax
Her cheeks like the dawn of day,
And her bosom white as the hawthorn buds
that open in the month of May.   **LONGFELLOW**

If put in the shoes it (flax) preserves from poverty. **OLD PROVERB**

Linum is derived from Greek **LINON** meaning flax; or from the Celtic **LLIN**, meaning a thread. Both are from Indo-European root **LINOM**, one of the oldest fabric words. English words like line, lint, and linnet are derivations.

Usitatissimum means "most useful", from the Latin adjective **USIFATUS**. Lewisii is named after Meriwether Lewis, of Lewis and Clark expedition. Flax is from the Old English, **FLEAX**, related to **FLECHTEN** "to weave or intertwine", from the Indo-European **PLEK**, meaning to twist, to braid, to plait or interweave.

Flax may derive from **FILARE**, meaning "to spin" or **FILUM**, a thread.

Album means white, pratense of the meadow, and catharticum, cathartic as in purgative. Fairy Flax stems from the Middle Ages, when the plant was associated with strong, powerful spirits of the country. Wild Blue Flax symbolizes domestic virtues, and is related to the birth date of September 19. It is associated with the 8th Norse Rune, Wyn.

Usually, when driving across the prairies, you see a patchwork of brown, yellow and green. Occasionally, you come upon a marvelous field of blue, waving in the breeze. This is flax. One day, I picture flying over the prairies and patch works of purple (echinacea and milk thistle), orange (safflower), blue (borage) fields will join the yellows and greens in a bold and vibrant blanket.

Already, Canada produces 40% of the world's flax, with 25 million bushels in 2001 and 70% of this from Saskatchewan.

Flax fibers have been woven into linen for over 10,000. Linseed oil has been used traditionally for paints, varnishes, and enamels, for slightly less time.

Archaeologists found prehistoric swiss lake dwellers spun flax, ten millennium ago.

Flax is mentioned in the Bible, and Talmud, both forbidding the blending of flax with impure wool.

In ancient Egypt, flax was grown along the Nile for clothing, bed sheets, diapers, sails and mummy wrapping.

Linen was a symbol of divine light, and purity associated with Isis, the mother goddess. A medicinal flax recipe from Egyptian literature dates back to the 14th century BC.

Pliny asked, "what department is there to be found of active life in which linseed is not employed? And in what production of the Earth are there greater marvels to us than this?"

Charlemagne encouraged the production of flax, finding it more sanitary than wool.

The medieval herbalist Bartholomew suggested dozens of applications, and said "none herbe is so needfull to so many dyurrse uses to mankynde as is the flexe."

Flax was believed to be a blessed plant, that brought good fortune, good health; even the flowers offering protection from witchcraft.

The Norse goddess Huldah (Hilda) was known as the Guardian of the Flax Fields, and reputedly taught mortals to spin and weave. It was believed Huldah had a mountain palace, entered from a cave. Twice a year she would pass through the valley, once when the blue flowers brightened the fields, and the other time during the 12 nights preceding the Feast of Epiphany, when gods and goddesses were believed to visit the earth.

German brides would put a few flaxseeds in their shoes to protect her fortune, or they might tie a flax string around their left leg to make the marriage thrive.

Sowing flax seed around the home in Norway and Denmark was a way of protecting against the spirit of the dead. Flax is the national flower of Northern Ireland.

Bohemians believed a seven year-old child who danced in a flax field would become beautiful, while in Mediterranean countries, a baby not thriving was laid in flax field and sprinkled with flaxseeds. In Brandenburg it was said that if you suffered from giddiness you should strip yourself naked and run thrice round a field of flax field after sunset.

In the Austrian Alps, men are not permitted to harvest the crop, as a hag spirit called Harpetsch will attack them.

Showing flax your buttocks to ensure a tall crop was practiced by the Pennsylvania German settlers. The term "dance for flax" was used at wedding feast dances to describe lifting your feet high above the floor, to help ensure a high crop yield.

In China, oilcloth was developed, over 2000 years ago. Linoleum (oil of linum) was developed more recently for floor coverings. Boiled linseed oil was mixed with cork and applied to burlap backing and rolled into sheets.

After cultivated flax was introduced in the 1700s, it spread westward with settlers, and was often one of the first crops planted on the homestead.

Oil cloth produced in North America in 1809, was made into tablecloths, shelf paper, floor and wall coverings, rain gear and carrying bags.

New processes for breaking down flax fibre include steam explosion and ultra-sonic technology.

The seed oil was a base for paints and varnishes to add waterproofing quality. It was used to treat wooden garden tools, shoes and leathers.

Flaxseed tea became a popular remedy for coughs and urinary tract disorders. Mixtures of linseed oil and lime-water were considered a laxative internally. Externally, the tea was healing to burns and scalds when applied externally (Carron oil).

When steeped in hot water, the seeds become soft and gummy and make a useful poultice, combined with mustard seed to soothe irritation and pain.

A single seed can be soaked in water, and inserted under the eyelid to remove tiny particles irritating the eyes.

In many parts of the world, flaxseed is powdered and taken with honey and hot water about a week before birthing due date. Since flaxseed contains prostaglandins, this may have helped an easier labor. Flaxseed can be roasted and used as a coffee substitute.

The seed has fungistatic activity, and can be used in various functional food formulas. Xu et al, *Int J Food Microbiol* 2008 212:3.

After the oil is expressed, the press cakes can be feed to cattle and poultry.

Today, flaxseed can freshly ground and sprinkled on cereal, especially hot oatmeal, baked in muffins and breads, used to thicken soups, or add a nutty flavour to crackers, pancakes,waffles and yogurt. The sprouted seed, when the tail is as long as the seed, is a richer source of omega 3 fatty acids.

Different cultivars have developed over the years, emphasizing either fibre or oil, similar to hemp. The fibres in the stem form a thin layer between the woody core and the outer skin. They have reached full length when flax begins to flower, but are still thin, delicate and weak. From flowering until the plant dies, the fibre becomes thicker, stronger, stiffer and more brittle. The best quality is obtained before seeds are fully ripe, so by harvesting three months after seeding, you sacrifice nearly all the seed crop. If you wait four months, and the seed is fully ripe, you get coarse fibre.

This timing difference is one of the main reasons farmers choose fibre or seed strains. Flax fibre was used in printing of Canadian money, until plastic was introduced. The straw can be used to make cigarette papers.

In October 2002, the Alberta Research Council entered an agreement with The Natural Fibre Association, and a German association to jointly study ways to add grain straw, flax and hemp fibre to a wide range of valued-added products. Agri-fibres are a billion dollar industry used in textiles, pharmaceuticals, resins, insulation panels, newspaper and even car brakes.

Researchers at the Institute for Plant Biochemistry in Halle have succeeded in isolating a gene from english marigold that if introduced into linseed plants, would make it possible to produce calenduleic acid.

Normally, flax is lacking a key enzyme, linoleoyldesaturase, needed to produce this fatty acid, widely used by cosmetic industry and as natural additive for dyes.

The enzyme creates a double link in a long chain of fatty acids, and turns a saturated fatty acid into an unsaturated one with potentially higher value.

Dr. Randy Weselake, U of Lethbridge, is working on bio-plastics from flax. This is not a big stretch, as linoleum illustrates. He is part of the Green Chemistry Network, a group of scientists using renewable resources that do not pollute.

Since the world consumes some 140 million tons of plastic a year, this has enormous potential.

The flowers with immature seeds contain 0.69% hydrocyanic acid; with only a half pound of the flowers ingested by cattle enough to cause death.

There is still to this day in England, an Act of Parliament that forbids the steeping of flax in rivers, or any water drunk by cattle, as it is poisonous to cattle, and fish in the water.

The unripe seed capsules are toxic to livestock, but used as a base for chutney in India.

In veterinary practice, the oil is used as purgative to sheep and horses, and a jelly formed from the boiled seeds is often given to calves in digestive distress.

The press cake is used for animal feed. This has a lysine content of about 4%.

Flaxseed, at 5% of rations, increases the number of pigs, conception rates, the production of more milk and bigger piglets. This is the conclusion of Dr. Baidoo, a swine nutritionist at U of Manitoba. He found, for instance, that by feeding a flax supplement at 5%, a 2,400 sow operation could be cut back to 1,800 sows, reducing feed requirements by 100 tonnes annually and still produce the same number of piglets at the end of the day. Omega-3 fatty acid content of meat was also increased.

Work at Kansas State University found feeding ground flaxseed to cattle 70-120 days before slaughter increased carcass value $10-15, and found 14% more animals graded higher, due to improved marbling. Researchers found lower back fat levels and up to 10 times increase in ALA, or alpha-linolenic acid.

Flaxseed helps ward off bovine respiratory disease, if feed for the first 35 days after moving to feedlots.

Chickens and turkeys have been shown to exhibit B6 deficiency from de-oiled meal, and ewes on a diet containing flaxseed meal have produced lambs with acute goiter, due to thiocyanate. Thiocyanate, even in humans, is formed in the liver to neutralize cyanide. In one experiment with two male adults, the urinary excretion of thiocyanate increased seven fold from only 60 grams of flaxseed daily.

The effect on thyroid and goitergenic activity is not fully understood but probably not of great concern.

Fish farming is another potential use. Dr. Murray Drew, U of Saskatchewan says, "annual world fisheries harvest about 30 million metric tonnes annually, and we expect this to triple in the next 10 years. Flax may be a suitable source of ALA, omega 3 fatty acid, now supplied by fish oil.

Atlantic salmon fed flax oil had omega 6:3 ratios lower than other fish oils.

Flaxseed contains cyanogenic glycosides and mucilage that are anti-nutritional to fish, however. Work is continuing, expecially for organic salmon market.

Omega 3 eggs are produced, by supplementing flaxseed in chicken diets.

Since flax contains a pyridoxine antagonist (1-amino D-proline) that occurs with glutamine (linatine), supplementation with B6 helps overcome this problem. The eggs contain 6-8 times more omega 3 than regular eggs, or equivalent to four ounces of fish.

Extruded, heated whole flax mixed 50:50 with peas provide the highest energy and lipid levels. Low mucilage flax would make protein more bio-available.

Flaxseed press cakes contain 75% arabinoxylan, an interesting high molecular weight compound. Warrand et al, *J Ag Food Chem* 2005 53 looked at possible new applications for these polysaccharide hydro-colloids.

In Ayurvedic medicine, the leaves are used for asthma and coughs, while the seeds are used for backache, biliousness, consumption, inflammation, leprosy, ulcers and urinary discharge.

Fumigation with seed smoke was recommended for head colds and hysteria. Bad idea!

Unani medicine uses seed oil for "bad blood", internal wounds, and ringworm and burnt bark as a styptic for wounds. The bark and leaves are for gonorrhea, while the seeds are considered aphrodisiac, emmenagogue and increase breast milk production.

The seeds and oil are official in nearly every *Pharmacopoeia* of the world, save Mexico.

Cherokee used introduced flax for violent colds, coughs and diseases of the lungs. They made decoctions that were poured over the body to cure fever attacks. The seeds were used for gravel or burning during urination.

Linseed infusions are used in veterinary medicine as a demulcent drink while the oil is a purgative for horses and cattle.

Various studies have indicated the importance of Omega 3 fatty acids for dogs and cats, for improving health of skin, coat, and nails. Merchant et al, *Advances in Veterinary Dermatology, Compendium* 1994 16. See seed oil.

Stabilized flaxseed is treated with zinc and B6, preventing rancidity in natural pet products.

Those interested in flax as a prairie crop can e-mail the Flax Growers of Western Canada at foodfocus@quadrant.net.

In the summer of 2009, GMO flax was found in a shipment from Canada to Germany. This genetically modified flax, known as Triffid, is problematic as 70% of flax is exported. This "accident" has created ongoing export problems to European Union.

Wild Blue Flax (*L. perenne/ L. lewisii*) seed is used in Europe and China as an emollient. In England, the fresh herb was boiled and taken for rheumatic pains, colds, coughs and dropsy. For diarrhea, a tincture of the entire plant can be useful.

Various native tribes roasted and ground the seed. The raw seeds contain small amounts of hydrocyanic acid, destroyed by roasting.

The Thompson and Okanagan of British Columbia infused flowers, leaves and stems as a wash for teenage and female skin and hair. The plant name roughly translates as "body or hair wash for pubescence".

Métis of western Canada know the plant as **PIKWÂCI WÂPAKWANIYWI-PAKWA**.

The Shoshone and Paiute used leaf poultices to reduce swellings, gallbladder trouble, or infused the whole plant as eyewash. In fact, the Shoshone name **BOO-EE NUT-AH-ZOOM** translates as "eye medicine". The root was preferred, but infusions of the stem, leaf and root were sometimes used. The stem was steeped for stomachache and gas.

Various preparations included whole plant, tops, or root in cold water or boiled preparations, depending upon the condition to be treated.

The Navaho decocted leaves to treat heartburn and headaches. Perennial flax seed was used in New Mexico, combined in a warm paste with cornmeal for swellings, lumps, boils and sore throats.

Various Native tribes gathered the fibers to make fish nets, and twine.

Purging or mountain flax, a native of Europe, is naturalized all over northeastern North America. It is purgative and depurative in nature; large doses are emetic and can cause cardiac concern. As a laxative, it is somewhat gentler than Senna, but with similar action. It combines well with peppermint to prevent griping.

Infusion of bruised stems, simmered in wine, was widely used in Europe as a purgative.

The effects were too powerful, with undesirable side effects, and use was discontinued.

Legend has it that the fairies use it to make their clothes and the small bells (seeds) make music that humans cannot hear. Maybe.

In Gaelic and Celt-speaking regions of British Isles, the herb was used for menstrual irregularity, and abortifacient. A minor use in Ireland was for urinary complaints, or boiled in beer for jaundice.

A combination of this herb and small meadow rue (*Thalictrum minus*) was infused to bring on suppressed menses.

Grieve wrote "dried herb has been found very useful in muscular rheumatism and catarrhal affections, the infusion of one ounce in a pint of boiling water being taken in wineglassful doses. In liver complains and jaundice, it has been employed with benefit."

John Quincy suggested this "only for very robust strong constitutions".

The plant is sometimes introduced to pastures, allowing animals to graze as they require.

Linola is a form of flax that produces high quality edible seed oil. It looks and grows like flax, but is more drought-resistant, with yellow rather than brown seed. Linola is available exclusively through United Grain Growers. The newest variety Linola 1084 seed has 45.4% oil content, used mainly in the margarine market.

The newly developed Solin flax variety contains around 70% linoleic acid with low levels of ALA.

White Flax (*L. album*) from Europe has been found to accumulate lignans, including podophyllotoxin. In dark and light-grown cultures, high yields of lignans (0.5%), mainly podophyllotoxin were produced. *Phyotochemistry* 1998 48:6.

Podophyllotoxin is the starting compound for the semi-synthesis of the anti-cancer drugs etoposide and teniposide. To herbalists, it is one of the active compounds in Mandrake or Mayapple *(Podophyllum peltatum)*.

Flax is a strong accumulator of cadmium, and the soil should be checked for this heavy metal before any crops are grown.

MEDICINAL

CONSTITUENTS- seed- mucilage (3-10%) pectin, enzymes, fatty oils (35-45%), protein (25%) lignans (SDG, matairesinol, (-)-pinoresinol digluco-pynanoside , cyanogenic glycosides (0.05-0.1%) linustatin, neolinustatin, linatine, lotaustralin, and linamarin; flavonoids such as herbacetin 3,8-0-diglycopynanoside, herbacetin 3,7-0-dimethyl ether and kaempferol 3,7-0-diglucopyranoside; and phenylpropane derivatives including linusitamarine. Also contain tocopherol, 0.7% phosphatide, cadmium and minerals.
leaf, flowers- linamarin and lotaustralin
aerial parts- C-plycoflavones lucenin-1 and -2, orientin, iso-orientin, vicenin-1 and -2, vitexin, and iso-vitexin, anthocyanidins, and glycosides and esters of p-coumaric, caffeic, ferulic and sinapic acids.
Root- vanillic acid, syringic acid, xanthine, vitexin, isovanillin, tachioside, berberine,

beta sitosterol, stigmasterol.

L. catharticum- various lignans including the bitter achromatin present in the fresh plant as a glycoside, linin, tannins, and volatile oils (0.15%). Also includes 5-methoxypodophyllotoxin, linamarin, and lotaustralin.

L. album- 5-methoxypodophyllotoxin

L. lewisii -aerial parts- linamarin, linoxepin lotaustralin.

seeds- linustatin, and neolinustatin.

Flaxseed is very useful for treating chronic constipation, irritable bowel, and colon damage caused by chronic laxative misuse or abuse. It is soothing and protective of the stomach and diverticular disease.

If seed is ground before eating, then essential fatty acids are available to the body. Some authors suggest that overweight patients use the whole seed, to limit caloric value.

This is only partially correct, as ingestion of higher quality essential fatty acids can actually help weight loss regimes.

Infusions are excellent for inflammation of mucous membranes of respiratory, digestive and urinary systems. Crush seed first for maximum benefit.

The stronger decoction is more suited to an injection enema for hemorrhoids, inflamed prostate, or as a douche for inflammation, leucorrhea, various odorous discharges, vulvitis and vaginitis. A tampon can be saturated and inserted at least one hour, repeated as necessary.

The crushed seeds make a good poultice for colds, pleurisy, and coughs, with or without mustard. Sometimes lobelia or hollyhock seeds are added to the poultice in the treatment of boils.

Flax poultices are excellent for enlarged glands, joints, swellings, carbuncles, pneumonia, pleurisy, sprains, bruises, contusions and inflammation (superficial or deep-seated) anywhere on the body. Be sure to coat the skin with oil before application.

The heated seeds can be applied to abscess. For mature furuncles, fill a linen bag with one-third flaxseed and sew shut. Then briefly boil until the bag is full, remove and gently squeeze to remove excess water. Wrap in clean cloth and apply to affected area, repeating as necessary. For severe inflammation, a cold arnica tincture compress is better.

Internally, seed tea is used for coughs, colds and urinary irritation, usually combined with lemon and honey.

With lemon, it is used in Lebanon for cystitis, gallstones, gravel, hepatitis, and kidney stones. Internally, fresh flax seed oil is given as laxative.

The roasted seed acts with more astringent property.

In the 1950s, a German biochemist Johanna Budwig, brought attention to flaxseed as part of cancer diet. Restricted foods were sugar, animal fats, salad oil, meats, butter and margarine; while whole foods, fruits, vegetables, and cottage cheese mixed with fresh flaxseed oil were encouraged.

Udo Erasmus, in his book *Fats that Heal, Fats that Kill*, recommends flaxseed oil as the only oil for cancer patients.

Linamarin is similar to glucoside found in lima bean (phaseolunatin), with a sedative effect on the respiratory system.

Dr. Muir and others at the Saskatoon Research Centre have developed a process for the extraction and purification of the lignan, secoisolariciresinol di-glucoside (SDG) from flaxseed. First identified in 1956, there was no thought to its biological activity.

In the late 1970s, research groups in Europe discovered two new compounds in urine thought to be new hormones. The level appeared to fluctuate with the menstrual cycle in females, and the level was low in women with breast cancer and high in vegetarians.

These were determined to be enterolactone and enterodiol, collectively known as mammalian lignans. It is soon discovered the lignans were of dietary origin and produced by healthy bacteria in the intestine. In 1991, Thompson showed that flaxseed was the richest food source of these lignans. Subsequently, numerous studies have linked flaxseed, and SDG, to prevention or risk reduction of breast cancer.

A clinical trial by Thompson et al, *Breast Can Res Treat* 2000 64:50 found 25 grams of flaxseed baked in muffins daily change tumour growth when tamoxifen is taken.

Dr. Muir et al, produced a model for lignan production, and found SDG accumulation in developing flax seed 5-7 days after flowering.

Studies on rabbits have shown SDG results in significant reduction in serum cholesterol and LDL levels, and significant increases in healthy HDL.

In one human clinical trial, by Rierenbaum et al, *Journal of American College of Nutrition* 1993, three slices of flaxseed bread and 15 gram of ground flaxseed daily decreased total serum levels of cholesterol and LDL.

Human studies indicate 0.6-2.0 grams of alpha linolenic (Omega 3 fatty acids) daily, decrease the risk of myocardial infarction. De Lorgeril et al, *Lancet 1994* 343.

The compound SDG slowed development of type 2 diabetes in Zucker rats. Prasad et al, *J Lab Clinical Medicine* 2001 138:1.

Plant lignans are soluble and insoluble fibres found at 100 times the density of other sources like wheat, oats, millet, corn, rye, buckwheat and barley.

Researchers have found these lignans enhance immune function and may reduce tumour development.

Flaxseed hull is evenly split between insoluble fibre and a highly soluble, pre-biotic mucilaginous fiber fraction. This makes the hull capable of high water absorption, moisture-binding capacity, and lubricity.

Allman et al, *European Journal of Clinical Nutrition* 1995 found ingestion of 40 grams of flaxseed oil daily more than doubled levels of platelet eicosapentaenoic acid (EPA).

Research shows patients with breast or colon cancers measure dramatic lowering of lignan content in body wastes. This suggests phenolic lignans assist in modulating immune response and detoxification of several metabolic processes. This may be of importance in moderating patients with food hypersensitivity.

Cunnane et al, *American Journal of Clinical Nutrition* 1985, found consumption of 50 grams of flaxseed for 4 weeks increased bowel movements by 30% and reduced LDL cholesterol by as much as 8% in healthy, young adults.

A study conducted at Victoria Hospital in London, Ontario found evidence flaxseed may help patients with lupus nephritis, associated with SLE.

Eight patients took daily doses of either 15, 30, or 45 grams of dried flaxseed for three months. Thirty grams performed best, and reduced the amount of total and LDL cholesterol. The results lasted for over a month after the study was complete. *Kidney International* August 1995.

A recent study at St. Boniface Hospital in Manitoba, found 30 grams of flaxseed added to diet of 55 peripheral arterial disease patients, showed, on averate, systolic and diastolic blood pressure reduction of 10 mm and 7mm Hg, respectively. The control group of 55 had no change. Results were reported at *American Heart Association Scientific Sessions* 2012.

Flax researcher, Dr. Lilian Thompson, U of Toronto, says, "Lignans subdue cancerous changes once they've occurred, rendering them less likely to race out of control and develop into full-blown cancer."

Researchers suspect flaxseed increases kidney filtration capabilities, and circulation in the kidneys' glomerular capillaries.

In SLE patients, these capillaries become inflamed, leading to dialysis and kidney transplant in some cases. Austin et al, *Seminars in Nephrology* 1996.

Flaxseed: a potential treatment for lupus nephritis. Clark et al, *Kidney International* 1995.

Other studies have examined potential anti-malarial effects of flaxseed and oils in the human diet. Levander & Ager, *Flaxseed and Human Nutrition* 1995.

Flaxseed may help offset the hot flashes of menopause. One study has shown that enterolactone substantially decreased the frequency and severity of hot flashes. Haggans et al, *Nutrition Cancer* 1999 33.

Flaxseed may alter female hormonal function. Phipps et al, *Journal of Clinical Endocrinology and Metabolism* 1993.

Eighteen healthy, normally cycling women found the second half (luteal phase) of their menstrual cycle lengthened when they supplemented 10 grams of flaxseed powder a day.

Flaxseed lignans are structurally similar to estradiol, diethylstilbestrol and tamoxifen.

An interesting study tested the flax derivative enterolactone on human breast cancer cells, which multiple when exposed to estradiol (human estrogen). When the researchers added enterolactone to the culture, it behaved like estrogen and stimulated cancer cell growth. But when they treated the cells with both estradiol and enterolactone, the cell growth was inhibited, much like tamoxifen in human patients.

It is interesting to note that oncologists suggest women taking tamoxifen avoid eating flaxseed.

Preliminary rodent studies suggest a role in preventing colon cancer and reducing growth of breast tumours. Thompson et al, *Carcinogenesis* 1996.

A systematic review of flax and breast cancer found a decreased risk. Protection against and reduced mortality of those with breast cancer was observed. Flower G et al, *Integr Cancer Ther* 2013 Sept 8.

A Canadian study found flaxseed intake associated with reduction in breast cancer risk. Lowcock EC et al, *Cancer Causes Control* 2013 24:4 813-6.

One study of post-menopausal women found addition of flax reduced estradiol and estrone levels and increased serum prolactin. Hutchins et al, *Nutr Cancer* 2001 39. The implications are uncertain.

Kettler, *Alt Med Rev* 2001 6:1 found omega 3 fatty acids, including flaxseed, may preserve bone density and slow postmenopausal bone loss.

Dew TP et al, *Menopause* 2013 20:11 did a systematic review, and concluded that bone density studies are too few to make a recommendation.

The news is good for men as well; research showing flax-derived compounds inhibit an enzyme that promotes growth of hormone-dependent prostate tumours.

In one study at Duke University Medical School, men with existing prostate cancer were given flaxseed for 34 days. At the end of study, they had reduced testosterone levels, lower rates of cancer cell growth and a trend to lower PSA levels- a potential marker for prostate cancer. Demark-Wahnefried et al, *Urology* 2001 58.

SDG was tested on 87 men with prostate enlargement in a randomized, double-blind placebo-controlled trial by Zhang et al, *J Med Food* 11:2.

At both 300 mg and 600 mg daily, improvement in urinary tract health associated with BPH was comparable to alpha1A adrenoceptor blockers and 5alpha reductase inhibitors.

A pilot study by Acatris looked at ten men between 20-70 years old with various stages of hair loss, or androgenic alopecia. They all took 250 mg daily of flax lignans for six months with 8 men showing benefit in Hodgkin's lymphoma and certain forms of cerebral tumours and bladder cancer.

When the roots of *L. flavum* are inoculated with agro-bacterium, the 5-methoxypodophyllotoxin production is 2-5 times that of un-transformed roots; and 5-12 times higher than cell suspension culture, as compared to natural roots.

White Flax (*L. album*) contains anti-tumour and cytotoxic lignans. Weiss et al, *Journal of Pharmaceutical Sciences* 1975 64:1.

HOMEOPATHY

Common Flax (*L. usitatissimum*) poultices have shown to produce in sensitive individuals severe respiratory disturbances, such as asthma; and hives. Its action in such cases is marked by intense irritation. The seed has been found to contain small amounts of hydro-cyanic acid, which may account for this intensity.

Decoctions can be helpful in inflammation of the urinary passage, cystitis, strangury, etc. It has a place in the treatment of asthma, hay fever and urticaria; as well as trismus and paralysis of the tongue.

DOSE-Lower potencies. The mother tincture is prepared from the freshly, crushed seed. Toxicology and clinical symptoms in Boericke, as well as poisonings noted by Clark and Allen.

Purging Flax (*L. cantharticum*) is indicated not only for respiratory symptoms, but also for colic and diarrhea.

The mind is dull and irritable, dreams of travelling by water with some danger, and vigil dreams of cholera.

Prolonged sleep, confusion of time, weight in forehead, fullness in ears, vertigo and congestion of head on bending head backwards. Congestive headache worse on left side.

Night time sneezing, dry mouth without thirst, bad taste in mouth. Urgent calls to stool, yet difficult with pressing down of rectum.

DOSE- as above. Proving by Gelston with one female and four males at tincture, infusion and 1C dilution in 1858.

SEED OIL

Flaxseed oil is one of the richest sources ALA with twice the density of salmon oil, another good source of omega 3 fatty acids.

As well as 55% alpha linolenic acid (ALA), it also contains 15% omega 6, 21% omega 9 as well as oleic acids, with less than 10% saturated fats. It should be noted that ALA requires conversion via the liver to form omega 3. This is not a pathway for those with impaired hepatic function.

The seed oil is rich in phospholipids that form cell membranes, promote nerve insulation, and improve immunity.

Flax provides sterols that are precursors of hormones such as estrogen and testosterone. These include delta 5-avenasterol, campesterol, cholesterol, cycloartenol, daucosterol, 24-methylene cycloartenol, sitosterol and stigmasterol.

Nutritionists believe cold-pressed, organic flaxseed oil results in smoother skin, improved immunity, better energy quicker wound healing and less anxiety and stress. Various personal care products such as Noxzema Original Skin Cream, and Ponds Fresh Start Daily Wash contain flaxseed oil.

Ingestion of the oil is great for hair. A study by Glanbia of 33 women aged 45-55 found 16 grams of flaxseed per day in nutrition bars for four weeks improved softness, smoothness, luster, shine, ease of brushing and combing and reduced oiliness.

It helps improve hormonal regulation, and lower cholesterol and triglycerides.

Alpha linolenic acid is believed to block the production of a protein called TNF, or tumour necrosis factor, that help create blood vessels tumours need to grow.

In order for alpha linolenic acid to be converted to omega-3 in the body, a number of biochemical reactions need to take place. In the healthy human, this occurs naturally, at a relatively in-efficient rate.

Work by researchers at U of Alberta and U of Lethbridge, as well as the Lethbridge Research Centre, is looking at ways to incorporate EPA and DHA, from fish oils, into flaxseed oil. Good progress is being made. Most people taking flaxseed oil boost their EPA levels but not the important DHA.

Omega 3 fatty acids appear to limit the production of prostaglandins, which in large amounts, can speed up tumour growth.

Omega 3 appears to reduce the incidence of blood clotting that can lead to heart disease and stroke. It lowers LDL cholesterol, and in one four-week study, taking five tablespoons of flaxseed oil daily lowered harmful LDL by 8%. In this regard it offers better protection against heart attacks than either canola or olive oil.

Most North Americans suffer from Omega 3 deficiency. It is believed that several generations of vegetable oil substitution, particularly those rich in Omega 6, hydrogenated and trans-fatty acids, has led to a plethora of health problems.

Work by Thompson et al, U of Toronto, found the oil reduced growth of established tumours in late stage cancers. *Carcinogenesis* 1996 17:6.

A study by Abdi-Dezfuli et al, *Breast Cancer Research and Treatment* 1997 45 verified flaxseed oil's ability to suppress tumour growth.

Allman et al, *European Journal of Clinical Nutrition* March 1995 compared the intake of 40 grams of flaxseed and sunflower oils for 23 days by healthy, young males. Results showed platelet eicosapentanoic acid (EPA) doubled in subjects consuming flaxseed oil compared to no change taking sunflower seed oil.

Flaxseed oil prevents cancer cells from sticking to other cell tissue, thus reducing the incidence of metastases.

Flaxseed oil may possess some indirect anti-inflammatory properties. In one study, it decreased expression of cell adhesion molecule-1 and E-selectin on blood vessel walls. Normally, these extend out into blood vessels during inflammation and grab immune cells passing by, provoking immune response.

This can exaggerate inflammation, and in fact, flaxseed oil decreases cell aggravation and inflammation. Thies et al, *Lipids* 2001 36:11. This may be part of the benefit experienced in lupus patients.

Work by Bhatia et al, *J Med Food* 9:2 found flaxseed oil protects the oxidative stress caused by cyclophosphamide chemotherapy.

The lignans and phyto-estrogenic activity of flaxseed extends to the oil, but in much smaller amounts. The lignans are both estrogenic and anti-estrogenic, helping reduce symptoms of menopause while also acting as weak estrogen antagonists, helping prevent hormone-sensitive cancers.

Flaxseed oil was found to make tamoxifen more effective in reducing growth of MCF-7 breast cancer cells at low concentration. Saggar et al, *Mol Nutr Food Res* 2010 54:3.

The fatty acids can help to remove heavy metals from the body, combining well with cilantro, ground ivy, parsley and other herbs.

In Ayurvedic medicine, flaxseed oil is considered sweet and a promoter of strength. **KSAUMA** is hot, pungent and aggravates pitta.

Ayurvedic physicians use flaxseed oil to treat urinary complaints, and a massage oil to help Vata types calm their nervous system, and reduce dry, inflamed skin conditions. Panic attacks may be due, in part, to deficiency of ALA. One study found three of four patients with a history of agoraphobia improved after 2-3 months of taking 2-3 teaspoons of flax oil daily. Rudin et al, *Bio Psych* 1981 16.

The freshly extracted oil is vulnerable to heat, light and oxygen, and is best packed in bottles that are dark and nitrogen packed. After opening, the oil should be used quickly, and kept refrigerated at all times.

Solin Flaxseed oil is a good substrate for the production of CLA, or conjugated linoleic acid, due to their naturally high levels of linoleic. CLA research was conducted extensively from 1938-58, but more recently in the 1980s when potent anti-cancer effects were reported. It is used in the areas of weight loss, and has shown ability to improve muscle mass in hogs.

In Russia, the oil is taken for stones, and amongst Afro-Caribbean people in Florida, it is used for bladder trouble, combined with cream of tartar internally.

The seed cake and oil help reduce pain and heal venous ulcers in twelve weeks. Skorkowska-Telichowska et al, *Wound Repair Regen* 2010 June 16.

Boiled linseed oil, also extracted from flaxseed is not edible, but used in making paint, varnish, furniture polish, waterproofing, enamels, primers, roof cement, linoleum (from linum and oleum) oil cloth, patent leathers, photography, coating silk thread, artificial rubber, printer's ink and more. People have been poisoned and died from applying boiled linseed oil, with its contaminants, to skin burns.

Linseed oil holds great potential in the area of synthetic nylons and bio-plastics.

OIL WAX

The seed oil of flax contains 0.01% of a wax, first discovered by Jacobsen in 1922. It has a specific gravity of 0.977, melting point of 65° C.

FLAX WAX

The surface of flax fibre is coated with waxy substances that can be extracted with solvents. The wax is composed of 18% stearic acid, 32% cerotic acid, 43% ceryl alcohol, and 7% hydrocarbons.

The yield is up to 2.5%, with between 8-13% in flax dust that falls off during combing.

The researcher, Gibson, found extraction of compressed blocks of dust leaves a material useable in the manufacture of insulating board.

It is a white to yellowish-green solid with the pronounced smell of flax, hard and brittle. The fatty acids of the wax consist of palmitic, stearic acids, and 12-28% oleic acid.

It has a specific gravity of 0.9083, saponification value of 77.5-101.51, and iodine value of 9.61. Melting point is 61.5-69 degrees C.

ABSOLUTE

Linseed oil absolute is a yellowish to light amber colour, with a mild, fatty oily odour, reminiscent of the freshly-expressed flaxseed oil. It is slightly fishy, like the odour of fresh cod liver oil and a refined oleic acid. The alcohol extract is not always available commercially, but easily made.

FLOWER ESSENCES

Linum (*L. usitatissimum*) is the angelic tailor. The flower essence rebuilds and reinforces the aura. This is most important for those individuals who constantly experience consciousness expansion through drug abuse, alcoholism, and other difficult and painful situations.   **FLORAIS DE MINAS**

Flax flower essence aids in assimilation of information and memory improvement. Reading skills improve partly from easing anxieties. It is a powerful cleanser for meridians, useful in acupuncture and acupressure. Emotional stress is eased.   **PEGASUS**

Flax flower essence is for stagnant energy and fear of spiritual self.
                                        BRYNAHERB

Blue Flax (*L. lewisii*) is a plant of compassion. While not a particularly fragile plant it is a sensitive and delicate plant. Blue Flax is a stimulant to the 3rd and 4th chakras and allows a basic rejuvenation of life force to speak truth in ways that are gentle and appropriate.   **HIGH SIERRA**

Blue Flax (*L. lewisii*) promotes good mental hygiene, discernment and intellectual flexibility. It helps create a balance with the seasons and life cycles.   **RAVENWORKS**

SPIRITUAL PROPERTIES

The spinster's spindle has long been a symbol of femininity. It became represented by St. Gertrude, who took most of the qualities of pre-Christian mother/goddesses such as Freja, Hulda, Perchta, and others. The spindle is also the symbol of the wise old woman and of witches. Flax was also regarded as having to do with feminine activities. In many countries women used to expose their genitals to the growing flax and say, "Please grow as high as my genitals are now". It was thought the flax would grow better for that. In many countries flax is planted by the women, for it is linked up with their lives. Therefore, sowing of the flax and spinning and weaving are the essence of feminine life with its fertility and sexual implications.   **WEIGLE**

In Prussia, the tallest girl, standing on one foot upon a seat, with her lap full of cakes, a cup of brandy in her right hand and a piece of elm or linden bark in her left, prayed to the god Waizganthos that the flax might grow as high as she was standing...If she remained steady on one foot throughout the ceremony, it was an omen that the flax crop would be good!   **FRAZER**

Flaxseed's keyword is illuminator. Flaxseed is the teacher that enhances your sense of rightness. It is excellent for anyone who is feeling off balance or useful for anyone who has fallen into addiction or bad company or a bad direction. Flaxseed will help bring these people back into resonance with their inner truth and their life path.
                                                                    MULDERS

Considering the presence of cyanogenic compounds and highly nutritious oils, both plants present a fine line between noxious and nourishing. Even the touted flax oil is tainted. It boon turns to bust since it becomes rancid after a few days. The oestrogen-like effects are also poised precariously on the knife-edge between help and harm.
                                                                VERMEULEN

BOTANICA POETICA

One stop shopping in a seed
Helps to keep your colon clean
All the laxative you need
Constipation you'll relieve
Get your lipids to behave
Arteriosclerosis you might stave
Osteoporosis won't you enslave
Omega 3, you'll get each day
It's a seed you ought to try
Crush it, eat it or apply
Inflamed skin will heave a sigh
Eczema will be less dry
And such a pretty flower, Flax
With other feathers in its cap
The fiber for your linen slacks
The oil of linseed for art class
It's been around for centuries
The Romans even used the seeds
To fight a cold, a cough, a sneeze
Or urinary tract disease
Oh Flax, you're quite a medicine
Can fight a cold with lots of phlegm
Some say cancer you condemn
Truth be known, you're quite a gem!

SYLVIA CHATROUX

RECIPES

LAXATIVE- Adults- 5-10 grams seeds, whole or crushed in water, up to 3 times daily. Children 6-12 years- Half dose.

FLAX SPREAD- Take one-third cup of hazelnuts, one-quarter cup flaxseed and grind in a clean coffee grinder or processor. Pour in one-quarter cup honey and mix. Store in fridge for up to one week. Use on toast or crackers.

Cardiovascular effect, probably due to hydrocyanic acid, has been recorded at various doses. However, no reports of cyanide poisoning from ingestion of up to 300 grams of raw flaxseed have been reported.

Benefits to the cardiovascular system far outweigh any negatives. Do not buy pre-ground flaxseed. The highly unsaturated fats go rancid within days. Grind at the last moment.

INFUSION- Put one ounce of organic flaxseed in a saucepan. Pour over it, 24 ounces of boiling distilled water. Let stand in hot place for ten minutes. Strain and add four ounces of honey. Mix by stirring, bottle and store in cool place.

Take 2-4 ounces three times daily. Add one ounce licorice root for more laxative product.

BULK LAXATIVE- Take 2-3 tablespoons of freshly ground seed with ten times the water in morning.

Mountain flax is extremely laxative, at doses of 2 grams of powder as a single dose in one cup of hot water, or better yet, warm mint tea. A good recipe for chronic constipation is to take equal parts of raspberry leaf, mountain flax, aspen poplar inner bark, and dandelion root and simmer slowly in water to half the original amount. Dosage is two tablespoons 3-4 times daily.

DECOCTION- Take two ounces of flaxseed to one litre of water. Boil 10 minutes, strain and squeeze out all mucilage and oil. Drink up to one half cup several times daily for constipation.

TINCTURE- *L. perenne-* 2-3 drops in water every hour for diarrhea. The tincture is made of 40% alcohol of the entire fresh plant at a 1:4 ratio.

ORGANIC FLAXSEED OIL- Take one to two tablespoons daily in cereal, or on salads. Do not heat, and avoid rancidity.

POULTICE- Add boiling water to 30-50 grams of ground flaxseed and apply as needed for a hot moist compress. Blend 50:50 with organic, unsalted butter for healthy spread.

SEALING WAX- Take 65 parts of resin (rosin), one part beeswax and one part linseed oil. Slowly melt together over low heat. Use for sealing corks or legal documents. A crayon will give you whatever colour you desire.

CAUTION- Immature flaxseeds may be toxic. In young chickens, growth inhibition after prolonged use is tied to B6 deficiency syndrome. Seeds are safe when cooked.

Flaxseed is an accumulator of cadmium, and levels up to 1.7 mg/kg have been found. In Germany, levels above 0.3 mg/kg are not permitted in food. Esophageal stricture, ileitis or any acute intestinal inflammation can be exacerbated by flaxseed, especially with insufficient fluid ingestion. Oxidized oil is unhealthy and increases, like all edible oils, liver toxicity. Flaxseed may affect the manner in which certain drugs are absorbed, particularly glucose absorption in diabetics. And like all bulk laxative, it should not be taken when there is risk of intestinal blockage. It may potentiate the effect of blood thinners, and best taken with caution by those on blood thinners.

Animal studies show flaxseed oil may increase gastric irritation when taken with NSAIDs. Turek et al, *Prostaglandins Leukos Essential Fatty Acids* 1993. Take two hours apart from medications to reduce chance of interaction.

BLACK HAWTHORN
(*Crataegus douglasii* Lindl.)
RED HAWTHORN
GOLDEN FRUITED HAWTHORN
(*C. chrysocarpa* Ashe)
(*C. rotundifolia* Moench p.p. non Lamb)
(*C. columbiana var. chrysocarpa* [Ashe] Dorn)
LONG SPINED HAWTHORN
FLESHY HAWTHORN
(*C. succulenta* Schrad ex Link)
CHOCOLATE HAWTHORN
(*C. erythropoda* Ashe.)
(*C. cerronis* Nels.)
ASIAN HAWTHORN
(*C. pinnatifida* Bunge)
LARGE FRUITED HAWTHORN
(*C. pinnatifida var. major* [NEBr.] W. Lee)
PARTS USED- spines, leaves, flowers, berries (haws).

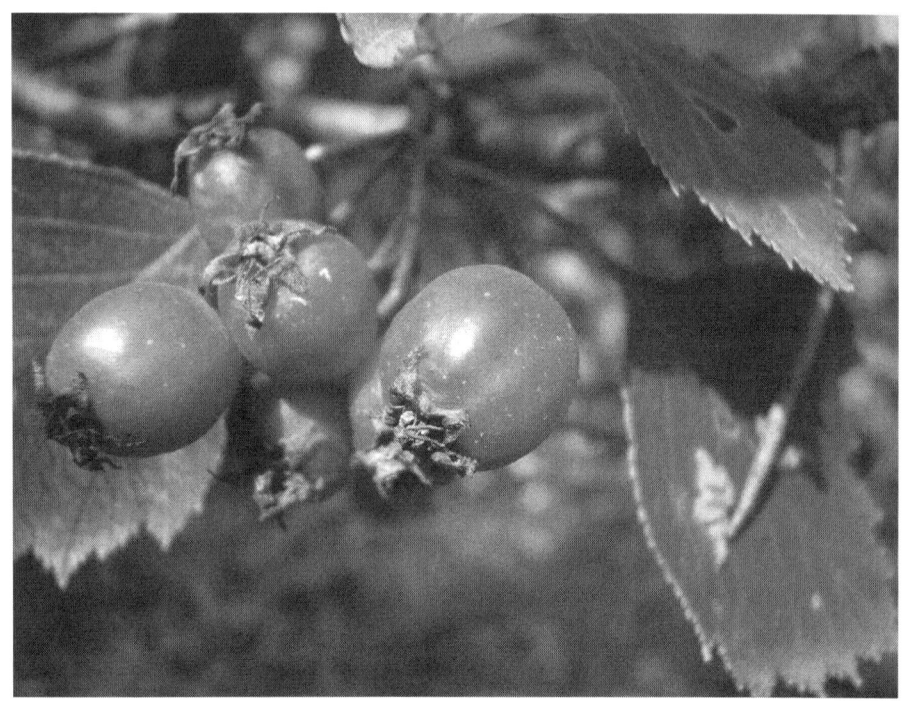

Red Hawthorn (*C. chrysocarpa*)

You are the Hawthorn bush; in spring you clothe yourself in white, at harvest time you dress in blood red.

You rip the fleeces of sheep which pass beneath you. In the same way you pluck any evil, impurity or wrath of the gods from this initiate, who walks through the gate of your hedge.   **HITTITE PRAYER**

A fair maid who, the first of May
Goes to the fields at the break of day
And washes in dew from the hawthorn tree
Will ever after handsome be.   **ENGLISH SAYING**

A thievish clown by cruel thorns opprest
Shows in the moon that honesty pays best.
The Hawthorn bush, with seats beneath the shade,
For talking age and whispering lovers made.

OLIVER GOLDSMITH

The risen cream of all the milkiness of May-time.   **H. E. BATES**

100

Crataegus is from Greek **KRATOS**, meaning strength, mainly due to strong nature of the wood. Words ending in Cracy, like democracy, and aristocracy, stem from the same root.

AGOS is from the Greek, and means bringing. Krataigos, the name given by Theophrastus, a Greek botanist of 3rd century BC means, "bringing strength". Or, Aegus may stem from the Greek **AKIS**, meaning thorn, or **AKE**, sharp point. Then, Krataigos means strong point or thorn, also a good description of the thorny tree.

The first century BC pharmacologist, Crateuas was honored with the nickname of Rizotomos. This refers to traditional herbalists known as Rizotomoi, or root cutters.

The common name Hawthorn is from Anglo-Saxon **HAGUTHORN**, meaning a fence with thorns, from early use as a hedge. Black is from the blackish-purple colour of the fruit when ripe.

Douglasii is named for David Douglas, Scottish botanist and explorer, who made several trips to explore British Columbia and Oregon in the early 1800s. He has numerous plants (Douglas Fir) named in his honor.

He returned to North America in 1830, traveled in California, made botanical trips in British Columbia, wrecking his canoe on the Fraser River and losing his journals and collections of plants. He visited Hawaii in 1834, accidentally fell into a pit trap, and was gored to death by a wild bull.

In ancient Greece, a spring bride would wear a corona of hawthorn flowers, while her daidouchos, or torchbearer, carried a wedding torch of hawthorn wood smeared with pine resin. Hawthorn was dedicated to Hymen, the god of marriage, as a symbol of hope.

In Turkey, the gift of a hawthorn branch implies a kiss is expected.

This was the May tree, and in England a hawthorn wreath served as the female symbol surrounding the phallic pole. The gathering of hawthorn blossoms was known as "going a-Maying". Traditional May Day festivities are times of courtship, dancing and love-making in the woods.

Some authors suggest the flower's heavy scent is somewhat erotic, and reminiscent of female sexual secretions, but I believe that is overstated.

The strange burnt rubber smell was believed to carry the Great Plague, according to some sources. In the 19th century, the sickly scent of hawthorn was identified with sickrooms and death. Today, there are many people that will not permit the flowers in their home. The scent of Hawthorn blossoms is due in part to trimethylamine, a by-product of tissue decay. Trimethylamine scent stimulates the pulse rate slightly and has a peripheral vasoconstrictor effect.

It is said that bringing a flowering branch into the house gives one year of bad luck.

Other legends say it grew from a branch of the Holy Thorn, brought to England from the Holy Land by Joseph of Arimathea. He thrust his staff into the ground, and it took root and leafed. It is said to bloom twice a year, once in spring, and at midnight on January 6th, the Orthodox date of Christmas. The tree is the *biflora* variety of *C. monogyna* that in fact does bloom winter and spring. A slip of the tree now grows on the grounds of the National Cathedral in Washington, DC.

In the Druid tree alphabet it represents the letter H (uath), fertility, and the 23rd Nordic Rune, Odal.

An old English name for hawthorn buds, when just expanding, was Lady's Meat. King Henry VII, the first of the Tudor dynasty, named the Hawthorn shrub his badge of honour.

Superstitious Roman mothers stuck hawthorn leaves in baby's cradles to ward off evil. The tree was sacred and related to Cardea, the goddess of childbirth, and guardian of the threshold between the past and future.

The Irish called the trees Fairy Thorns, a place for wee folk to meet. Hawthorn was considered, in medieval Europe, to be a witch's favourite spot to rest, especially on Walpurgis Night.

One of the first hawthorn goddesses was Olwen, daughter of Yspaddaden Pencawr to Celts of Wales. She was the virginal aspect of the White Goddess, and it was said that white trefoils (clover?) grew where she walked. The Welsh goddess Blodeuwedd was associated as well, and formed from nine types of flowers for the Celtic Sun God.

In Brittany, Viviane enchanted Merlin to sleep under the tree until he re-awakened in another age. In the *Mabinogion*, Culhwych, the nephew to King Arthur, has to fulfill 39 tasks set by the Giant Hawthorn, to marry his daughter Olwen—"She of the White Trace".

In Iceland, hawthorn is known as **SVEFNTHORN**, or sleep thorn. Odin used a thorn to send Brunhilde into a magical sleep.

The Christians, of course, counteracted the sexual significance by having Jesus wear the crown of thorns from hawthorn. Some beautiful woodcarvings of hawthorn leaves and flowers can be found in churches.

Before 1899, only 65 species were known, but today there are more than a thousand. Red Hawthorn is the official state flower of Missouri, *C. monogyna*, the official emblem of Estonia.

Boiled hawthorn roots have been used in many cultures for back pain, by helping "bring strength" to the spine. In the Doctrine of Signatures, a spine from a plant must indicate support for our spine.

Spines of Black Hawthorn were used by Native americans to pierce ears, pop boils, lance splinters, make fish hooks and game pieces.

The wood is very hard grained and durable, for tool handles and weapons. Digging sticks were sharpened into a chisel point at one end and fire hardened to temper.

Black Hawthorn was known to the Cheyenne of Montana as bear branch berry. They were gathered when ripe and dried for winter use.

In fact, one Haida name for the thorns, **STLII.N**, means literally spine, thorn or quill of a porcupine.

Hawthorn and other members of rose family contain proanthocyanidins discussed below. When tent caterpillars, for example, attack one side of a grove, eggs laid on the other side when hatched were denied a source of food by inedible anthocyanidins excreted at the other side. This helps prevent total foliage destruction, another example of plant's protecting themselves.

An interesting genetic experiment was conducted with gypsy moths in 1966. The colony was about to die from in-breeding and a diet of alder leaves, and made a complete recovery when fed hawthorn leaves, becoming stronger and larger.

The Cree named the relatively rare round-leaved Hawthorn **MISIKAMIN-AKASKOSE** meaning "large thorn plant".

The Nlaka'pamux or Thompson, used the fruit, and bark decoctions for relieving diarrhea; making sure the bark was collected from the side facing the rising sun. They made a decoction of sap, bark, wood or root as a stomach medicine; the bark or cambium layers, inner side down, for chest pains.

Other tribes used root tea for backaches, and soaked the flowers and leaves in boiling water for cough medicine.

Red or gold-fruited Hawthorn comes about because the fruit is either red or yellow orange in colour, sometimes both on the same tree.

The Blackfoot know *C. chrysocarpa* as Foot Blister Berries or Fire Berry, as well as **L'KAASI'MIIN**.

The Kwakiutl chewed the leaves, and applied them to swellings. The Bella Coola believed that eating too many berries would attract visitations from supernatural beings.

Further east, the Chippewa gathered the ripe haws of **MINE'SAGA'WUNJ** and squeezed them together into cakes without cooking. The cakes were dried on birch bark and then stored for winter cooking. A decoction of roots of C. *aestivalis* was used for back pain, up to a quart daily.

The Forest Potawatomi used the fruit to cure stomach complaints. They call it thorn bush or **MINESAGA'WIC**.

The Meskawi used un-ripe fruit to treat bladder conditions.

The Mohawk used *C. punctata* wood chips with *Malus* species shoots and bark as a hypotensive remedy to stop menstrual bleeding.

The Cayunga peoples used *C. submollis* with pigweed (*Amaranthus retroflexus*) as magical antidote for the lovelorn, according to Diana Beresford-Kroeger.

The leaves were dried and smoked, or flavored with fruit juices and dried again for a more pleasant pipe.

The pips or nutlets inside the fruit were dried and ground to make a coffee-like beverage. Diana Beresford-Kroeger, in *The Global Forest*, suggests these nutlets contain high amounts of caffeine. The seeds may be roasted for additional flavour.

The first recorded, written use of hawthorn was for gout by Petrus de Crescentis in 1305.

From then, until the 1890s, Hawthorn was used mainly for dropsy, kidney stones and as a digestive aid.

An Irish physician, Dr. Green, first used a tincture of the fresh berries for cardiac problems. In Devon and the Isle of Man, flowers and berries were used as a heart tonic. In the Scottish Highlands, hawthorn tea was taken to balance blood pressure. One report from East Anglia indicated leaf decoctions ease labour pain, in the manner of raspberry leaf. In Ireland, the dried bark is steeped in black tea as a toothache cure.

In 1917, the famous Eclectic herbalist John Uri Lloyd published a Treatise on *Crataegus*. He and his brother prepared tinctures from an American species they never identified, but declared it superior to any others. This followed the work of Dr. Jennings in 1896, and Dr. Ellingwood in 1907.

Under outer bark is a layer of white inner bark suitable for cords, and ropes. Fishing nets made of interwoven hawthorn bark are strong and rot resistant.

The young leaves are edible raw, and can be added to salads, or cooked as greens. In Germany, the leaves are dried and made into a tea that is considered as pleasing as Chinese Green Tea. Sometimes the leaves are mixed with those of Black Currant as a refreshing infused hot beverage.

The green buds can be added to salads, especially good in new potato salad. In England, the buds are used to make a suet pudding, with a light crust rolled out long and thin and the surface dotted with the buds and thin strips of bacon. This is rolled up, sealed and steamed for an hour or more.

The young flowers have an unusual smell, and can be added to desserts and drinks, including a delicate wine. In England, it was believed that hawthorn flowers preserved the stench of London during the Black Plague. Others consider the smell sexy, and hence its association with spring and weddings.

The scent is actually created to attract fertilization by carrion insects. They are attracted by its perfume, and later hatch their larvae in decaying matter.

The fruit was an important food for various tribes. They would dry and grind them into a meal that could be mixed with flour to make a mush, or with animal fat to make pemmican. A jelly made from equal parts of mountain ash berry and haw berry is quite tart and tasty.

In Europe, a liqueur is made from the berries. When collecting berry clusters, a convenient spine is usually left on the stem, making it easy to tack them to a cork or cardboard base.

An old weather proverb says, "Many Haws, Many Sloes, cold toes." If the berries are thick on the hawthorn, you had better get ready for a cold winter.

Hawthorn, as a cardiovascular tonic, is helpful for racehorses and working dogs under blood pressure stress.

Later in life, of course, it can be used for support of older animals with congestive heart failure, damage from heartworm, or various viral and bacterial infections.

Hawthorn tincture made from fresh berries can be given to livestock to prevent miscarriage.

Hawthorn bark has an interesting property, useful for survival skills. The bark is peeled off the tree when wet and allowed to dry. When needed, the bark is moistened and placed by a fire to absorb heat.

When warmed, the fibre can be stretched, making it pliable and easy to work. It can then be applied to areas of fracture after the bones are set, and as the bark cools it shrinks and forms a durable cast.

Hawthorn wood makes excellent fuel, producing the hottest wood fire known. It is more desirable than oak for oven heating, and the charcoal made from wood is said to melt pig iron without the aid of a blast furnace.

The leaves contain hormones that influence growth and development of caterpillars, as well as bio-chemicals that produce adenosine triphosphate or ATP.

The substance RN 30/9 stimulates growth hormone in caterpillars, helping them grow into stronger butterflies for migration.

Cosmetic and hair care products containing hawthorn extracts are used for anti-seborrheic and anti-inflammatory activity, and to increase hydration and elasticity of skin. This is based, in part, on a study conducted by Longhi et al, *Fitoterapia* 1984 55:2.

Hawthorn extracts are often made from the stems, with a pH of 5-7.

In one study of twenty male teens, prone to acne and oily skin, the group was divided in two. One group of ten applied ethanol/water extract twice daily for four days; while the others used a 20% hawthorn extract. The latter group showed a 35% decrease in total acne lesions, with a 69% decrease in *P. acnes* bacteria on skin.

UV-induced erythema was reduced 25% in another study.

The introduced Asian Hawthorn (*C. pinnatifida*) is fully hardy to the prairies, with a hardiness rating of 10 from Morden Research Centre. The large fruit variety, major, is especially interesting.

The fruit is used in Traditional Chinese Medicine for circulatory issues, and digestive complaints. Known as **SHAN ZHA**, the uncooked fruit is used for postpartum abdominal pain due to blood stasis with retention of the lochia, the uterus not returning to normal position after birthing; amenorrhea due to blood stasis, inguinal hernia, or swelling of the scrotum or testicles associated with Qi stagnation.

The stir-fried fruit is warmer and more astringent, and used for food stagnation, loss of appetite; combining well with stir-fried radish seed and germinated barley. The fruit is used locally in soft drinks.

High-end restaurants in New York and Paris are adding hawthorn berries to their menus.

Two common, spineless cultivars, Toba and Snowbird, were developed years ago at Morden, crossing English Hawthorn (*C. laevigata*), and our native *C. succulenta*.

The latter is highly susceptible to cedar apple rust, which can co-host with apple trees. The hybrid is very resistant to this rust and is called *C. x mordenensis*.

Other hardy species are *C. crus-galli, C. chrysocarpa, C. chlorosarca, C. cerronis, C. arnoldiana* and *C. mollis*.

Chocolate Hawthorn is a small native tree that derives its name from the fruit colour, not its flavour. Unfortunately!

MEDICINAL

CONSTITUENTS- flavonoids, including vitexin 4'-xyloside and other C-glycosyl flavones, 1-3% oligomeric procyanidins or pycnogenols, including 1-epicatechol, procyanidin B2 and C1, various triterpene acids including oleanolic, ursolic and crataegolic acids, purines, cholines, acetylcholines, sterols tri-methylamine, chlorogenic acid, as well as Vitamin C, sugars, rutin.
bark- esculin (6-glucoside of esculetin)
leaves- cratemons, amygdalin, luteolin-7-0-glucosides, hyperoside, hyperin, rutin and other flavonoids, including highest source of vitexin, as well as isovitexin, orientin and isoorientin.
flowers- hyperosides, 2-0-rhamnosylvitexin (a flavone C-glycoside)
C. monogyna- seed- 85.7% alpha tocotrienol.

Hawthorn berry, leaf and flower are all heart tonics, slow and gentle in action, but strengthening the heart function overtime. The herb is a mild vasodilator, increasing the supply of blood to heart muscles, thus reducing the chance of spasms, angina and shortness of breath in the elderly. Studies have shown berry extracts help decrease lactic acid during angina attacks.

Many stage one patients of cardiovascular risk have no symptoms at rest, but experience shortness of breath with exercise. These individuals will find much benefit from daily hawthorn preparations.

In moderate hypertension, when pulse and blood pressure are slow to return to normal after workouts, snow shoveling, or walking up flights of stairs, hawthorn will help.

It will gradually lower the diastolic (the lower of the two numbers) pressure and calm the pulse, and soothe arrhythmia associated with functional weakness. Tachycardia, or episodes of rapidly beating heart are well suited to daily administration of hawthorn.

Its greatest use is in slowing down and preventing degenerative heart disorders in a safe and gradual manner. It enhances myocardial contractibility, and yet dilates coronary arteries.

It does possess beta blocking activity, and ACE inhibition, both of which are of real value in cardio-protection.

Hawthorn widens coronary arteries by increasing nitric oxide production, perhaps due in part to the procyanidin content.

One randomized, double-blind, placebo-controlled trial of 72 patients with exercise induced cardiac disturbance, was conducted for eight weeks. Oxygen uptake and anaerobic threshold increased compared to controls. In another trial, 600 mg of extract daily for 4-8 weeks, taken by 78 patients showed significant improvement. Another study of 85 patients taking only 300 mg daily showed no statistical difference, suggesting the range of effective therapy.

Trimethylene, ethanolamine and ethylamine open urinary circulation and secretion of ACE, while coumarins produce urination, hypotension and reduced anxiety.

This is of use in obesity with hyperlipidemia and menopause, when excessive sweats, lack of sleep, and aches, pains and weight gain are problematic.

In Parkinson's tremor, hawthorn helps calm anxiety and gives support for a vegetative parasympathetic activity to reduce muscular spasms. It is worth a trial with multiple sclerosis, due to its muscular and circulatory influence.

The flavonoids dilate coronary and external arteries, and like other members of the rose family, hawthorn is astringent and useful in diarrhea and heavy menstrual bleeding.

Procyanidins, most prevalent in August leaves, slow the heart beat and are antibiotic. Bersin et al, 1955. These are similar to the procyanidins in grape seed extracts.

Crataegus is a natural calcium-channel blocker due to phosphodiesterase inhibition. The increased intracellular calcium levels lead to sustained myocardial contractibility. Early work suggested a mechanism known as phosphodiesterase 3 inhibition. PDE-3 breaks down cAMP, and you can slow its breakdown by inhibiting the PDE-3 that disables it. This is the mechanism in heart drugs such as Primacor and Inocor. In the heart, cAMP allows calcium stored there to be released and increase active calcium concentrations inside heart muscle cells. This causes them to contract, and pump blood more forcefully. In blood vessels, increased cAMP relaxes muscles and allows the blood to flow more easily and blood pressure drops.

New evidence suggests that hawthorn may block the flow of potassium ions in the heart and is therefore a potassium channel blocker.

Calcium, sodium and potassium ions are all involved in heart rhythm regulation. Hawthorn may delay the recharging action of potassium ions like a type III anti-arrhythmic drug. The heart takes longer to recharge, preventing abnormal, fast arrhythmias of the heart.

Matthew Wood relates a story in his book The Earthwise Herbal about Jennifer Tucker, an herbalist in Pennsylvania. A woman came to her with a 4-5 month old boy with a small aorta that needed surgery. She gave the baby hawthorn and at the next checkup the doctor exclaimed, "what did you do to this baby?" He quickly explained the artery was now normal in size.

Recent work on leaf and flower extracts suggests inhibition of extracellular calcium entry into calcium-depleted neutrophils. Dalli et al, *Pharmacol Res* 2008 May 8.

Work by Rodriguez et al, *J Med Food* 2008 11:4 examined the influence of berry, leaf and flower extracts versus berry only, on rat cardiomyocytes. The former showed initiation of robust calcium transients and overload, whereas the fruit only increased calcium sparking, initiation of calcium transients and increased beating rate with no calcium overload. The implication for humans is uncertain, but suggestive.

A meta-analysis of eight double-blind trials on 632 patients with chronic heart failure concluded hawthorn significantly improved the heart's "maximum workload" as well as heart rate, blood pressure, dyspnea and fatigue. Pittler et al, *Am J Med* 2003 114:8.

Hawthorn may modify left ventricle remodeling. Huang et al, *Cardiovas Drug Ther* 2008 22:1.

Both beta-phenethylamine and O-methoxy beta phenethylamine are alkaloids that provide sedative action on the CNS. This makes it valuable for patients who fear flying, agoraphobia, or individuals with fear of death.

A study by Della Loggia et al, *Rivista di Neurologia* 1981 suggests hawthorn may help Attention Deficit Disorder/Attention Deficit Hyperactivity Disorder (ADD/ADHD). Hawthorn extracts relieve anxiety, restlessness and acting out in children.

The herb not only increases circulation to the brain, but stops the inflammation caused by allergies; which give the brain more information than its can process efficiently.

Hawthorn and Green Flowering Oats are a good combination for mood swings associated with menopause, as well as some bipolar conditions.

It combines well with rose hips for varicose vein weakness associated with cardiovascular weakness.

Hawthorn berry combines well with Lobelia for recovering heroin or alkaloid addicts; and with yarrow and linden flowers for those suffering hypertension, associated with atherosclerosis and plaque in arteries.

Combine with Prickly Ash bark to treat poor peripheral circulation and exhaustion, and with cedar (Thuja) for cardiac weakness associated with chronic bronchitis.

It should be noted that the berries help lower blood pressure, while the flowers increase circulation but can be used safely in those suffering low blood pressure. Hawthorn may be useful in hypotension, if the picture pattern fits.

The leaves contain amygdalin, that is sedative and increases the parasympathetic tone of the heart.

Berry syrup can strengthen connective tissue that is weakened by excessive inflammatory response. The high levels of flavonoids are probably responsible for reduction of chronic inflammation, and stabilization of collagen in cartilage, reducing joint damage. Collagen is the principal protein in bone, suggesting use to prevent or repair fractures.

Combine with horsetail and cattail pollen for bone and joint problems and with gravel root, marshmallow root and oak bark for ligaments, tendons and other degenerative connective tissues.

Flower extracts prevent the formation of thromboxane A2, a hormone involved in inflammation.

Hawthorn berry contains a bioflavonoid, procyanadin B2, which helps stabilize connective tissue, and prevent capillary fragility. Collagen strands in connective tissue are bridged by procyanadin B2, which preferentially interacts with blood vessels.

Both leaves and berries are heat sensitive, so boiling probably reduces their effectiveness. Bladder infections and kidney disturbances are helped with dried flower or fruit teas. The saponins in fruit cause reduction of bowel surface tension and improved transport of nutrients. The high emulsifying effect improves excretion of uric acid, one-third of which is broken down in the bowel.

Hawthorn combines well with goldenrod in the treatment of kidney failure, by improving blood circulation through renal arteries, without increasing blood pressure.

I formerly did some work with New Era Nutrition for a nutraceutical company, Prairie Sun. We developed a hawthorn berry-rich food bar, and hot cereal designed for cardiovascular health. It never made it to market.

Crataegus is probably a general cell stimulant. Dr. E. Holtzem, Pharmacological Institute of Bonn University Germany, checked feeding experiments with the fruit fly and hawthorn leaves. Compared with the control group, he found in a group of five generations, a distinct increase in offspring. Feedings with pure oleander acid, one of the triterpene acids of hawthorn, produced the same result.

Oleandrin, also present in Oleander leaves, is an aglycone closely related to the digitoxin of foxglove. It is toxic in large amounts.

Fourteen clinical studies on therapeutic efficacy of hawthorn in 808 heart patients were published between 1981 and 1994. Almost all of the studies showed improvement in clinical symptoms, even in doses less than 300 mg/day.

A Cochrane review of 14 studies showed it worked significantly better than placebo with mild or no side-effects. Pittler et al, *Cochrane Databases of Systemic Reviews* 2008:1.

A meta-analysis by researchers at the Universities of Exeter and Plymouth, England, looked at 8 trials with 632 patients suffering chronic heart failure, and found hawthorn significantly better than placebo.

A recent placebo-controlled study of 143 men and women with average age 64, and mild congestive heart failure, looked at fresh hawthorn berry extracts or placebo, three times daily for eight weeks. Significant exercise tolerance was realized by hawthorn patients versus those taking placebo. *Phytomedicine* 2003 10.

A two-year German study of 952 patients revealed palpitations, stress dyspnea and fatigue reduced by hawthorn extract.

Hawthorn combines well with Valerian root for high blood pressure, or as a sedative for nervous heart conditions.

Hawthorn extracts may protect the heart, liver, and pancreas from effects of a glucocorticoid drug, Isoproterenol sulphate, commonly prescribed for asthma. It may help reverse tissue damage in asthma patients caused by hydrocortisone and steroid drugs. Ciplea et al, *Arzneimittel-Forschung* November 1988.

In fact, Hawthorn inhibits the enzyme, histadine decarboxylase, that transforms histidine to histamine; giving an anti-histamine effect. Small amounts, say 30 drops of tincture, can be tried instead of an inhaler, helping patients reduce or eliminate their use in episodes of chest tightness, or dyspnea.

Ethanol extracts of berries exhibit anti-inflammatory, gastro-protective, free radical scavenging and anti-microbial activity. Tadic et al, *J Ag Food Chem* 2008 56.

Moderate activity was noted against gram-positive bacteria such as *Micrococcus flavus, Bacillus subtilis*, and *Lysteria monocytogenes*.

Lipase, crataegolic acid and saponins help increase gastric activity and digest fats. Austrian researchers found decreased free fatty acids and lactic acid in the body. Oriental herbalists use hawthorn berry for food stagnation, as well as nourishing the heart and spirit.

The leaf paste or poultice can be applied to injuries, skin cancers, rashes, ulcers and tumours, helping reduce pain and swelling. Hawthorn berry infusions make a great gargle for sore throat, and vaginal douche when needed.

Hawthorn, like Echinacea, inhibits hyaluronidase, decreasing the ability of viruses to spread.

Hawthorn appears to strengthen endothelial surface layer resistance, explaining in part, the benefit to tissue health. Peters W et al, *PLoS One* 2012 7:1.

Hawthorn contains compounds that de-activate plasmin, a chemical in the body that allows cancerous tumours to spread. In one study, hawthorn aerial extracts stopped 93% growth of human larynx cancer cells. Saenz et al, *J of BioSciences* 1997 52:1-2.

Hawthorn leaves, as a hot water extract, lower blood sugar levels in STZ rats. Jwad et al, *J Herb Pharm* 2003 3:2.

Both mistletoe and non-infected aerial parts demonstrated significant cytotoxic activity that was more potent than 6-mercaptopurine solution.

Hawthorn contains rutin that kills leukemia and Burkitt's lymphoma cells, and compounds that deactivate plasmin that allows cancer cells to spread through the body.

Work by Thirupurasundari et al, *J Med Food* 8:3 found Hawthorn tincture protected myocardial infarcted rats, and improved liver health as well.

The leaf contains various flavonoids with strong alpha glucosidase activity. Li et al, *J Am Soc Mass Spectrom* 2009 20:8. Application to blood sugar levels is unclear.

Hyperoside, found in hawthorn leaf and St. John's wort, may be beneficial in atherosclerosis and inflammatory conditions associated with high blood sugar levels. Ku SK et al, *Inflammation* 2014 March 9.

In Russia, both the dried flowers and fruit are used medicinally, while in Switzerland, the dried leaves are preferred. I like them all!

Leaf extracts of related *C. pinnatifida* show potent inhibitory activity against HIV-1 protease at a concentration of 100 mcg/ml. Two active compounds, uvaol and ursolic acid, were found active at 5.5 and 8 microM, respectively. Min Byung Sun et al, *Planta Medica* 1999 65:4.

The leaves contain eriodectyol, that inhibits production of thrombus. Song SJ et al, *Planta Medica* 2012 78:18 1967-71.

The berries are soothing to Vata types, neutral to Pitta and aggravating to Kapha types in the Ayurvedic tradition.

The ripe berries are used for abdominal distention and pain, associated with digestive complaints. The unripe fruit relieves diarrhea, the charred fruit stops abnormal bleeding and dysentery.Work by Erl Shyl Kao et al, *J Ag Food Chem* 2005 53 found the dried fruit reveals significant anti-inflammatory potential.

Kao et al, *Food Chem Tox* 45:10 found potential in fruit as cancer chemo-protective agent against tumor formation.

The bark contains esculin, the same constituent found in bark of horse chestnut. It has been found to inhibit chemical-induced carcinogenic action, and bacteria *Bacillus subtilis*. The bark can be collected, even in winter, and made into a hot decoction to reduce fevers.

The bark of *C. oxyacantha* has been shown to regulate procyanidin-mediated anti-oxidant/detoxifying effects in healthy hepatocytes, suggesting the Nrf2/ARE pathway may be important in liver protection and anti-carcinogenic activity. Krajka-Kuzniak et al, *Phytother Res* 2014 28(4):593-602.

HOMEOPATHY

Crataegus (Hawthorn berry) produces giddiness, lowered pulse, air hunger and reduction in blood pressure. It acts on the muscle of the heart and is a heart tonic. It has no influence on the endocardium.It is used for myocarditis, failing compensation, and irregularity of heart. It relieves insomnia of aortic sufferers, anemia, edema, high arterial tension, and cold extremities. It acts sedative in cross, irritable patients with cardiac symptoms.

There may be painful sensation of pressure in the left side of chest below the clavicle; and is said to be a solvent of crustaceous and calcareous deposits in arteries.

The patient may be very nervous and irritable, with pain in the back of the head and neck. It is useful when there is sugar in the urine, especially in children.

It is mainly for the heart, in cardiac dropsy, fatty degeneration, and aortic disease. The heart muscles seem flabby and worn out. The pulse is accelerated, irregular, feeble and intermittent. Angina pectoris, and valvular murmurs may be present.

The circulation is poor, with blueness of the fingers and toes, all aggravated by exertion or excitement. Hawthorn sustains the heart through viral infections. The patients symptoms are made worse by a warm room, better from fresh air, quiet and rest.

DOSE- Mother tincture to 30C. Take 1-15 drops of MT. Must be used for some time in order to obtain good results. The mother tincture is prepared from the fresh, ripe fruit at 1:10 ratio. First proving by Cowperthwaite and Brown with 14 provers and tincture in 1900. Proving by Hinsdale with three provers and tincture in 1910. Proving by Assmann with nine provers with tincture, 1x, 3x in 1930. Proving by Monika Stoschitzky with six provers at 30c in 1992-93, and proving by Chetna Shukla with three females at 30c in 2003.

GEMMOTHERAPY

The young shoots of Hawthorn have a bypass type action. In cases of hypertension, it lowers blood pressure, acting as a blood pressure regulator. It also gently works to moderate low blood pressure.

DOSE- 50 drops of the 1D macerated glycerite of the young shoots of various Hawthorn species, including *C. oxyacantha.*

SEED OIL

The seeds from the hawthorn berry contain 9.63% oil with a pleasant scent, and a yellow to orange yellow colour. It is composed mainly (81%) of oleic acids, with minor amounts of linoleic, linolenic, palmitic and stearic acids.

It has a specific gravity of 0.9161, a saponification value of 172.8 and iodine value of 152.8.

On exposure to air, at a temperature of 50° C, the oil dries after seven hours to a hard, almost colour-less skin. At ordinary room temperature, it thickens after seven days, and dries after ten days.

Hawthorn blossoms have an unusual odour similar to that of Mountain Ash. An "essential oil" of Hawthorn is on the market, but is almost certainly the synthetic chemical anisic aldehyde.

HYDROSOL

CONSTITUENTS- linalool 45%, dimethyl sulphide 42%, terpinen-4-ol 3%, and some minor constituents.

The distilled water of the flowers stay the lask. If clothes or sponges be wet in the distilled water, and applied to any place wherein thorns and splinters, or the like, do abide in the flesh, it will notably draw them forth.   **CULPEPPER**

Viaud suggests the hydrolat is useful for calming the heart, a muscle regenerator and as an anti-depressive.   **VIAUD**

FLOWER ESSENCES

Holly Thorn (*Crataegus* sp.) flower essence opens our hearts to love and the acceptance of ourselves, and others allowing intimacy and the expression of our truth and creativity.

It is indicated whenever there is blocked self-expression and creativity, withholding of one-self, lack of involvement, creating of barriers to friendship, fear of rejection or repression of the true self.

FINDHORN

As a flower essence, Hawthorn protects the heart in times of extreme stress, pain, or grief. It stimulates the healing power of love and cleanses the heart of negativity to restore hope, trust and forgiveness. Use this extract to free the spirit and follow you own path in life.

HARVEY

Hawthorn flower essence is very physical in its effects. It eases the spread of cancer, especially tumours. But it is not very effective against leukemia or bone cancer. In cancerous tumours, it eases the thickening of the cellular structure and its spread.

Precancerous emotional states such as extreme stress or grief over the death of a loved companion can be treated with this remedy.

GURUDAS

SPIRITUAL PROPERTIES

Hawthorn has the ability to create greater attunement to the choices of life, and is one of its most important spiritual characteristics. And it has the ability to assist individuals in understanding how they manifest God in their lives. The way some of these properties are transferred naturally leads to a greater focus of energy on the heart center.

What occurs as a result of this is that an energy is formed in the heart that can be quite warming and remains long after the herb has been used or has fulfilled its function of aiding the blood or the heart.

The etheric signature of the plant appears to have a pulsation that is close to the tempo of a heartbeat. Before taking hawthorn, it is wise to tune into your heartbeat for a few minutes to activate its spiritual properties.

The ability to let go is greatly enhanced with hawthorn. Negative thought forms lodged in a person's own aura may be dislodged or even utterly destroyed. Therefore, there is some benefit in using this herb. This implies forgiveness, but it is not quite so; it is more forgiving yourself than anyone else.

In Lemuria, the plant was often used as a symbol; the fruit or berry was used as a decoration or gift and a way of sharing. In Atlantis, one gave hawthorn to a friend just as one might today give someone a quartz crystal. Love was imbued deeply by the Lemurians into this plant. The devic order was gradually affected by this. This was not the more conscious direction of energy, but one that developed alongside the civilization. This is why the energy of hawthorn today is relatively subtle, yet is may have a powerful effect with certain individuals very attuned to Lemuria. The karmic lesson here is to again allow this energy into the Earth, if people wish to choose it.

The heart chakra is energized. The pericardium meridian is energized, and the etheric and emotional bodies are cleansed. It is sometimes wise to give hawthorn to an animal when the animal has done something wrong.

GURUDAS

Crataegus is indicated any time there is stress that has the potential to cause the patient to close down emotionally, for example, in times of betrayal or terrible loss, divorce, death of loved ones, trauma or abuse. In these cases, *Crataegus* can help to keep the heart open, yet protected both emotionally and physically.

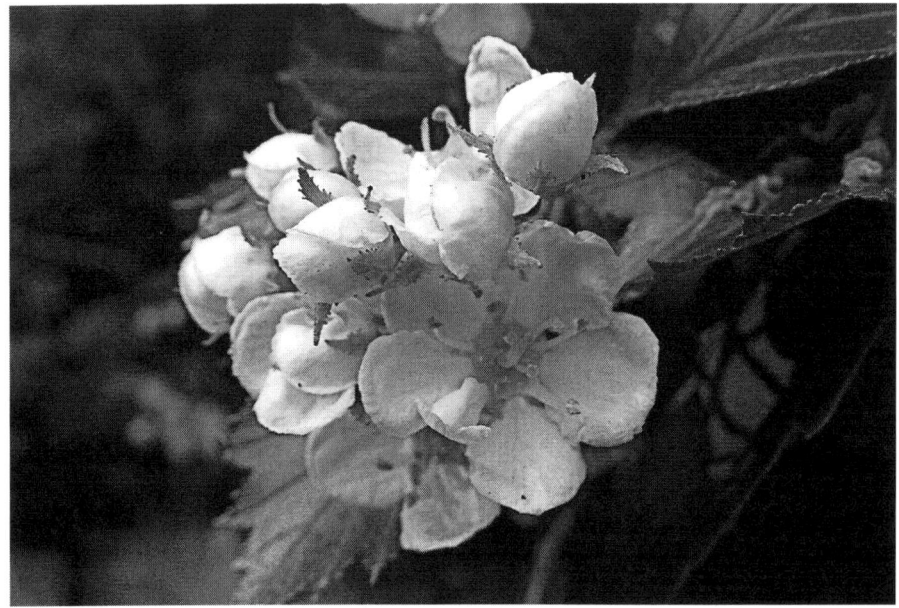

Hawthorn flowers

Crataegus can be of help in alleviating the pain of grief, not blocking the feelings, but rather enhancing the flow of feeling such that the patient does not get stuck or overwhelmed by the grief process. Patients who are out of touch with their feelings and wanting to connect more deeply with their emotions may find *Crataegus* a helpful ally. It can be helpful for patients who find it hard to be receptive, or trust. **DEBORAH FRANCES ND**

As the twilight descends I come upon the Thorn Apple covered with pomes and I notice a flickering of light beneath the tree. I look to see what could be reflecting light but find nothing. As I get closer the light disappears but around the base of the tree is a circle beaten down as if someone were dancing under the tree...

The spirit of Hawthorn can bring balance to the heart organ, the official of the fire element within the Five Element modality, and can also clear the heart chakra.

But the most important use of Hawthorn in Plant Spirit Healing is the ability to put the heart back in its rightful place as the pilot, allowing the mind to serve as the copilot. **MONTGOMERY**

PERSONALITY TRAITS

Hawthorn, also called the May tree, represented the White Goddess Maia, who was the mother of both Hermes and Buddha, as distinct versions of the Enlightened One.

She was the Goddess of love and death; representing the young virgin giving birth to a god, or the Grandmother helping him age gracefully.

She was therefore, the tree associated with both female sexuality and destructive spells.

In England, the blossoms were gathered and place around the Maypole on the first day of May, the wreath the female symbol surrounding the phallic pole.

According to Celtic tradition, the tree was sacred to Olwen; and represented fertility in the Druid alphabet, or the letter H, uath.

WALKER

The Maypole...is a happy, innocent amusement, a symbol of the joy of spring; but few recognize that the Maypole and its dance is one of the oldest and most sexual of public ceremonies involving the Tree of Life.

It was to Earth Mother that people prayed for good crops, human and animal fertility. If Earth Mother was with child, so would be the fields. But gods were forgetful and had to be reminded annually of their responsibilities to the faithful.

Decked with flowers, the tree was ritually worshipped with dances that included sexual orgies…and thus not accepted in Judeo-Christianity.

The spring ritual began in Rome on March 22. The music of cymbals, drums and flutes became wilder as the day progressed. Frenzied by the dance, participants lacerated themselves and dripped their blood upon Diana's epiphany. The dance culminated in self-emasculation of young men wishing to become Diana's priests. The excised organs were thrown at the tree to hasten the resurrection of the earth and its impending fertilization.

With minor variations, the festival was similar throughout Europe. A May Queen was selected, and she and the King of the Woods- called Green George, Father May, Bark King, Grass Lord, or Leaf Man-presided over the dancing. As night fell, the queen and king mated in the fields, and this act was affirmed by the faithful.

The Morris dances of England were May dances, and May Queen Mary only later became Robin Hood's Maid Marion.

One is struck by the universality of concepts which flow around the Tree of Life. Life, death, and the perils of everyday existence must somehow be understood...Carl Jung seized upon this as one of the arguments to support his theory of the collective unconscious, an attempt to integrate the universal symbols humans use to relate themselves to their environment.   **R KLEIN**

The Hawthorn personality is melancholic, pessimistic, irritable and frequently ill tempered. They feel worse in a warm room and improve in fresh air.   **BIANCHI**

Red Haws are associated with the "Monster Woman of the Woods". She lives in a hawthorn grove, and it was she who created the red haws.

If anyone even so much as tastes of their fruit, they come under her spell and are drawn into the grove...

If a person dreams of her, he turns crazy. A dying man will hear her cry from the top of a mountain, "He! he! he!".

If a person passes a hawthorn or enters a hawthorn grove, he must immediately cry out: "Thou are Asin, thou shalt always live in the woods, thou art nothing." Then he may go on his way unharmed.

                    GUILLET

The heart of the hawthorn person may be broken from grief, sorrow, or long-sufferings. Despair and fragility are keynotes. The individual may develop strategies for keeping people at arm's length, just as the plant itself maintains boundaries with its sharp thorns.

The person with chronic heart afflictions tends to close down from a painful world and desires to keep completely quiet, yet even this shows a resistance between the self and a threatening world. This resistance sets up a tension between the flow of blood and the walls of the vessels that contain it. When the walls of the blood vessels are too constricting, the result is hypertension. Hawthorn strengthens the heart muscles, clears the arteries, and makes the blood vessels more elastic in order to withstand heart irregularity.

CLARE GOODRICK-CLARKE

Hawthorn's keyword is courage, especially good for those undertaking a difficult or daunting task. Hawthorn is the keeper of vital energy.

MULDERS

Mangialavori…observed Crataegus patient to have a 'double face' in terms of having an undeveloped, immature side combined with difficulties to 'develop a mature and adult side'.

This immature side enables them to play with kids and to have a strong relationship with children. In addition there is an attitude of service, a duty to help others. It is interesting to note that Janus originally was pictured with one clean-shaven and one bearded face, representing the middle ground between youth and adulthood. He was frequently used to symbolize the progression of past to future, of one condition to another, of the growing up of young people. Hence, he was worshipped at marriages, births and other beginnings. **VERMEULEN**

MYTHS AND LEGENDS

A cunning stepmother wanted to get rid of her husband's son. She prepared lunch with half cooked rice, hoping he would die of indigestion. After a few weeks, the child began complaining of indigestion and losing weight.

One day, the child found a tree with plenty of berries, which he picked and found delicious. He began to feel better and ate them every day, gradually putting on weight.

The stepmother thought what is happening, maybe God is protecting the child? She stopped making lunches with half cooked rice and when the husband returned he found out about the berries from his son and decided to market them to herbalists in town. **HENRY C. LU**

Roman goddess Cardea is often considered identical with Carna. Cardea refers to Latin **CARDO** a hinge, with a suggestion of Greek **KARDIA** heart, the protector of well-being. She presides over door hinges and also over house, family and physical well-being. She was originally an elusive nymph dedicated to virginity.

She would trick any amorous pursuer by sending him ahead of her into a shady cave, under the promise to enjoy the delights of love with him there, meanwhile taking to her heels and hiding in the forest. The trick always worked, except at one time with Janus, the god with one face looking forward and one backwards. She couldn't fool him, so that he had his way with her and in return as a reward for her favours, appointed her the protector of door hinges, giving her a branch of flowering hawthorn to keep out all evil spirits.

Consequently Cardea or Carna is closely allied to Janus's task of presiding over all beginnings, which the Romans believed crucial to the success of any undertaking. This is the reason that the name of the first month of the year is January.

Cardea's alternative name Carna comes from Latin *carnis*, flesh. Combining her influence over beginnings and flesh, she especially protected newly incarnated souls, infants in their cradle, life's beginnings embodied, from striges sucking their blood at night. Striges are described as nocturnal vampire-like birds of ill omen. To assist her, hawthorn leaves were laid in the cradle.   **VERMEULEN**

OTHER INTEREST

Several species of birds called shrikes use hawthorns as killing spikes. The loggerhead shrike snatches large insects on the wing.

If the bird finds its new acquired dainty to be a hard chew, for example, a plump beetle with a chitinous exoskeleton, the enterprising shrike finds a hawthorn bush, and impales the wriggling victim on a long, sharp thorn.

Then? Yum yum!

Shrikes also impale mice and smaller birds on hawthorns. In spite of their facial mask markings, which give them a gruesome mien, shrikes are highly beneficial birds, helping rid large parts of their range of vermin and insect pests.   **CASSELMAN**

When De Lorean set up his car factory in Ireland, there was a lone hawthorn standing in the centre of the site the builders had refused to destroy. Apparently De Lorean finally bulldozed it to the ground himself, and there was little surprise among his workers when the car plant turned out to be a total disaster. **GIFFORD**

ASTROLOGY

The sun warms, relaxes, releases, and stimulates growth. It powerfully affirms all life, and, as the most generous being in our solar system, it unceasingly spends itself for the benefit of living things. In alchemical imagery, the heart is the sun of the body. The heart must be warm in order to relax and to release tension. It can stimulate spiritual growth by opening to love and compassion—for the suffering self as well as for others. When we describe someone as open or warmhearted, we contrast this with the closed, coldhearted person. These warmhearted people are approachable, life-affirming, loving, and giving. They too may have suffered grief and sorrow, but their "sun" remains open and giving.

Just as the hawthorn has a thorny side, Mars, associated with aggressive behavior and suppressed anger, can be an important factor in heart arrhythmias. Nevertheless, in the Greek myth, Mars is disarmed by love. **CLARE GOODRICK-CLARKE**

BOTANICA POETICA
The Hawthorn is a lovely tree
And of its uses all agree
From China to the Eiffel Tower
Its berry, leaf and its flower
All agree it's with the heart
That Hawthorn really plays its part
A cardiac tonic quite renown
Helps to bring blood pressure down
For congestive failure, palpitation
It can improve the circulation
Decrease cholesterol as well
And angina it might quell
It can depress or stimulate
It normalizes any state

Helps the heart to perform
Where it's ailing, here's reform
Collect the berries in the Fall
When the Frost has covered all
A tincture of the leaf and flower
Also has the healing power
When you consider Hawthorn's gift
Think of the heart that needs a shift!
SYLVIA CHATROUX

RECIPES

FRESH PLANT TINCTURE- 15-30 drops. A fresh plant tincture of the flowering tops, twigs, leaves and spines is made of a 1:2 ratio of 60% alcohol in early summer. The fresh berry tincture is made with ripe berries in fall using the same ratio. Combine. The leaf procyanidins are richest in August. Flower polysaccharides are maximal at 15% ethanol. The lower the alcohol content, the more precipitation later.

The flavonoid content of the leaves and flowers is 1%; while only 0.1% for the berries. Standardized leaf and flower products contain 2.2% flavonoids, or 18.75% oligomeric procyanidins. Hawthorn berry was originally used, but higher concentrations of the flavonoids have been found in the flowers and leaves when in full bloom. White blooming hawthorns are medicinal, while the red blossomed trees have not been studied well enough to recommend. One study, by Costa et al in 1986, found young spring shoots the most active. Hawthorn tincture is very safe, and one would have to consume over one gallon at a time to experience acute side effects.

GOLD DROPS- Combine 3 parts Hawthorn, 2 parts Valerian root, and 1 part Squill. Take for heart attack symptoms such as acute chest pain, shortness of breath, sweating and irregular pulse; 20 drops every two hours until symptoms stabilize. Later take 20 drops after meals three times daily as lifestyle is improved.

DRY PLANT TINCTURE- 10-20 drops. A dry herb tincture is made with 1:5 of a 40% alcohol using the previously dried leaf and flowers and/or dried berries.

INFUSION- Use a teaspoon of dried flowers and leaves, and/or crushed, dry berries to one cup of hot water. Steep for half hour.

Take three cups daily for a few weeks, and then decrease to twice daily morning and evening.

Standardized extracts in a range of 300-600 mg daily are considered a therapeutic and clinical dosage of hawthorn. It is extremely useful where digitalis is not tolerated, or where chronic poisoning has resulted from long-term usage. It may potentiate the effects of digoxin type glycosides but appears to be safely taken together. Tankanow R et al, *J Clin Pharmacol* 2003 43 637-42.

It has been used clinically as an intermittent with digitalis (Van Hellemont 1985). Hawthorn preparations may increase side effects of beta-blockers. Maybe.

CAUTION- the seeds, just before germination, release large amounts of cyanogenic glycosides (HCN), or plant cyanide. This poison helps protect the seeds from attack by insects, and stimulates growth and energizes chlorophyll production. Eaten in large quantities, a toxic reaction can occur germinating berries. Always use fresh from the tree, or sun-dried fruit. Boiling will also dispel the cyanide.

Researchers have calculated the toxic dose of *Crataegus* to be 500-1000 times the therapeutic dose in humans. Hawthorn potentiates the action of barbituates.

HORSE CHESTNUT
(*Aesculus hippocastanum* L.)
OHIO BUCKEYE
(*A. glabra* Willd.)
SMALL FLOWERED BUCKEYE
(*A. parviflora* Walt.)
PARTS USED- nuts, bark, leaves

A woman's tongue gives not half so great a blow to the ear as will a Chestnut in a farmer's fire.   **SHAKESPEARE**

These nuts strew the roadside. Very handsome-colored but simple formed nuts, looking like mahogany knobs with the waved and curled grains of knots.   **THOREAU**

But I have peeled away your anger down to its core of love
and look mother
I am a dark temple where your true spirit rises
Beautiful and tough as a chestnut.   **A. LORDE**

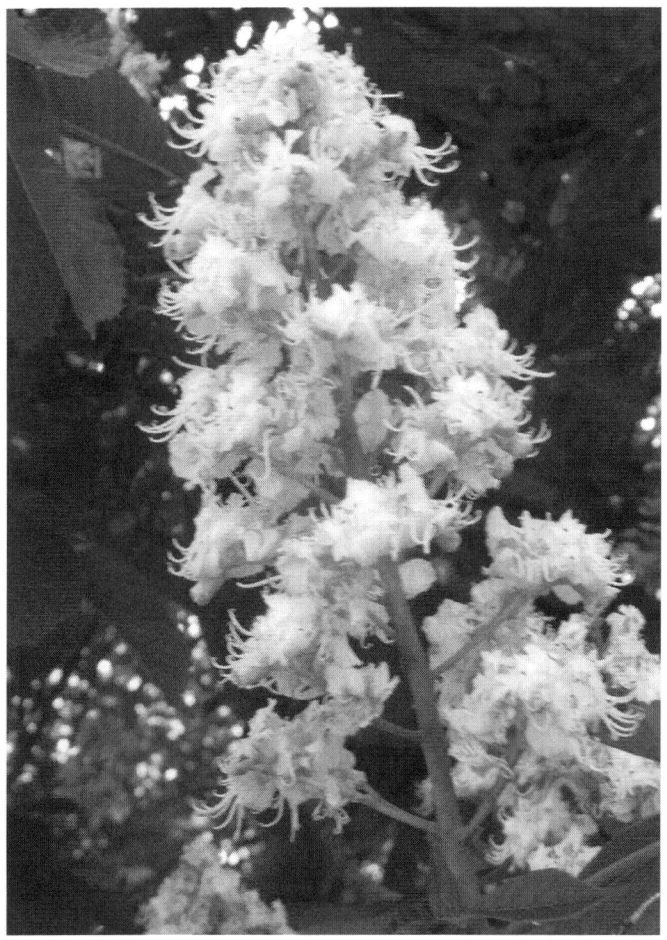

Horse Chestnut flowers

Aesculus is from the Greek name for an Oak. Esca is from the Greek, meaning nourishment, in reference to the seeds.

The word **IPPOS** means horse from the Greek. Castanum is from the Latin, **CASTANEA**, meaning Chestnut. The generic name is possibly related to Balkan horsemen using the saponin rich decoction for soap to wash their animals.

The Common name may be related to the fact that during the middle ages the fruit was fed to horses with coughs. The Arabs fed powdered nuts to horses affected by pulmonary disorders, hence the common name. Other authors feel it is the resemblance of the nut to the eye of the animal. More likely it is related to Horsetail, Horseradish and other references of size and coarseness.

One ingenious author suggested the cicatrix of the leaf resembled a horseshoe, with all the nails evenly placed.

Another likely origin is the Welsh word **GWRES**, meaning "heat" or "fever" due to the seed's pungent taste. This may have turned into Horse. The Buckeye gets its name from the white scar on the nut.

The first Horse Chestnut tree introduced to North America was planted in Pennsylvania in 1763.

Today, it can be found across the whole continent, and flourishes in the zone 3 climate of my present hometown of Edmonton, Alberta. One of the city's Horse Chestnut trees is right downtown, at 106 Street and Jasper Ave. It is over one hundred years old, and one summer one thousand seeds were harvested, with 100% germinating. These seedlings are being offered by Sunstar Nurseries to support a fund to maintain the old mother tree.

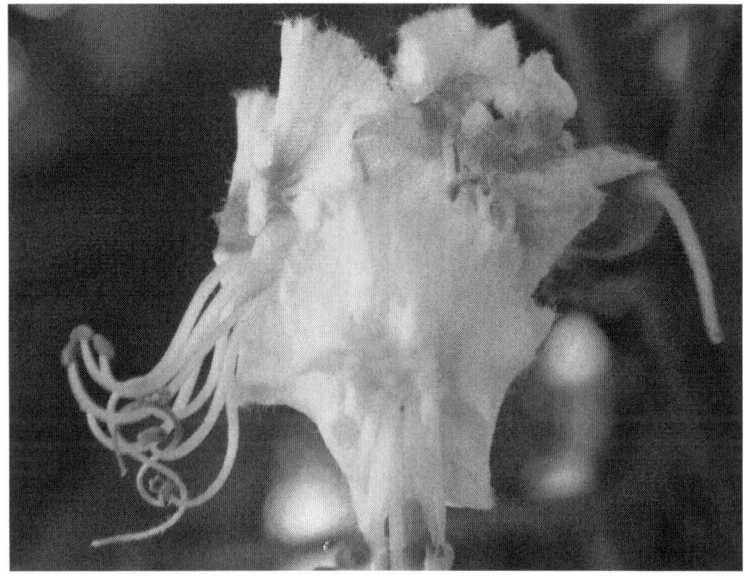

Individual Horse Chestnut flower

When the honey-perfumed flower petals fall, six small nutlets are formed. One grows more quickly than the others, and crowds the rest out. This crowder is the only one to develop.

The flowers have a distinctly masculine, sperm-like, musky smell that can be captured in sun infused oils for perfumes and such.

As a child growing up in Halifax, my brother and I enjoyed the game of conkers.

In the fall, we would go into the cemetery across the road and find the biggest horse chestnuts and string a shoelace through it. When dry, the hard, round objects were whirled through the air, to smash into each other, with only one winner, or conqueror, and the other "conking out". Bilbo Baggins mentions conkers in new film *The Hobbit*.

Each October, in Ashton, England the annual World Conker Championship is held. In Australia, they are known as Bullies.

Traditionally, the nuts were carried in the front pants pocket to ward off arthritis, rheumatism and hemorrhoids. When the nuts dried and cracked, the healing powers went into the human body, and were replaced with fresh specimens. The Horse Chestnut flower represents amusement and the birth date of September 7th.

The Cree of northern Alberta call the introduced tree **WEYIPASATIM, or WIYIPASTIM**.

Farmers in Germany and elsewhere in Europe observed that bulls eating the nuts in large amounts seemed to increase prostate size and usefulness.

The use of Horse Chestnut for medicine dates back to the writings of Matthiolus.

Zannichelli promoted its use for intermittent fevers, for which it was considered equal or superior to Peruvian bark.

The usual dose was one to four scruples of the powder, repeated 2-6 times in 24 hours.

Seed oil was produced in Europe with ether, for use in neuralgia, including internal organs, and rheumatism.

Infusions of the bark or nuts were used for indolent and gangrenous ulcers as a wash.

The seed is narcotic and according to Dr. McDowell, ten grains are equal to 3 grains of opium in effect.

It was used as a fish poison throughout Europe, in a manner similar to mullein seeds or soapwort.

A powder of the light-colored centre was recommended traditionally for ophthalmia and headache.

In Europe, the saponins of the seeds were highly esteemed for cleaning and fulling woolens, especially in France and Switzerland.

The extracts are used in shampoos, foam baths, and various skin care products like hand creams, lotions and toothpaste.

In fact, an early use of the extracted glycoside, aesculin, was a sun blocker, to protect the skin from prolonged exposure to UV rays. Extracts are found in Vitabath Bath and Shower Gelee Moisturizing Bath Gel.

Work by Fujimwa et al, *Int J Cosm Sci* 2007 29:2 found seed extracts generate contraction forces in fibroblast cells, suggesting anti-ageing activity.

Cellulite creams contain aescin, as do sports creams for tendonitis, sprains and other injuries.

The leaf extracts have been used to treat eczema, varicose veins, phlebitis and swelling of tissue, but are less powerful. A new cosmetic product from Indena, an extract from horse chestnut branches, has been found to protect capillaries and preserves the integrity of peri-vascular tissue.

In areas where the tree is plentiful, the nutmeat is given to horses, pigs, cows, goats and sheep after boiling it in potash, and then washing with water.

Germination also renders them a pleasant food, through change of the bitter principles to saccharine, similar to that produced by malting barley. The starch is said to be of finer quality than that of any cereal, and that a paste of the powdered nuts is very tenacious and not attacked by vermin and moths.

Most of the whitish pink flowers are male, but a few are female or androgynous.

The petals have a yellow spot that turns red, and then a green spiny fruit forms containing 1-3 red brown seeds.

They may remind you of Lychee fruit, which is from a related tree of the same Order. Honey from the flowers can be toxic. The young aromatic buds have been used in place of hops for making beer. What hasn't, for that matter?

One component of the seeds, cyclamin, is particularly toxic to fish and has been used in India to paralyze fish in order to catch them more easily.

In China, the fruit and seed of *A. hippocastanum* is used for medicinal purpose. It is called Seven Leaves Tree, or Monkey Chestnut, or **SUO HUO ZI**.

Studies by Yoshikawa et al, *Chem Pharm Bull* (Tokyo) 1996 indicated various escins in the seed have hypoglycemic activity, worthy of further exploration.

The pollen from the flowers, however, causes allergic reaction (IgE) in over 12% of urban children.

Ohio Buckeye is a similar beautiful tree hardy to zone 3. It has a long lifespan, and can grow 30-50 feet tall and wide. It is so common that is has become an emblem of the "Buckeye State". There are several nice specimens at our University in Edmonton, and another at the George Pegg Garden near Glenevis, Alberta.

The creamy yellow flowers in late spring give rise to edible fruit similar in appearance to Horse Chestnut. They contain saponins that are eliminated by boiling in water. They can be eaten only after several changes of water and then chopped up and ground to a meal.

The buds, young leaves and seed have poisoned livestock, especially cattle, resulting in loss of motor control, convulsions, stiff legs, and falling.

The wood of both trees is valued for making superior violins.

Small Flowered Buckeye is semi-hardy to the prairies and produces a beautiful display of dainty, frilly flowers. It is native to southeastern United States.

MEDICINAL

CONSTITUENTS- leaves- castaprenol-11, 12, 13, triterpene saponins, various hydroxycoumarins including aesculin, fraxin and scopolin; flavonoids including rutin, quercitrin and isoquercitrin, and tannins, traces of aescin (escin).

bark- coumarin glycosides aesculin (3%), fraxin, and scopolin and their aglycones aseculetin, fraxetin and scopoletin; flavonol glycoside quercitrin and its aglycone, saponins aescin, allantion, sterols, leucocyanidin, leucodelphinidum, catechol tannins, alkanes

seeds- Aescins, flavonoids, including biosides and triosides of quercitins; oligosaccharides including 1-ketose, 2-ketose, and stachyose; triterpene saponins (13%) known as aescin; (alpha aescin is an equilibrium mixture of beta aescin and cryptoaescin.

Polysaccharides (starch-50%); oligomeric proanthocyanidins; condensed tannins (in the seed coat, mainly cinnamtannins and aesulitannins); fatty oil, allantoin; barringtogenol, escigenin, phytosterols, plastoquinone B.

Aescins (escins) are the total saponins and are a mixture of several glycosides derived from two triterpenoid aglycones from the olean-12-en series; namely protoaeseigenin and barringtogenol C.

The seed tegument, formerly eliminated from the commercial preparations, contains proanthocyanidins which are oligomers of epicatchol.

Aescin not found in seeds at beginning of development, increases to 12-13% by August, and then declines to under 8% by maturity in October.

A. parviflora- cis-alpha-amino-2-carboxycyclopropane acetic acid.

Horse Chestnut leaves have been used as a cough remedy, including whooping cough and to help reduce fevers. Their narcotic activity has been used for treating insomnia.

They are used to reduce the pain and inflammation of arthritis and rheumatism. Very often, dried leaves are found in various vein or hemorrhoid teas.

Leaves are used in Europe for eczema, varicose veins, phlebitis, thrombophlebitis, hemorrhoids, menstrual spasms, soft tissue swelling from bone fractures and sprains; sometimes combined with bark and seed extracts.

The leaves, flowers, fruit and stems have all been tested for anti-microbial activity. Both ethanol and water extracts show activity against gram-negative and positive bacteria, as well as viruses.

The flowers can be prepared as a liniment for neuralgic, rheumatic and gouty conditions. The tincture can be used to relieve abdominal cramping and fainting.

The seeds can be crushed and poulticed and used topically to treat skin ulcers and cancers.

Topical preparations are used for treating varicose veins, hemorrhoids and phlebitis. Externally, in sitz baths, it combines well with witch hazel, stone root and comfrey.

Rudolf Steiner suggested a mild infusion of the husks to re-mineralize teeth.

Orally, the saponins are poorly absorbed, but it appears that the saponin aescin is hydrolyzed by intestinal flora into active metabolites.

Aescin is actually the conglomerate of some 30 different active saponins that have been shown to promote circulation of the veins, having both anti-exudative and vascular tightening effect.

Horse Chestnut stabilizes lycosomes, limiting the release of glycoaminoglycan hydrolyses, the enzymes that influence capillary rigidity and pore size.

That is, by increasing the ability of the inner walls to draw fluids, it enhances the ability of the tissue to drain.

Although the extract mechanism is unknown, it is believed that the seed extract reduces the activity of lycosomal enzymes (glycosaminoglycan hydrolases) that are increased in chronic pathological conditions of the veins, so that breakdown of mucopolysaccharides in region of capillary walls is inhibited. The filtration of low molecular proteins, electrolytes and water in the interstitium is inhibited through a reduction of vascular permeability. Aescin may act as an angiogenesis inhibitor, preventing tumors from building blood vessels to help them survive.

In lab studies, aescin stimulated both the generation and release of prostaglandin (PGF2a). One of the effects is "sealing" of the capillary walls and antagonizing of bradykinin, which increases vascular wall permeability.

Increased levels of leukocytes in affected limbs, suggests an enzyme activation that is reduced by the herb.

Aescin may increase prostaglandin F2-alpha that causes contraction in certain involuntary muscles such as those surrounding veins and arteries. This may increase vascular tone, and prevent vein swelling that leads to varicose veins. It may keep blood vessels from leaking by preventing histamine and serotonin from making them more permeable to fluid.

One other mechanism may play a role. In animal studies, the extracts prevent expression of immune response in blood vessels, so that white blood cells do not stick around and cause more harm.

Aescin inhibits hyaluronidase in a manner similar to echinacea, but not elastase. Facino et al, *Arch Pharm* 1995 328:10.

This same mechanism is part of the reason horse chestnut extracts and creams help inflamed joints, carpal tunnel syndrome, Bell's palsy, and other injuries.

Contraction of arteries and veins by horse chestnut extracts is mediated by 5-HT_{2A} receptors. Felixsson et al, *Phytother Res* 2010 Feb 10.

In cases of liver cirrhosis, or where esophageal varicosities present themselves, combine equal parts of horse chestnut and milk thistle seed extracts internally.

This is particularly important after traumas associated with sport, surgery or head injury. Topical creams are very popular in Europe for acute sprains of sporting events, including amateur and professional soccer venues. Escin reduces the number or size of tiny openings in capillary walls, help prevent outflow of fluid into surrounding tissue.

For varicose veins, it combines well with Cowslip (see above).

In one randomized, double-blind, placebo-controlled study of 70 patients with hematomas, a 2% topical gel reduced sensitivity to pressure on the affected area. Calabrese & Preston, *Planta Medica* 1993 59. Care must be taken to avoid irritating and infiltrating open wounds and weeping eczema.

Allantoin, also present in corn silk and comfrey, is considered a cell proliferant and healing agent.

It somehow ensures that as cell death occurs, new cells are accurate carbon copies. Allantoin appears to have an inhibitory effect on the continued existence of random or badly formed cells, and a stimulatory effect on the normal DNA-RNA code, encouraging accurate new cell growth.

One Japanese study looked at 65 herbs and found horse chestnut one of seven with anti-oxidant potential against skin wrinkles.

It promotes the normal tone in the walls of the veins, promoting return of blood to the heart. Horse chestnut stimulates the production and release of prostaglandin F2alpha, which in turn increases the tone of the venous system and increases blood return to the heart.

Horse Chestnut lowers blood cholesterol and is anti-coagulant. It strengthens the cell walls of red blood cells, but does not influence iron content.

Congestions of the prostate and varicocele formation are relieved in the male, with both internal and external application.

Work by Fang et al, *Phytomed* 2009 Aug 17 divided 219 males with varicocele associated infertility into three groups: control, surgery and aescin supplementation at 30 mg twice daily.

After two months, control group improved 38%, surgical group by 68% and herbal group by 57%. Sperm motility was measured and was 46%, 77% and 55% improved respectively, and it was noted that in mild to moderate cases the herbal therapy was superior.

Double-blind studies have shown that oral extracts help chronic venous insufficiency.

Those suffering edema after surgery have found topical extracts provide relief. The extract helps excrete excessive sodium, which is helpful in edema, but can be hard on those suffering kidney disease.

An exception can be made for treating kidney stones, as the herb's anti-edema properties enlarge the internal diameter of the ureter. This helps the stone pass more easily.

Heaviness of legs, nocturnal cramping in the calves, as well as itching and swelling of the legs call for the seed extract. Phlebitis and thrombo-phlebitis, as well as hemorrhoids call for this herb. Menstrual cramps and swellings associated with fractures and sprains will find relief.

Prophylactic doses of horse chestnut were found to prevent many of the leg problems commonly found in healthy individuals after long airplane flights.

Traditionally, horse chestnut was used in the absence of quinine for malaria. Today, it is still a useful herb for regulating body temperatures and controlling hot flushes.

The saponins are used in cough remedies.

One placebo-controlled trial of 137 post-menopausal women with chronic venous insufficiency-grade 2 was conducted. They were on placebo for one week and either oxerutins (1 gram daily) horse chestnut seed extract (HCE) at 600 grams/daily, or HCE at one gram daily.

This was followed by 500 mg/day of oxerutins for 12 weeks and further observation for six. Oxerutin at 500mg/day was found equivalent to HCE.

A randomized, partially-blinded, placebo-controlled parallel study was done with 240 patients with chronic venous insufficiency-grade 2 over 12 weeks using compression stockings, HCE (50 mg aescin twice daily), or placebo.

Lower leg volume was significantly decreased on HCE (43.8mL) or compression (46.6mL) compared to placebo (9.8mL).

In another randomized, placebo-controlled, cross-over, double-blind trial, 22 patients with chronic venous insufficiency (CVI) were given two capsules (50 mg aescin). Three hours later the capillary filtration coefficient had decreased by 22% with horse chestnut and increased slightly with placebo.

In a meta-analysis of Horse Chestnut extract up to December 1996, it was concluded that in all studies it was superior to placebo for alleviating signs and symptoms of CVI.

It was effective at reducing lower leg volume, protective against edema and decreased capillary filtration, reducing leg pain, itch, and feelings of fatigue and tension in the legs. Pittler & Ernst, *Archives of Dermatology* 1998 134.

At least 13 double-blind, placebo-controlled studies on the use of horse chestnut for chronic venous insufficiency have been published since 1973.

A case observation study involving 800 practitioners involving over 5000 patients concluded that HCE was an economical treatment with much better compliance than compression stockings.

Perhaps that is part of the reason for horse chestnut seeds benefit after surgery, reducing post-operative swelling and the risk of ulceration.

For arm lymph edema created by breast cancer surgery, a combination of horse chestnut, poison hemlock, henbane, and calendula in a neutral ointment base can be helpful. Apply it after performing exercise, before applying compression bandages, and to affected areas both morning and evening.

Escin was found to improve sperm quantity in a DB, PC study of 219 males with varicocele associated infertility. Fang et al, *Phytomed* 17 3-4.

Ricci et al, *Angiology* 2004 55 supp 1 found an aescin-phospholipid topical mixture applied three times daily to the ankles of patients with venous hypertension, varicose veins, or venous micro-angiopathy, showed a statistically significant decrease in free radicals.

In vitro anti-tumour activity has been observed from both hippoaesculin and barringtogenol-C-21-angelate.

Studies in Advances in Chinese Medicinal Materials Research show that beta-aescin can cause a ten-fold increase of plasma adrenocorticotropic hormone in rats and a 20 fold increase in plasma corticosterol levels. This means that horse chestnut extracts may help produce more ACTH and corticosteroids, which are anti-inflammatory hormones.

In one study, aescins were found to increase magnesium absorption. The authors conclude that neither the sympathetic nervous system nor prostaglandins are involved, but point perhaps to parathyroid hormone and/or vitamin D as the mode of action.

Recent work by Xiu-Wei Yang et al, *Journal of Natural Products*, focused on the various triterpenoid saponins (aescins) in the seed of

A. chinensis. They were found to show moderate anti-HIV-1 protease activity.

Aesculin, a coumarin derivative, possesses microvasculo-kinietic activity and is useful for treating cellulitis and hair loss. It has a similar structure to coumarin, and can prolong bleeding times. Mojzisova et al, *Phytother Res* 2013 27:2 observed anti-proliferative and anti-angiogenic properties against variety of cancer cell lines, Jurkat at 93.7%.

Lab studies have found aescin saponins cytotoxic against 9KB, human nasopharyngeal carcinoma, and possess anti-fungal activity.

Aescin has been shown to possess anti-ulcer activity, due in part to inhibition of gastric acid and pepsinogen secretion; as well as increasing blood flow to the stomach region.

Beta aescin is a potent inhibitor of acute myeloid leukemia cell lines inducing apoptosis as well. Niu et al, *J Pharm Pharmacol* 2008 60:9.

Recent work by Yalinkilic et al, *Photochem Photobiol* 2008 84:1 found saponins from this seed, and to a lesser extent, saponins from alfalfa and spinach, protect the immune system against X-rays.

In one twenty-year human clinical study, over 900 million doses of horse chestnut extract were prescribed, with only 15 patients reporting side effects.

And aescin is not dependent upon the release of corticosterone for inflammatory benefit. Zhang et al, *Fitoterapia* 82:6.

Escin sensitizes pancreatic cancer cells to cisplatin, suggesting a synergistic solution to this difficult disease. Rimmon et al, *Biochem Res Int* 2013 Oct 27.

Injectable forms are used in German trauma centers for the treatment of acute head injury or brain trauma. Unfortunately, the FDA and Health Canada are not as progressive.

The bark of the tree is more astringent, bitter and cold than the seed. It can be decocted or prepared as a tincture for similar conditions as the seed, as well as treating remittent fevers. It was formerly used, as mentioned, as a quinine substitute.

It treats diarrhea and hemorrhoids, and decoctions have been used as an external wash for skin problems including *Lupus erythematosus.*

The bark contains a catechin dimer, proanthocyanidin A2, which exhibits protection against UV damage. This is due mainly to its very strong anti-oxidant properties. It is found in suntan products.

Ohio Buckeye bark is astringent, and tonic, and similar to *Cornus* species, according to Dr. Cook. The nut, at ten grains per hour, was used to gently relax intestinal colic. Triterpenoid saponins from the seed are cytotoxic against various cancer cell lines including PC-3 and A549. Wei Yuan et al, *Phytochemistry* 2011 December 16.

The seeds of *A. chinensis* contain flavonoids with significant anti-viral activity, especially influenza virus type A. Wei et al, *J Nat Prod 2004* 67:4.

Beta-escin inhibits cell proliferation and induces apoptosis in HL-60 acute myeloid leukemia cancer cell lines. Niu et al, *J Pharm Pharmacol* 2008 80:9.

HOMEOPATHY

Aesculus hippocastanum is used mainly for venous stasis, and congestion of the portal system, leading to hemorrhoids, and lumbar sacral pain.

There may be great sleepiness during the day, and a dull, heavy sleep with irritable mood. Complaints are aggravated upon waking from sleep, and ameliorated by movement in open air.

Headaches have a heavy sensation, as if numbed, above the eyes, with vertigo and occipital pain, sometimes accompanied by flickering of vision.

There is a typical constant pain in the sacrum and hips, particularly pronounced on bending down and on rising from sitting. It improves with walking.

The left arm and hand, as well as the knee and lower leg are prone to paralytic sensations.

Burning and stabbing pains in the precordium, are found with constriction of the chest.

Fever, with hot, dry hands, running nose, with burning discharge and irritation of nostrils is noted. Inhalation of cold air causes discomfort, and tickling of the larynx and air passages with coughing and expectoration. Chills are experienced at 4 pm.

The tongue is coated yellow white with a bitter taste, nausea and pain extending to the right shoulder blade indicate this remedy.

Blind, knotty hemorrhoids may be present.

There may be irritation of the male and female uro-genital organs, including seminal emissions, and leucorrhea. Contraction like pains radiate from the sacrum to the uterus.

Matthew Wood, in *The Earthwise Herbal*, relays a study of a woman suffering glaucoma. "She had a bounding pulse with a lack of space between the beats so I asked a few questions. Yes, she had obsessive/ compulsive thinking, insomnia, and hemorrhoids.

Aesculus hippocastanum 12X homeopathy brought a flood of tears to her dry eyes and rapid elimination of the glaucoma.

This condition, in her case, was evidently due to venous congestion in the eyes. Remember, glaucoma should be treated like a 'high blood pressure of the eyes'."

DOSE- Tincture to 200th potency. The mother tincture is prepared from the fresh nutmeat. In work by Parimal et al 1991, the undiluted mother tincture was found to have no effect on hemorrhoids, but various dilutions relieved symptoms. The 200 C potency produced best results, with 48 hour intervals best for acute, and 96-120 hour intervals best for milder, but chronic hemorrhoids.

Provings reported in the *New Materia Medica* by Colin Griffith, found 30C potency useful for emotional issues such as opening patients to seizing opportunities to heal damaged innocence.

Ohio Buckeye (*A. glabra*) is indicated for inflammation of the rectum, with very large painful, dark purple, external hemorrhoids. There may also be constipation, portal congestion and the vertigo that accompanies poor blood quality and flow. The speech is thick, with a tickling in the throat, impaired vision and inflammation of the brain.

Professor E. M. Hale did a proving of this remedy, as reported in Millspaugh's *American Medicinal Plants*. He claimed it is an irritant of the cerebrospinal system and alimentary tract. Other symptoms include confusion of mind, vertigo, stupefaction and coma, nausea and vomiting, cramp like pains of the stomach, lameness and weakness of the lumbar region, spasms and convulsions.

DOSE- Tincture to third potency. The mother tincture is prepared from the fresh nutmeat, producing a honey-like odour; but slightly bitter and pungent taste.

GEMMOTHERAPY

Horse Chestnut buds are used in gemmotherapy for treating hemorrhoids, including acute hemorrhoid thrombosis.

DOSE- Use 50 drops daily of the 1D macerated glycerite.

SEED OIL

The seed kernels contain from 3-6% oil composed of 67.2% oleic acid, 22.7% linoleic acid, 2.2% linolenic acid, 4.4% palmitic acid, and 3.6% stearic acid.

Alpha tocopherol is $402g/kg^{-1}$, and gamma tocopherol is $591g/kg^{-1}$. The oil has a saponification value of 194.5, an iodine value of 95.4.

In France, the oil is extracted and used externally for the treatment of rheumatism, and cellulite. A gel or ointment can be prepared from the seed flesh and found useful in slipped disc, by helping disperse the extruded nucleus pulposus, the cushioning gelatinous mass lying within the inter-vertebral disc.

FLOWER ESSENCES

White Chestnut (Horse Chestnut) *A. hippocastanum* flower essence is helpful for the worrisome, repetitive thoughts and chattering mind. It will help to calm and allay the racing gramophone of the mind, and help produce inner quiet, and a calm, clear mind.   **BACH**

White Chestnut flower essence is prepared by the sun method.

Chestnut Bud *(A. hippocastanum)* green buds essence is for those who have been poor observers of live, and have failed to learn from experience. They continue to repeat mistakes, but with help from the flower essence can begin to understand the laws of karma, and lessons of life experience. **BACH**

Chestnut bud is prepared by the boiling method from immature leaf buds.

LEAF ESSENCE

White Horse Chestnut *(A. hippocastanum)* helps to alleviate the numerous distressing symptoms from the movement of kundalini. It may also be given for up to two years after kundalini abates to help integrate the massive changes that the energy can bring.

FALLING LEAF

SPIRITUAL PROPERTIES

Ohio Buckeye is a "self esteem strengthener" when you have let self doubt about an experience contribute to a lack of assertiveness, oversensitivity to criticism, or difficulty in putting things in perspective. **CHASE & PAWLIK**

For centuries, it was believed that if a man carried Buckeye nuts in his pocket, it would improve his sexual performance and he would have better luck seducing a woman. He would also be sure to win in cards.

SUSAN GREGG

PERSONALITY TRAITS

The Horse Chestnut person picture is physically active, with good muscular co-ordination in the lowest part of the body. These people love walking, and tend to be adrenal cheerful first thing in the morning.

All this energetic leaping about in early life can lead to adrenal over-charging and a constant strain on the other endocrine glands.

In the male, especially, there often seems to be a great development in the physical and athletic use of the adrenal glands, sometimes as the expense of the sensual and sexual uses for the prostate gland.

Such males can be gladiators in the sporting world, but find great difficulty with the softer and gentler hormones used in emotions, sexual activity, and in physical comfort.

They are martyrs to physical perfection, and even regard sexual activity in a performance sense, notching up the quantity, and not necessarily aware of the quality- especially for their partner.

The female Horse Chestnut can be fearsome, with large arms that pummel you on the massage table, and you can bet she'll run around the block at the end of day to use up that excess hip and thigh energy. She can have serious pelvic tension, with painful periods and slow or uncontrollable flooding. Pregnancy can be traumatic for such women, with varicose veins appearing early, and remaining and worsening after birth.

Hemorrhoids are the classical affliction of Horse Chestnut. Constipation can be a consequence, and it's only a small step from there to severe prostate congestion, inflammation, and enlargement.

The long term negative Horse Chestnut may face either ovarian or prostate cancers, chronic or severe constipation, or even lower bowel tumours. Varicose veins like twisted tree roots, and of course, intermittent or chronic hemorrhoids- 'the grapes of wrath'.

The positive Horse Chestnut person is physically and sexually active until at least 80, if not 90 years of age. A strong sense of humour and the ability to laugh off the inevitable failures and weakness we all suffer at times, no matter how perfect we'd like to be.

It's a happy and healthy octogenarian yodeling his way up the mountainside who can also relax by the fire at night with his beloved. The lesson to learn is that perfection does not exist in this world; weaknesses flaw even the strongest of us; but it takes real strength to admit it and laugh. **DOROTHY HALL**

In the long ago, the little animals of the woods held a council and expressed indignation at the "Crowder". They voted it unfair for one nut to take all of the room in the shell, so they decided to boycott the big nut. So the squirrels and chipmunks and other small creatures of the woods leave the lovely shiny nuts unheeded in the grass, but sometimes the pigeons peck at them. The birds also held a council and voted the crowding cowbird a nuisance, but they did nothing further about it. **GUILLET**

DOCTRINE OF SIGNATURES

The flowers of White Chestnut, *Aesculus hippocastanum*, lack defined shape or design. Single flowers, thirty to forty of them, are held in a loose pyramid on a central stem. A complex spiral of small side branches hold sets of two, three or four flowers. The effect is made more irregular by the fact that on these smaller stalks the blooms open randomly through the weeks of early summer. Bursts of varying intensity pulse through the massed light of the flowering candles. Each single flower has five amorphous white petals, delicate and beautiful, but uneven in form. The centre of each flower is splashed with yellow, which quickly turns red on pollination.

Fringed with hair, the petals grow larger as the bud opens...In a perfect White Chestnut flower there are five sepals, five petals, seven stamens, one pistil and a three chambered ovary containing two rudimentary seeds.
BARNARD

BOTANICA POETICA
Originally from Asia
Now it's everywhere
We have this big shade tree
With qualities to share
The bark is quite astringent
A hemorrhoid relieves
Or in case of diarrhea
That symptom it can ease
The seeds are quite specific
Improving vessel tone
Venous insufficiency
Reduce, if you are prone
If you suffer from phlebitis
Horse Chestnut is a friend
Leg edema lessens
Capillaries mend
Apply to sprains and bruises
Make a tea with the leaves

Don't ingest the crude herb
It has toxic properties!
But if your legs are heavy
With fluid or an ache
Horse Chestnut is a gift
A healthy choice to make!
SYLVIA CHATROUX

RECIPES

SEED TINCTURE- 1-4 ml 3 times daily, or 5 drops every hour in acute phase. Use the hard brown fruit without the rind. The tincture is made at 1:5 and 50% alcohol.

Another recipe involves one part dried seed powder to ten parts of 45% alcohol. Dosage is one teaspoon daily. Better to buy standardized extract below.

BARK TINCTURE- as above.

FLOWER TINCTURE- 10-15 drops as needed.

AESCIN EXTRACT 50-100 mg daily. Horse chestnut seed extracts standardized for aescin content (20-22%) are recommended in doses of 50-75 mg. twice daily. Or put another way, 250-313 mg extract twice daily corresponding to daily dose of 100 mg aescin. Slow release forms are best. The good quality products have removed aesculin. *Venovar* is a superior product available in stores.

CAUTION- In standard dosage there are no contraindications, except in serious kidney disease. However, rare cases may cause itching, nausea and upset stomach.

Bark tincture should not be combined with aspirin or anti-coagulants due to possibility of anti-thrombin activity of esculetin that is not in seed.

Do not use before surgery, or bleeding disorders, with one proviso. It is sometimes given, in Germany, to women undergoing uterine surgery, if they have excessive varicose veins, with attendant risk factor of blood clots. In humans, after surgery, a daily intravenous dose of 340 mg/kg produced no effect, but 510 mg/kg caused acute kidney failure. Commission E gives no restrictions during pregnancy or lactation, but some authors do so. It could elevate prostaglandin F2, which is labor inducing. The LD50 in mice is 990 mg/kg, and 130 mg/kg in the dog.

Beta aescin combined with aminoglycoside antibiotics can precipitate renal insufficiency. A recent report by Snow et al, *J Emerg Med* 2012 43:6 is of a patient with angiomyolipoma, a fat-containing mesenchymal tumor of the kidney. She was taking horse chestnut extract for venous insufficiency and suffered a life-threatening rupture of kidney.

LILY OF THE VALLEY
(*Convallaria majalis* L.)
PARTS USED- roots, leaves, flowers

No flower amid the garden fairer grows
Than the sweet lily of the lowly vale,
The queen of flowers.   **KEATS**

The Naiad-like Lily of the Vale,
Whom youth makes so fair and passion so pale,
That the light of its tremulous bells is seen
Through their pavilions of tender green.   **P B SHELLEY**

And stooping Lilies of the Valley,
That love with shades and dews of daily,
And bending droop on slender threads
With broad hood-leaves above their heads
Like white robed maids in summer hours,
beneath umbrellas shunning showers.   **JOHN CLARE**

Convallis is from the classic Latin meaning a valley enclosed on all sides; **VALLUM**, an earthen wall or palisades. Hence **VALLUS**, meaning stake or pale, then onto Old French **VAL** meaning, valley. The plant was originally named *Lillium convallium*.

Majalis suggests the month of May; named after the ancient Italic Earth Goddess **MAIA**. This, in turn, is from the Latin **MAIOR**, meaning greater.

May is the month of increase, greater and renewed growth, and hence major. May 26 is the birth date of the herb. In the language of flowers, it depicts the return of happiness and unconscious sweetness associated with May.

146

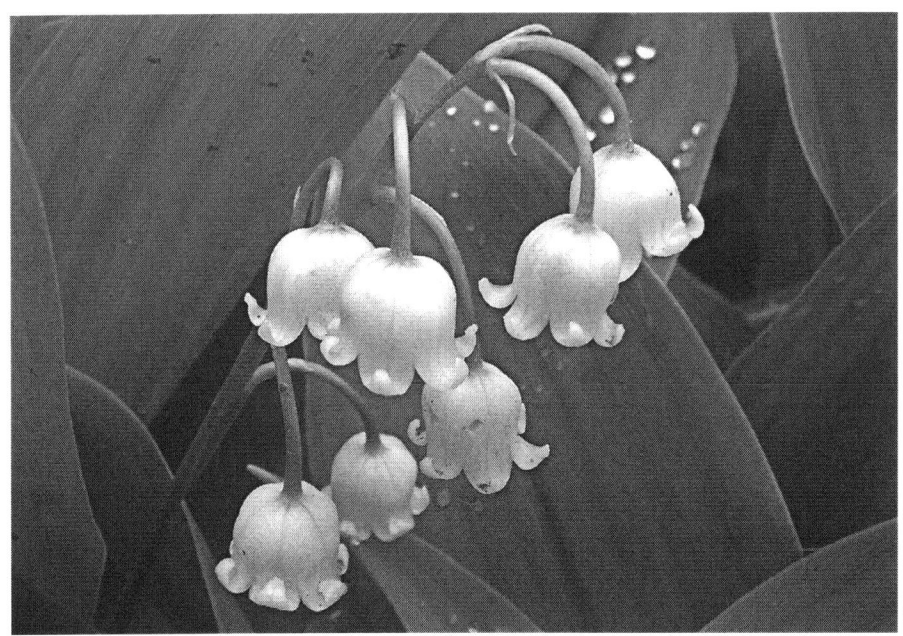
Lily of the Valley

The plant and fragrance are sometimes called Muguet, also from French meaning valley. The flowers are a customary May Day gift in Paris. It is the national flower of Finland and former Yugoslavia. In old astrology books, the plant is placed under Mercury or Hermes.

Legend has it the fragrance of the Lily of the Valley draws the nightingale from hedge to bush, and leads him to choose his mate in recesses of the glades. Another legend suggests chaste white flowers are a symbol of the Virgin Mary, appearing in many painting.

An older legend relays the plant sprang from the wounds of St. Leonard during his battle with a dragon.

The even, step-like arrangement of the flowers along the stalk inspired medieval monks to name it Ladder to Heaven.

Lily of the Valley flowers are small but sweetly perfumed, and over the centuries came to be associated with spring festivals and Whitsuntide. An old custom in Germany was to gather bunches on Whit Monday, and were called May Bloom, or **MAIGLOCKCHEN**.

Earlier, the plant was sacred to Ostara, the Anglo-Saxon and Germanic goddess of spring.

A famous carnival near Rambouillet, France, held in May has carts, and floats all elaborately decorated with the flower spikes.

At one time, bonfires were lit and flowers thrown into the flames as an offering.

In the 4th century *Herbarium of Apuleius*, it was known as Glovewort, and prized for care of the hands.

In the 16th century, herbalists recommended infused flowers for gout; the whole plant steeped in wine to strengthen the memory and soothe inflamed eyes.

William Cole (1657) wrote the plant, "recrutes a weak memory".

Culpepper agreed that the distilled water of the flowers in wine, "restores lost speech, helps the palsy, and is excellently good in the apoplexy; comforts the heart and vital spiritual."

Matthiolus observed it strengthened the heart and alleviated spasms and palpitations. Porcher wrote the flowers, "have a delightful odour, resembling that of musk, and when dried and powdered are much employed as a sternutatory, acting sometimes quite violently." The dried, powdered flowers are today still used as snuff.

Russian peasants relied on it for dropsy caused by pulmonary edema and other cardiac insufficiencies.

Early Ukrainian settlers in Alberta ate the fresh flowers or made an infusion of the dried flowers for breathing problems.

Traditionally, the herb was used for weak contractions in labour, epilepsy, conjunctivitis and leprosy, uses no longer having much scientific basis.

For relieving headaches, including migraines, a few flowers dipped in wine, and eaten are said very effective. "An infusion of the flowers constantly taken instead of tea is an excellent remedy for nervous headaches, trembling of the limbs and other similar complaints."

In parts of Germany, a wine is made from flowers and raisins, while the root was traditionally powdered as a snuff.

Golden water, the hydrosol was stored in golden or silver containers.

The whole plant can be utilized for healing farm animals, according to Juliette de Bairacli Levy. She considered the flowers most potent for helping quiet heart disorders, and the mild narcotic properties for nerves, hysteria and epilepsy. The leaves cool skin inflammation; the seeds reduce fevers and kill round and thread worms.

The roots are mildly aperient and soothing to the intestines.

During Victorian times, the forced flowers were a popular winter decoration, and exported from Germany as Berlin Crowns.

The plant is hardy to zone 2, in protected nooks. Work by Oinonen, *Acta For Fenn* 1969 97 estimates plants can live more than 670 years.

Un-developed plant growth can be sped up by use of anaesthetics such as chloroform. Simply wet a cotton swab with a few drops and let the winter buds absorb vapors for a few hours. Plant the bulbs and you'll be amazed at how much sooner they develop leaves and flowers.

This is interesting as during the First World War, it was used to treat soldiers who had suffered from the effects of mustard gas, due to a strengthening of the nervous system. Leaf infusions were traditionally used in Wiltshire, England as a nerve tonic, to strengthen the memory and restore speech after stroke.

MEDICINAL

CONSTITUENTS- whole plant- convallarin desglucocheirotoxin, convallosaponins, convallogenin B, thymidine, rhodexin A, rhodexoside, sarmentosigenin A, bipindogenin, convallatoxin (40-45% of total alkaloids) locundioside, nearly 40 cardenolide glycosides, associated with nine different aglycones (23 in aerial parts) have been isolated so far; as well as 8 flavonoids, saponins, essential oils, asparagine, convallarinic and chelidonic aicd, malic acid, citric acid, caffeic acid, carotene.
flower- 0.1-0.4% cardiac glycosides (cardenolides), isorhamnetin (quercitin), convallamarin (glucoside). The main glycoside is convallatoxin, which converts to strophanthidin and (-)-rhamnose.
seeds- 0.5% cardiac glycosides (highest content of cardenolides in plant.
leaves- 0.2-0.4% cardiac glycosides, flavonoid glycosides, vitamin C, silver, trace of progesterone (57 mcg/100 grams) in fresh leaf.
leaves, flowers and seed- lokundjoside. saponins.
root- canarigenin-3-0-alpha-rhamno-pyranosyl (cardenolide); saponin convallamaroside.

Lily of the Valley is most useful for treating cardiac arrhythmia due to mitral stenosis and coronary diseases, such as pericarditis.

It vasodilates, and opens capillary circulation, making it invaluable in chronic nervous depression, memory loss, and peripheral artery deficiency.

Strokes, concussions, paralysis and cerebro-vascular ischemia may all benefit from doses of this herb. Infusions are useful for restoration of speech after cardiac arrest.

In the case of cardiac asthma, left-ventricular heart failure, and congestive heart failure, the diuretic activity of the herb is excellent.

It lowers the elevated left ventricle diastolic pressure, and pathologically raised venous blood pressure. It is worth noting that vitamin E supplementation is contra-indicated in left ventricular disorders.

The herb slows the ventricular rate in atrial fibrillation or flutter, and acts only on the heart muscle, and not the vagus nerve, like digitalis.

Work by Hoffmann and Bigger, in Goodman and Gilman's *The Pharmacological Basis of Therapeutics*, 8th Edition 1990, suggest both mechanical and electrical modification of the vascular system. The cardiac glycosides exert a number of effects on neural tissue and thus indirectly influence the heart and modify vascular resistance and capacitance.

Chronic nervous depression and catatonic states may respond to Lily of the Valley leaf and flower.

Pulmonary edema and severe heart failure in the elderly can be greatly relieved. This is without the toxicity of digitalis, or foxglove, and acting more rapidly.

Nausea and vomiting may present itself in some patients, but this is generally mild and rare. It combines well with hawthorn for treating arteriosclerosis and gout; and with dandelion leaf for dropsy (left-sided heart failure).

The principal glycoside is convallatoxin, but the plant contains many minor cardenolides.

Convallatoxin is poorly absorbed as a pure product, but according to Weiss, other compounds aid in its absorption.

Strophanthidin, as a degraded constituent, has been found in animal studies to increase contractility of right ventricle, increase diastolic relaxation of both ventricles and increase pressure of the pulmonary artery. Frantsuzova et al, *Farmakol Toksikol* 1985 48:4.

Like linden flowers and hawthorn, the herb softens accumulated deposits in the arteries, and blood, as well as joints and muscles. It possesses anti-tumour activity, including those of a cancerous nature, by promoting drainage processes in metabolic organs.

For arterial hypertension combine it with gentian root, while for excitation combine with motherwort.

Lily of the Valley relieves urinary tract infections, and when kidney and bladder stones are present. Leaf infusion, taken cold, when the flower is in bloom, is a good diuretic.

Convallamaroside possesses anti-fungal and antibiotic activity. Work by Tschesche, *Pharmacognosy and Phytochemistry*, 1971 suggests these effects are not therapeutically useful, since it forms a complex in the body with cholesterol.

Convallamaroside is a steroidal saponin that shows significant inhibitory effect in angiogenesis. This prevents new blood vessel growth from kidney tumour and sarcoma cancer cells. Nartowska et al, *Acta Pol Pharm* 2004 61:4.

Study by Sauter and Wolfensberger found the berry contains cytotoxic activity, as well as preventing replication of the avian influenza virus. However, the berry is toxic.

The rhizome contains cardenolide glycosides, cytotoxic to human submandibular gland carcinoma. Higano et al, *Chem Pharm Bull* 55:2.

All parts of the plant, except berry, can be used. The flowers are picked in full bloom in May or June, the leaves in June-August, and the rhizomes, if desired in the fall after the tops have died down. Late harvests in July and August give higher yield (0.5%) of glycosides.

The pulp of berries contains traces of cardenolides but the seeds contain about 0.45% of water-soluble glycosides, mainly cardenolides.

An interesting ouabain-like compound (cardenolide) has been identified in humans. Discovered by Nakanishi et al in 1996, this cardiotonic factor appears to be involved in renal function, and in the pathogenesis of hypertension.

The cardiac glycosides are only 10% absorbed and 50% eliminated in 24 hours.

An older US publication found in 2639 cases of lily of the valley ingestion, that although 6.1% of patients had symptom side-effects, only three had severe symptoms, and none died. Krenzelok et al, 1996.

See Frohne & Pfander, *Poisonous Plants* volume 2 for more information.

HOMEOPATHY

Lily of the Valley increases the energy of heart's action, and renders it more regular. It is of use when the ventricles are over-distended and dilation begins, and when there is an absence of compensatory hypertrophy, and when venous stasis is marked.

The patient may be irritable, with a dull headache and intellect, and some degree of depression. The headache moves from the vertex to the temples.

The nose and lips are raw and sore, with a distortion of vision of an imaginary gray spot three inches square. When reading, all letters look the same, and there is a heaviness of the upper eyelids, with a dull right eye pain and a pulsating pain in the left ear with pain.

There is grating of teeth and a copper taste in the mouth upon waking. The tongue may feel scalded or sore, with a thick, heavy, dirty coating.

The back of the throat may feel raw upon inspiring.

Clothing feels tight, with movement in the abdomen like the fist of a child. The digestive tract involves fatty-tasting eructations, nausea after meals with mucous vomiting, and a dull colic like pain in umbilical region.

The bladder feels distended, with frequent, scanty, offensive, cow-like odor upon urination.

The female may suffer great soreness of the uterine region, with sympathetic heart palpitations. There may be pain of the sacro-iliac with sciatic pain running down the legs.

Pulmonary congestion and dyspnea while walking, may be accompanied by a feeling as if the heart is beating throughout the chest. Sensation as if the heart ceased beating, then starting very suddenly. Tobacco heart, especially when due to cigarettes, with angina pectoris, and rapid, irregular pulse also present.

Back and extremities are painful, with trembling hands and aching in wrist and ankles. The patient is chilly down the spine, followed by fever, and little sweat.

One distinct symptom is the presence of tiny nodules on the front of the thigh, like insect bites, that itch strongly.

The patient feels better in open air, and worse in a warm room, feeling sleepy and restless during sleep.

A split or dissociation from one's own feelings, helps make one invulnerable to dangerous situations. Indifference takes the place of unpleasant feelings like fear, pain, grief and pain.

DOSE- Third attenuation. In cases of heart involvement use 1-15 drops of the mother tincture. This is prepared from the whole fresh plant in flower. Proving by Lane and self experimentation in 1883-4, and Sutherland in 883 with tincture. A dream proving by Santos & Konig of 20 females and 8 males at 30c was done in 1994.

FLOWER OIL

The fresh flowers may be picked and sun infused in cold pressed canola oil. If the summer temperatures are below normal, you may have to use a gentle simmer on the stove. The scent is extremely subtle, and after two days of sun infusion, you must squeeze them out and replace with new flowers. Repeat 6 to 10 times, until desired scent appears, or until you run out of patience.

ESSENTIAL OIL

In early days, Lily of the Valley fragrance could only be captured by sun infusion of the flowers in olive or sweet almond oil. This is known as enfleurage.

In modern perfumery, the flowers are extracted by volatile solvents, into a concrete or absolute. No essential oil is distilled.

It is usually mixed with synthetic hydroxy citronellal up to 50%, and the resulting product sold as Muguet.

This in turn provides perfumers with the most exquisite fragrance used in some 14% of all modern perfumes of any quality. Opium, Roma and Florissa are some examples.

When diluted in ethanol, the oil was 94.6% effective in repelling mosquitoes in field tests in Sweden. Thorsell et al, *Phytomed* 1998 5.

The leaves of Lily of the Valley have been distilled and yield 0.058% green-brown oil with a pleasant odour.

The oil melts at 40.5° C and begins to boil at 120° C. After expressing the liquid, white shiny crystals melt at 61° C and composition $C_{20}H_4O_5$ is obtained.

It is composed of 49.5% hydroxy-citronellal and 10.8% citronellol.

HYDROSOL

The distilled water of lilies of the valley, taken in one or two spoonful doses, will strengthen a weak head and heart, promote difficult delivery, withstand the falling evil, apoplexy, and dizziness, and restore lost speech. Those small children who are plagued by fits, colic and worms should be given a tablespoonful from time to time.

During this distillation, the first waters to condense are trifling and normally thrown away, but the spirit that follows is especially valued. If it is rectified again, the inherent volatile salts will go off and collect on the sides of the glass.

After this comes a very smooth, fine spirit that, as well as the salts, can be stored away for future use. Administer the spirit in 15-20 drop doses each time.   **SAUER**

The distilled flower water is used as an astringent and skin-whitening agent, known as **AQUA AUREA**, or Golden Water. It was considered worthy of preservation in vessels of gold or silver.

The water can be taken internally to reduce fluid retention caused by heart problems, and is given as a tonic in China.

Culpepper recommended the flower water for inflammation of the eyes. "Water of the flowers of the Lilies of the valley, strengthens the brain and all the senses."

Brunschwig recommended a water of the flowers only for bee and wasp stings, trembling of the hands, flecks in the eye, trouble in labor, epilepsy, stitches of the heart, heat of liver, comforting mind and brain, excessive menstruation, loss of milk in breasts, and swollen penis and testicles.

The water doth strengthen the Memorie and comforteth the Harte.

DODOENS

The flours of the Valley Lillie distilled…the water doth strengthen the memory that is weakened and diminished; it helpeth also the inflammations of the eies, being dropped there into.   **GERARD**

FLOWER ESSENCES

Lily of the Valley essence brings us back to that state of child-like innocence and wisdom where we only know how to respond with loving behaviour. It puts us in touch with that place within ourselves that existed before our lives were complicated by "shoulds" and all the other layers of conditioning we learned in order to survive and get love and approval.

Lily of the Valley is an emotional tonic which helps us see "through the eyes of a child". People who live their lives bound by convention and seeking social approval can benefit.   **PACIFIC**

Lily of the Valley essence helps one begin to express their emotions.

CHOMING

Lily of the Valley essence helps bring joy and lightness and prevents self-deception and unattainable goals.   **MIRIANA**

This is the essence for yearning, for those who desire things that are unattainable. Perhaps they are in love with someone and those feelings are not returned.

Lily of the Valley helps to create "the empty cup" so that what we truly need can find the space within us and enter it.   **BAILEY**

PERSONALITY TRAITS

A herbal remedy such as Lily of the Valley leaves contains several cardio-active glycosides that are released sequentially in the body, the result is a lengthening of the cardiac response and the avoidance of an abrupt and undesirable peak in plasma concentration.

Certain non-cardioactive glycosides also present increase almost 500 times the water solubility of convallatoxin and convallatoxol. Other glycosides act synergistically by occupying protein-binding sites and thereby effecting a high plasma concentration of active glycosides with correspondingly increased bioavail-ability. The combination occurring in the leaf has many therapeutic advantages over the isolated glycosides…   **F. FLETCHER HYDE**

MYTHS AND LEGENDS

There are many Russian fairy tales about the lily of the valley. In one tale, a young woman called the White Snow Maiden ran away from her wicked stepmother. As she ran, the necklace she wore fell apart. The fallen pieces became the lily of the valley.

In another tale, Volhva, the Water Queen, was in love with Sadko, a handsome musician. When found out that he was deeply in love with a young girl who lived in a village near the river, she left the water to hear him play and sing to his beloved. When Volhva heard him play, bitter tears welled up in her beautiful blue eyes. They fell onto the ground and became the aromatic white flowers we know as lilies of the valley.   **ZEVIN**

An English myth involves St. Leonard, who slayed a dragon that was troubling the whole countryside. After an epic battle, the exhausted knight collapsed and lay near death. The fairies used tiny buckets and brought one drop of water at a time from a nearby creek to moisture his lips and after much work revive the hero. The fairies in their haste to remain unseen quickly disappeared, but left behind their tiny buckets on stems of grass. These became the flowers of Lily of the Valley. Ancient myths depicting patriarchal saints destroying dragons represents the move from matriarchal societies to male dominated ones.

RECIPES

INFUSION- 2-7 grams twice daily. The aerial parts are collected as the flowers begin to open and are dried or tincture.

TINCTURE- 5-20 drops twice daily. Use a 1:5 tincture at 60% alcohol of the recently dried root. Both leaves and roots can be used, but wait until after flowering. If fresh, use 1:2 ratio. For 1:8 tincture use 1.2 ml 3 times daily. A flower tincture is made 1:8, with dosage of 5-15 drops in water three times in 24 hours.

STANDARDIZED EXTRACT- 600 mg (0.2-0.3 % glycosides).

POWDER- One gram of lily of the valley equals 120 digitalis units in potency. Toxicity occurs more rapidly but is non-cumulative. Maximum allowable dosage in Britain is 150 mg with a daily maximum of 450 mg.

CAUTION- Overdoses can cause diuresis and purging.

Use emetics, or activated charcoal, atropine if necessary, and watch potassium imbalance and treat serum insulin if needed. Take for ten days, and then ten days off. Avoid in Yin deficient conditions or where fatty heart degeneration is already present.

Do not use simultaneously, according to Commission E, with quinidine, calcium salts, saluretics, laxatives or glucocorticoids. Do not combine with gotu kola!

LITTLE LEAF LINDEN
LIMEFLOWER
LIME TREE
(*Tilia cordata* Mill.)
(*T. parviflora* Ehrh.)
BASSWOOD
(*T. americana* L.)
DROPMORE LINDEN
(*T. X flavescens*)
MONGOLIAN LINDEN
(*T. mongolica* Maxim.)
SILVER LINDEN
SILVER LIME
(*T. tomentosa* Moench.)
MANCHURIAN LINDEN
(*T. mandshurica* Rupr. & Maxim)
BROAD LEAVED LINDEN
(*T. platyphyllos* Scop.)
(*T. grandifolia* Ehrh.)
(*T. rubra* DC.)
PARTS USED- leaves, flowers, sapwood

If thou lookest on the lime-leaf, Thou a heart's form will discover.

Therefore are the lindens every chosen seat of each fond lover.
HEINRICH HEINE

The linden in the fervours of July, hums with a louder concert.
W C BRYANT

Now, tell me thy name, good fellow, said he, under the leaves of Lyne.
SHAKESPEARE

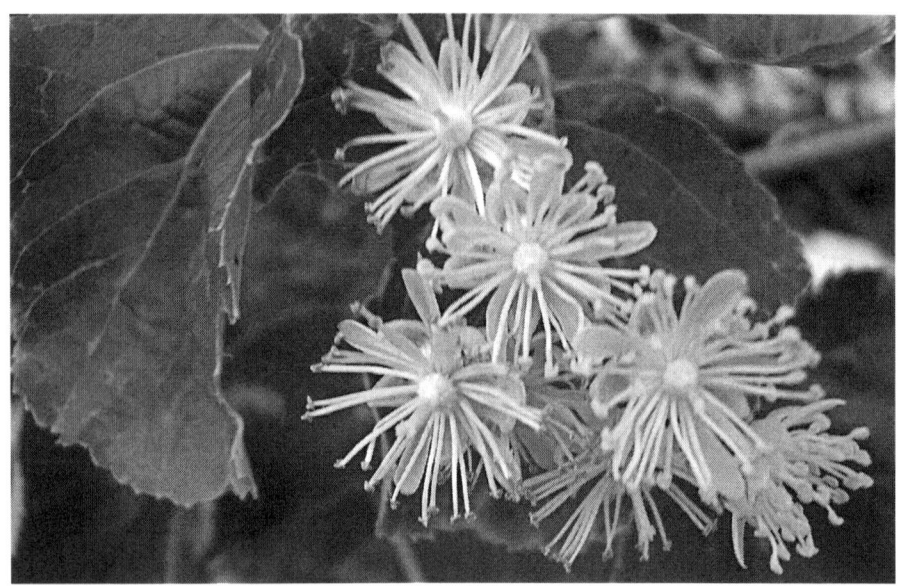
Linden leaf and flower

Tilia is from Greek **TILLEIN**, "to pluck or extract fibre". Other authors suggest it is an alteration of **TELIA**, in turn from **TELUM**, a dart, in reference to use of wood. And yet, other authors suggest it derives from **PTILON** meaning feather, in reference to the floral leaf appearance.

Basswood is from bast, the fibre from inner-bark of linden, later applied to other fibre like hemp or flax. Linden was originally an adjective of Old English or Norse **LIND** tree. The root **LI**, from the Indo-European root means flax thread, with **LENTUS** coming to mean "flexible". Linné, the father of taxonomy, was Swedish and **LINN**, meant linden. Lyne may later have become lyme.

The German verb **LINDERN** means, "to soothe". Cordata means heart-shaped, referring to leaf. Lime tree is related to the plants usefulness as an antacid or systemic alkalizer of the body system. Maybe.

According to Greek legend, the nymph Philyra was raped by Saturn, disguised as a horse. She eventually gave birth to the famed Centaur, Chiron. Philyra was so devastated that she begged the gods not to leave her among mortals. The gods granted her wish by transforming her into the mother spirit of the linden tree.

Linden has been a shade tree since the time of the Egyptians. It was a holy tree in Greece, sacred to Venus due to heart-shaped leaves, and Germans and Slavs, who attributed the power to ward off destruction by lightning. Linden is female, and Oak is male in the Teutonic tradition.

The trees are long-lived, in part due to an interesting stem production. As one stem matures, the next begins to form below it, so that it can replace the older one when it dies.

Siegfried, a famed mythical hero, was dipped in a magical river by his mother to make him invulnerable. But a linden leaf clung to his heart, leaving one vulnerable spot that later proved his undoing. Sound familiar, Achilles?

In many cultures, linden was believed to absorb disease by simply being touched.

In Lithuania, for example, women made sacrifices to linden as part of religious rites. It was believed bark of linden, if carried, would prevent intoxication, while the leaves and flowers were used in love spells. In Poland, the inner bark was said to be able to tie up the devil.

In Sweden, many surnames such as Lindemann, Tiliander and Linné derive from the guardian tree.

Pliny noted in ancient Rome that bast fibre, known as **LIBER**, was used to make paper, and hence the origin of words such as library.

In Russia, the corky outer bark forms a sole, and strips of the plaited bast were used to form the top of a shoe. This footwear was short-lived and so were the lime flower forests.

Linden oil is a personal favourite fragrance of my wife Laurie. Whenever the various trees boom in July, we make a point of visiting and sniffing the fragrant emissions.

In Germany, the flowers were never brought into the house due to their ability to induce erotic dreams.

The tree was associated with Freya, the guardian of life and goddess of fortune, love and truth. It was believed the tree would un-earth the truth, so town meeting were held under the trees in central squares. Over 850 place names can be traced back to linden.

Honey produced from the blossoms is regarded as one of the most delicately flavored in the world.

Little Leaf Linden is the national emblem of Slovakia, Slovenia and the Czech Republic.

Both American Basswood and Little Leaf Linden are hardy to the prairies, the former to zone three and the small import from Europe, to zone two.

Dropmore Linden is a hardy hybrid of the two, resistant to the linden mite, and well adapted to dry prairies.

Mongolian Linden is a much shorter tree, only getting to five metres, about half the average of others. Silver Linden is not quite as hardy (zone 4) in our region. It is native to Turkey and Eastern Europe, with fragrant flowers that are somewhat intoxicating to bees. Manchurian and broad-leaved linden have been grown successfully at Morden Research Station.

All Linden flowers have exquisite perfume. American Basswood scent is similar to grape flowers, while *T. cordata* and *T. tomentosa* are more honey-like, and *T. platyphyllos* flowers are sweet like watermelon with a touch of clove and fringe tree flower.

Green Sunday, or the Feast of the Pentecost, held in the Russian Orthodox Church, is decorated with linden blossoms to symbolize new life in the Spirit.

It is said that eleven different varieties are grown in Russia, with an estimated 27 million acres of linden tree plantations (Zevin, 1997).

The bark was removed in spring and soaked in water until soft by various Native peoples. The tough outer bark then easily separates from the desired inner bark, separated into mainly one-inch strips, and coiled for future use.

Sometimes the bark was boiled with wood ash and peeled off the soft fibrous inner bark and cut into lengths. This was used to make belts, fishing nets, snowshoe webbing; and when cut thinner, as thread to sew robes, moccasins, pouches, birch bark containers, fishing line and even sutures for severe skin cuts.

False face masks were carved by the Iroquois on the living tree, and when finished cut off to hollow out the back.

Wide strips were cut by Chippewa to weave mats and tie large and small packets. The width of fibre determined the strength, but also the softness; and it was often re-boiled after separation to add additional toughness.

Pehr Kalm, traveling through Quebec in 1749 wrote, "I could have sworn it was a fine hemp cord."

The inner bark of American Basswood was infused by the Cherokee for dysentery, or mixed with cornmeal as a poultice for boils.

They used the inside bark and twigs in pregnancy to relieve heartburn, morning sickness, weak stomach and bowels.

A jelly was made from the bark and used for cough of tuberculosis.

The Fox tribe used inner bark poultices for drawing boils, while a twig decoction was reserved for lung trouble.

The Iroquois infused the bark to increase urination, and the shoots for those feeling worn out. The bark was part of a compound decoction for internal hemorrhage, and part of a leaf poultice for broken bones and swollen areas.

The Mi'kmaq used the roots as treatment for worms, while the bark was used for suppurating wounds. The Onondaga decocted the bark to promote urination.

The Mohawk drank the flower tea to induce sweating and relieve spasms, and the twigs, when combined with staghorn sumac bark, were considered a tonic tea during pregnancy.

Linden has been used for timber, and the fibrous inner bark or bast has been used for baskets, ropes, and mats. The Swedes used the fibre as a source of thread for fishing nets, while the Polish used inner bark to make rough shoes called **CHODAKI**, baskets and hats.

Archeological digs have un-earthed woven basswood necklaces, strung with copper beads from before the time of Christ.

The wood is prized for carving, being close-grained, white and very smooth. Over three centuries ago, Grinling Gibbons used it for many of his exquisitely detailed carvings; and because linden wood is never worm-eaten, well-preserved today. Good luck charms are often carved from the wood.

The wood carvings found along Gaspe Peninsula are often made of basswood.

The keys and sounding boards of musical instruments are often made from linden wood; as well as yardsticks and Venetian blinds. During the Second World War, the Mosquito fighter planes were crafted from this hardwood.

The wood is burned without oxygen to produce medicinal grade charcoal, useful for dyspepsia and other digestive complaints.
The twigs can be placed in a burning fireplace, and later removed, powdered and put into empty gelatin or vegetable capsules in an emergency.

A sticky black substance that drops onto parked cars is produced not by the tree, but a aphid that lives on the tree. This honeydew sugar can cover one square metre of ground with as much as one kilogram of syrup.

As mentioned above, honeybees are particularly attracted to the sugary sap. This sap quickly ferments, so they often drink an alcoholic cocktail, resulting in meandering paths back to the hive. Collisions with trees and their own hives are common. Guard bees are on the outlook for disorderly bees, and like night club bouncers forcibly eject drunks from the premises. Persistent offenders may have their limbs bitten off, resulting in a most unpleasant hangover. Linden flowers of *T. tomentosa* have a hypnotic constituent that causes drowsiness in bees.

The tree can be tapped, for a sweet, sugary juice in the spring. In Europe, an electuary from linden was highly prized during the middle ages, especially when combined with linden blossom honey. The fermented sap was drunk as wine.

A mucilaginous sap from inner bark is very useful for healing skin burns.

The seeds, or berries can be collected and powdered, and used for treating diarrhea; or put into a pepper grinder and used as a salt substitute. The fruit, commonly called "monkey-nuts" contains rich oils.

The French chemist Missa discovered in the 1700s that grinding the fruit, with linden flowers, produced a substance with the scent of chocolate. It was even commercialized in Prussia for a short time, but did not preserve well.

The roasted fruit can be used as a coffee substitute.

The leaves when young and translucent, added to salads, or cooked to thicken soups and stews.

The leaves are simmered down to half the water, becoming quite mucilaginous when cooled, and used for chapped skin, cuts, sores, burns and other minor problems.

Linden extracts are used in hair products such as Freeman Botanicals Hair Rescue and Intensive Conditioner.

During the Second World War, the older, tough leaves were dried, pulverized and powdered to make a nutritious "green flour" to supplement bread and cakes. The leaves contain inverted sugars, easily used by diabetics. Elsewhere, the leaves can be dried like hay, and used for winter feed for livestock.

In France, and elsewhere, afternoon tea is served under scented linden trees helping calm hyperactive children, and creating a quiet, peaceful moment of time. Linden leaf tea is a good choice for those with poor protein digestion, due to lack of tannins.

It was linden flower tea into which Proust dipped his madeleine, evoking the nostalgia of his childhood and inspiring the masterwork *A LA RECHERCHE DU TEMPS PERDU*. I haven't taken the time to read it. My loss, no doubt.

MEDICINAL

CONSTITUENTS- *T. cordata* flowers- organic acids p-coumaric, caffeic and chlorogenic; tiliacin; proanthocyanidins, tannins and especially flavonoids (1%), mainly quercitrin, isoquercitrin, tiliroside, hyperoside, hesperidin, rhamnosyl-7-kaempferol, etc; essential oil (see below); and mucilage composed of D-galactose, L-arabinose, L-rhamnose, and uronic, malic, acetic and tartaric acids. Also contains the amino acids phenyalanine, alanine, cysteine, and cystine. Fresh flowers contain 40 mg/100 g of vit C, carotene, and benzodiazepine-like compounds.
sapwood- phenolic acids, tannins, fraxoside, esculoside, cichorioside, amino acids, 1.5-7% polyphenols.
leaves- 16.5% protein (11.9% soluble), relatively high calcium (2.79%), iron (198 ppm), and boron (52 ppm).
fruit- squalene
T. tomentosa leaves- flavonoids: quercitroside, kaempferine, astragaline, quercitol 3, glucose 7 rhamnoside, tiliroside quercitroside, soquarcitro-cide; scyllitol; coumarin derivatives, tillroside amino acids including aspartic acid, proline and indol-3-acetic acid;

Linden flowers and bracts are gathered and used in herbal teas for their sedative and relaxing quality, and cooling and drying nature.

The stalks of dried linden flowers are used in France for Tilleul tea.

The flowers have been used traditionally in France, and elsewhere for the symptomatic treatment of neurotic states, especially minor sleep disturbances, nervous vomiting and heart palpitations. This may be due to the binding of GABA receptors, similar to valerian.

Just walking or sitting under the trees can be soothing to nervous people.

The flowers are poulticed or infused for treating itchy skin, or other dermatological irritations. Cold infusions, gently-warmed and added to baths, are said useful for hysteria, and overly-excited nervous states.

As a febrifuge, linden is especially good for cooling the entire system, in cases of excessive heat, or acute fever states. Linden flower is better than Catnip for this purpose. Peter Holmes puts it best "The remedy excels for heavy-set, tense-muscled people with acute upper or lower respiratory infections manifesting heat and lack of sweat."

Matthew Wood says the tongue calling for linden flower is usually red, sometimes flame-shaped, and usually somewhat moist.

In Germany, the flowers are specific for children with influenza. They are anti-catarrhal and used in various respiratory infections. Recent research in India indicates linden extracts are effective against various virus cultures.

Isoquercitrin, and tiliroside are some of the flavonoids responsible for its diaphoretic effect. The former compound inhibits lens aldose reductase (prevents cataracts), and is active against *Pseudomonas maltophilia* bacteria.

Tiliroside shows liver protective activity. Matsuda et al, *Bioorg Med Chem* 2002 10:3.

A study, by two pediatricians at Chicago University, involved 55 children with flu symptoms, treated with bed rest, linden blossom tea and at most one or two aspirin. Thirty-seven other children, in addition to above, were given sulfa drugs, and another 67 antibiotics only. The authors were surprised children taking linden tea and bed rest not only recovered quicker, but had the fewest complications. Children given antibiotics needed longer to overcome the condition, with more complications.

The flowers and leaves are used to treat disorders associated with Earth, Wood and Fire Yang. To use traditional Chinese terms, by draining the Fire of the Heart, it is useful for treating insomnia, anxiety, anguish, neurosis, hysteria, epilepsy, vertigo, migraines and apoplexy.

The flowers and bracts are useful for Wind Heat in lungs, with cough, chronic bronchitis and yellow phlegm.

Taken hot, the flower or leaf infusion will often stop head or respiratory infections from fully manifesting. This is External Wind Heat.

Steam containing linden flower extracts has been shown superior to steam alone in alleviated un-complicated colds.

Linden, or Lime Flowers, as they are sometimes called, remove excess uric acid from the system, and slowly dissolve cholesterol from the arterial walls.

In the treatment of hypertension, for example, the slow steady influence of linden flower can be helpful on several levels. Linden balances the central nervous system, calms the nerves and scrubs the buildup of plague and/or calcification of arteries. Add to this a stimulation of sluggish renal function and elimination, and you have a good hypertensive tonic. The vaso-dilating action reduces constrictor tone in the peripheral blood vessels.

Linden flowers are effective in conditions of abnormally high blood viscosity and hyper-coagulation. Tiliroside induces anti-hypertensive activity through an L-type Ca^{2+} influence on smooth muscle. Grazielle C. Silva et al, *Planta Medica* 79:2 1003-8.

Extracts show anti-thrombin activity. Goun EA et al, *J Ethnopharm* 2002 81 337-342.

There appears to be a synergistic effect between the saponins and flavonoids on the blood vessels. It shares a similar saponin with horse chestnut, and thus is useful in varicose veins, phlebitis, migraine and arteritis.

Tinctures or cool infusions are best for conditions of hypertension and neuro-cardiac concern over the long term. It is similar to, and work well with chrysanthemum flower.

Slanc et al, *Phytother Res* 2008 Dec 23 found linden leaf (*T. platyphyllos*) possesses lipase inhibition. Experimental work supports it reputation as an anti-spasmodic and relaxant, and demonstrated estrogenic effect.

Like bupleurum root, it relieves headaches and blood pressure associated with Liver Yang. Water extracts of *T. cordata* flowers have been found, in vitro, to stimulate lymphocyte proliferation. Anesini et al, *Fitoterapia* 1999 70:4.

They found the same effect from two different agonists of peripheral benzodiazepine receptors, leading to speculation that *Tilia* extracts bind to these sites.

Work by Arcos et al, *Phytother Res* 20:1 found flowers of *T. cordata* exhibit anti-proliferative activity against tumour cells.

The flowers are one of our few stomachic herbs with very low levels of tannin. This, of course, favors digestion, as tannins, even in ordinary tea, inhibit true protein digestion.

The leaves create some astringency useful in diarrhea, or bleeding from the nose and mouth, due to protocatechic leaf tannins. The leaves are mildly diuretic.

The flowers combine well with hawthorn for high blood pressure, with hops for nervous tension and anxiety, and with elder flowers for colds and flu.

Think of linden flowers for hyper-adrenal conditions, combining well with burdock root.

Various French physicians do not consider the flowers of American basswood to be useful medicinally. They suggest the flowers are hexamerous, not pentamerous, like *T. cordata*, and do not contain adequate concentration or proportions of the active principle.

I don't know if this is geocentric or scientific in basis, as both have pronounced odiferous properties. There appears bias with some authors suggesting the flowers of American Basswood can cause nausea. This has not been my experience, however.

In fact, linden flowers with higher tannin levels and low mucilage content as found in *T. cordata* and *T. platyphyllos* are more flavorful teas.

Schmidgall et al, *Planta Medica* 2000 66:1 found polysaccharides from *T. cordata* show moderate bio-adhesion to isolated epithelial tissue.

Tiliroside appears to interact, at least *in vitro*, with CYP3A4, CYP2C9 and CYP2C8 pathways, suggesting influence on possible herb/drug interactions, or absorption of drugs with the herb. Sun, DX et al, *Phytother Res* 2010 24:11.

The sapwood decreases bile flow in humans. This is useful in the treatment of biliary dyskinesia, or when dandelion root is contra-indicated. Work by Debray showed this was due to inhibition of T.G.P transaminase.

At the same time it is a uric acid dissolver and hepato-biliary drainage remedy.

It combines well with horse chestnut, fleabane, meadowsweet and goldenrod for the treatment of cellulite.

Laboratory studies in early 1960s have found sapwood to be anti-spasmodic, serotonin antagonist, diuretic and hypotensive agent. It is a coronary dilator, acting to ease tension in the whole cardiovascular system.

Sapwood tea, decocted from the dried strips of wood, is useful for epigastric bloating, and impairment of digestion.

It can be us eful in certain types of migraine associated with coronary syndromes, such as angina and maintenance treatment, after infarction.

The decocted bastwood can be used in relief of rheumatism.

The wood charcoal, made from dry linden twigs or bark, is used internally for intestinal disorders, including hyperacidity, gallbladder and liver complaints and cases of poisoning. Externally, the charcoal has been used for skin ulcers.

Coumarin anti-coagulant content in *T. tomentosa* decreases from the stalk toward the leaf. When compared with amino acids and particularly flavonoids, the quantity of active ingredients is higher in buds.

The flowers, bracts and developing seeds of *T. americana* show activity against *Staphylococcus aureus*. Borchardt et al, *J Med Plants Res* 2008 2:5.

The bark shows activity against methicillin-sensitive *Staphylococcus aureus*, and *Mycobacterium phlei*. Omar et al, *J Ethnopharm* 2000 73 161-70.

Squalene is an intermediary in cholesterol synthesis, found in shark liver oil and some plants such as olive and linden. Squalene is anti-bacterial, anti-tumour and immune stimulating.

HOMEOPATHY

Lime Tree/Linden is indicated for uterine prolapse, passive hemorrhages and urinary incontinence. It is of value in muscular weakness of the eyes; neuralgia that is first right sided and then left; and a dimness of vision as if a veil is over the eye.

The patient may find difficulty using binoculars, for example.

The female may suffer intense soreness of the uterus with bearing down pain, and sweating with no relief. Profuse slimy leucorrhea is produced while walking. The external genitalia are sore and red; while the skin suffers intense itching and burning, made worse by scratching. Eruptions of small, red, itching pimples may occur.

Sweating is profuse and warm soon after falling asleep, with the sweating increasing as rheumatic pain increases.

The patient feels worse in the afternoon and evening, or in a warm room or bed. Symptoms are better from cold, and motion. Feeling separated from family, laughing and joking about death, injury and suffering-black humor.

Strong desire to smoke, vertigo with tendency to fall backwards or to right. Deep cracks in skin of heels. Dreams of fire, flood, military, shooting, black water and yellow colours.

DOSE- Mother tincture to 6th potency. The mother tincture is prepared from the fresh flowers of the Tilia species, particularly *T. cordata* and *T. platyphyllos* in Europe. On the prairies, use *T. cordata* or *T. americana*.

The first proving with *T. cordata* was by Robert Bannan with 31 provers at 30c in 1995.

GEMMOTHERAPY

The buds of Silver Leaf Linden *(T. tomentosa)* are rich in farnesol, a terpene with neuro-regulating sedative properties.

Experiments in laboratory animals confirm that it clearly holds sleep-inducing capacities.

It is not a hypnotic, but a sleep-inducer without toxicity, and non-habit forming. It is particularly recommended for treating the nervous system of fragile persons, such as children, pregnant women and the elderly.

Not only is Tilia sedative, but it anxiolytic. In too high a dose, it has the reverse effect and will prevent sleep.

It works well with *Pinus montana* 1D for neuralgia and other nerve related pains. However, do not combine gemmotherapy drops, but alternate from the individual bottles.

DOSE- Bud macerate 1D, 50-100 drops at bedtime or after the evening meal. For children, 25 drops, depending upon age, both with water.

ESSENTIAL OIL

CONSTITUENTS- bracts- rich in phenylacetyaldehyde and other aldehydes. flowers- dominated by monoterpenoid hydrocarbons, tricosane, isocyclocitral, notrienol.
Both contain oxygenated mono- and ses-quiterpenes such as linalool, geraniol, farnesol, camphor, carvone, and cineole; aromatic alcohols like phenyl-ethanol, benzylic alcohol, phenols, and aliphatic compounds.

Linden blossom oil is strongly affected by urban pollution. In one study the content of oxygenated compounds reduced from an average of 47-55%, to 20-27% in dirty city environments.

The oil is used in nervous tension, insomnia, and anti-depressant. It combines well with rose, and some citrus notes, as well as jasmine and frankincense. The oil is produced from absolute.

Work by Buchbauer et al, *Arch Pharm* 1992 325 April, found linden species oil sedative to mice upon inhalation.

HYDROSOL

Linden hydrosol is slightly floral and heady, like yeasty beer in odour. It has a pH of 4.3-4.6, is slightly unstable, but good for at least one year.

The distilled water of linden blossoms, taken in spoonful doses, is highly praised for treating the falling evil, convulsions, dizziness, and other cold distempers of the head. It is also good for colic, and will benefit injured bowels following bloody flux. If someone has been struck by convulsions, administer often a spoonful of linden blossom, lily of the valley and black cherry water mixed together. When young children are afflicted with the fits, give them often a tablespoon dose of one part peony water and one part linden blossom water.

Linden blossom water is used by women to remove spots on the face. It will also heal blisters in the throat and a scurvied mouth.

If young children develop a large, bloated belly (cardiology), they should be administered a tablespoonful of linden blossom water from time to time.   **SAUER**

A hydrolat may be prepared from the leaves. Viaud says this distilled water is stimulating and a vasodilator, low doses calming and higher doses more stimulating.

Jeanne Rose suggests the hydrolat in a spray for shingle pain, as it is very soothing. She finds it calming, relaxing and sedative, helping to relieve anxiety and depression.

Catty finds it useful in headaches, including migraine, and nervous exhaustion. It may be put to good use in dry eczema, itchy skin eruptions, or puffy skin.

A hydrolat prepared from the wood is used for arthritis, gout, and rheumatoid arthritis, according to work by Viaud.

A water from the blossoms is good for falling sickness, pain in gut, trembling heart, sunburn, clearing sight, cold uterus or womb, causing to speak and for much milk.   **BRUNSCHWIG**

SEED OIL

The seeds of American Basswood yield oil that solidifies at -10° C. It has a specific gravity of 0.938, a saponification value of 178.1, and an iodine value of 111.

Linden seed oil has been used for consumption, in days past, as well as oil lamps.

FLOWER ESSENCES

Linden (*T. platyphylla*) flower essence is for helping develop receptivity to human love. It strengthens the relationship between mother and child. It eases communication and exchanges with respect and cordiality. It helps bring out qualities of protection, nourishing warmth, softness and calmness.   **DEVA**

Basswood or Linden flower essence will help make you more outgoing. It will also help people to notice you instead of having to always be the one to stick out your hand first. Linden will help you to lighten up at a party and if you want to let go and be romantic, it will help you do so. Linden essence is excellent for cultivating love for humanity and in overcoming prejudices.   **JADE MTN**

Linden essence is for people who feel alienated and never welcome anywhere. It is symbolized, by Hestia, the Goddess of Hearth and Temple.   **HORUS**

Limeflower (*T. platyphylla*) flower essence helps us open our hearts to the light and loving of our universal being. From this awareness we experience our inter-relatedness on earth and create harmonious relationships in our lives.

It is indicated when individuals are too introspective or focused on self; or there is over identification with lower self/personality.

Limeflower essence supports us in overcoming feelings of separation from our spiritual self or others, and can empower and encourage us to work for peace and spiritual harmony on earth.   **FINDHORN**

Linden (*T. x europea*) leaf essence is a great pick-me-up after a period of stress or illness. It can also be taken continuously to deal with ongoing stress.   **FALLING LEAF**

Linden (*T. cordata*) leaf essence releases the pattern of "male chauvinism"- being authoritarian, domineering, controlling, or insensitive in intimate relationships with females.   **FALLING LEAF**

Lime essence helps to decrease an oversensitive cross energy, allowing the body to focus on a spiritual endeavor. It is useful for when you want to shift levels of consciousness without disorientation, helping to lessen past behavior programming, erase doubts and fears, and calm the anxiety related to the practical use of your psychic and healing potential.   **OLIVE**

PERSONALITY TRAITS

When Zeus and Hermes visited Phygria in human form they were refused hospitality ...until they came to the cottage of Philemon and his wife Baucis, who entertained them kindly. Zeus gave them practical thanks by taking them to the top of a high hill where they survived while a flood devastated the lowlands. There was a temple of Zeus on this crest, and he made them it guardians. The only wish the old couple had was that they should die at the same moment, and this was granted to them by Zeus.

As they died he changed them into trees- Philemon into an oak, and Baucis into a linden, the emblem of conjugal love.   **POWELL**

On a cold winter day the tall Mississauga chief, Niniboju was tramping the shores of a frozen lake. He stopped suddenly and inspected a large basswood tree that stood on the shore. He peeled off a strip of the bark and with it tied two stones to his heels. Then he tried leaping on the ice and laughed at the tinkling sounds that the stones made as they hit the ice. Attracted by the tinkling sounds, a little fish came up through a hole in the ice.

Quickly Niniboju caught the fish in his hands and ate it. Then he danced vigorously and the sounds of the stones grew louder. Soon more fish came up through holes in the ice and Niniboju caught them all.

He tore the basswood strip down the centre and strung the fish as he caught them. By night he had a long string of fish which he carried back to camp. All the Indians had a good laugh and helped to eat the fish. Niniboju praised the basswood tree and called it Niniboju's helper. Other Indians tried dancing on the ice, but they caught no fish.

GUILLET

Confident with who they are from an early age, Lindens will be determined to follow the path they set for themselves, carrying on regardless of any opposition to their plans. These are open and up-front people, helpful when the mood takes them. They are a very interesting personality as they can change and wear many guises.

Lindens are perfectly happy to reside in the shadow of their partner or family, nurturing their growth and encouraging their ambitions…Due to lack of ambition, Lindens are often found in jobs that do not suit their temperament.

In negative mode, Lindens are possessive of their partner or children, always reminding everyone of what could go wrong. They become the worriers. **WORWOOD**

The southern American basswood likes its taste of flesh. *Tilia tomentosa* sneaks a hypnotic potion into its floral nectaries because it is hungry for nitrogen. The pollinating bees take a hit. They slowly die in the cool shade, their bodies supplying just enough nitrogen for the trees to make maternal protein for another season of sex.

BERESFORD-KROEGER

MYTHS AND LEGENDS

Old words for dragon — the German **LINDEWURM**; the Old English **LINDWORM** – and the name of the tree have a common root, the Indo-European **LENTOS** (flexible). In all cultures the dragon is a personification of the Earth's life force, which flows along the dragon or ley lines. A person encountering a place of intense Earth or dragon energy is charged both physically and spiritually.

HAGENDER

RECIPES

TINCTURE- 2-4 ml as needed. The tincture is made with fresh flowers at 1:3 in 35% alcohol.

INFUSION- One tsp of dried herb to one pint of boiled water for 15 minutes.

When collecting the flowers, they should be picked early with the whole flower cluster including the bract. They are dried in the shade.

NIGHT CREAM- Take 25 grams of beeswax, and blend with 100 ml of cocoa butter in a double boiler. As it is cooling, add 5 drops of linden blossom absolute or its essential oil. Bottle, label and cool. Store in a cool, dark spot.

CAUTION- Linden flowers may bind up iron supplements. They should be taken 2 hours apart. Do not use in low blood pressure.

MOTHERWORT
(*Leonurus cardiaca* L.)
SIBERIAN MOTHERWORT
(*L. sibiricus* L.)
ASIAN MOTHERWORT
(*L. artemisia* [Lour.] S. Y. Hu)
(*L. japonicus* Houtt.)
(*L. heterophyllus* Sweet.)
PARTS USED- aerial parts

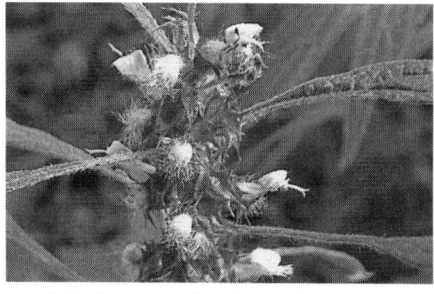

Motherwort leaf and flower

In the midst of the valley is Tui (Motherwort)
All withered and dry.
A girl on her own,
Bitterly she sobs,
Bitterly she sobs,
Faced with man's unkindness.   **ANCIENT POEM**

Drink Motherwort tea and live to be a source of continuous
astonishment and frustration to waiting heir.   **JAPANESE SAYING**

Leonurus means lion tail, and cardiaca, of the heart. Motherwort
suggests its use in conditions of the womb.

Motherwort is an introduced perennial that has sporadically
established itself throughout the Canadian prairies. It thrives in well-
drained, alkaline and sandy soil,

It is a member of the Mint family, with the familiar square stem,
opposite leaves, and flowers in the upper leaf axils. The flowers are
white to pink, with purple spots. The pink lips of the flower, according
to the Doctrine of Signatures, look like a vagina, and hence are useful
for menstrual problems.

It does not, however, have any mint odour, but a mildly unpleasant
scent that only bees appear to appreciate. The leaves are large, toothed
and palmate, most un-mint like.

Various native tribes integrated Motherwort into their repertory
including the Cherokee. It was given as a stimulating tea, and for
nervous and hysterical affections, including fainting and nervous
stomach unease.

They believed the plant a gift from the Iroquois and called it **E TSI**, meaning mother, using it for "cramp and weak hearts of women."

The Mohegan, Mi'kmaq, and Delaware all used the plant for female conditions, including amenorrhea, and uterine spasms.

The ancient Greeks valued the herb not only for heart problems, but to relieve pain during childbirth, or help those suffering anxiety during pregnancy.

An ancient tale tells of a town where the water source came from a stream surrounded by banks of motherwort. It is said that many in the town lived to be 130 years old, or more.

Culpepper said. "Venus owns this herb and it is under Leo. There is no better herb to drive melancholy vapors from the heart, to strengthen it and make the mind cheerful, blithe and merry." To translate, motherwort is for women and the heart.

John Gerard, the 16th century English herbalist said many "commend it against the infirmities of the heart: it is judged to be so forceable that it is thought it took this name Cardiaca, of the effect."

Herbalists of the time such as Leonhart Fuchs wrote, "motherwort is excellent for the beating of the heart." Adamus Lonicerus added, "with its root crushed and laid upon the chest, it removes constraint of the heart. And used thus, it makes the breast roomy."

Various Eclectic physicians, including Dr. Cook appreciated motherwort. "The nerves receive the most benefit of its influence, whence it is called as a nervine tonic and antispasmodic. In warm preparations it maintains a gentle outward circulation, and promotes the menstrual and lochial flow; and in this form proves of value in recent suppression...painful menstruation, and hysterical forms of nervousness and palpitation.

In cold preparations, it promotes appetite and digestion, strengthens the uterus."

Asian Motherwort (*L. artemisia*) is an annual, or sometime biennial, that grows well on the prairies. The plant prefers rich, warm, moist sandy loam, but I have seen it growing on dry and extremely poor alkaline soil.

The Japanese traditionally drank a beverage of **YAKUMOSO** flowers to ensure long life. This species (*L. sibiricus*) is an Herb of Life, and has its own festival.

On the ninth day of the ninth month, **KIKOUSOUKI**, meaning Month of the Motherwort Flowers, a celebration is held. The flowers are eaten with rice, stirred in saki cups, and blessings for a long life are exchanged.

Siberian Motherwort is mentioned in the ancient Book of Songs, the Chinese Shih Ching written ca. 1000-500 BC. It was called **T'UEI**.

Asian Motherwort is known in Traditional Chinese Medicine as **YI MU CAO** meaning, "good for mother", or **CHONG WEI**, "full and flourishing" because the stem, leaf and fruit are thick and abundant. At one time, the seeds, **CHONG WEI ZI**, were eaten as a substitute for sesame seeds. One common name is Benefit Mother Weed, another Bloody Mother Herb.

In Vietnam and Japan, the plant is used to promote menses, while in Cambodia, Laos and Vietnam it invigorates the flow of blood.

The dried leaf of *L. sibiricus* can be rolled as smoked as a hemp-like substitute. In Mexico, it is known as **MARIJUANILLO**, meaning Little Marijuana. It is popular in Malaysia as a substitute smoke.

In Vera Cruz, the herb is used in folk magic to make the groom return to the marriage.

It is believed that the true Asian Motherwort is *L. artemisia*, and that *L. sibiricus* is a separate, clearly defined species. Other authors believe they are variations of the same species.

Motherwort seed germinates within 10-14 days, and can be thinned to 8 inch spacing after developing four or five leaves.

The whole herb is harvested in early fall in full flower, and dried in partial shade with good ventilation. The full flower herb is richest in active ingredients, with a significant lack of benzoic acid and other constituents, before blooming, and after seed formation.

Seeds are harvested when ripe.

Motherwort is hardy to zone 3, and will easily self-sow when established. It prefers a well-drained soil with a pH of 7.7, with lots of sun. Germination takes 2-3 weeks, with high variability and low germination rates.

Seed seven to eight pounds of seed per acre, with up to 1000 pounds of dry leaf and flowers expected at end of first year. Subsequent years can double or triple in production.

In one Romanian trial, seeds were sown in November, mid-March, mid-April and late April. The highest yields were obtained from sowing in fall or early spring at over 2000 kg/ha, and seed yields of 217 kg/ha from sowing in fall.

The addition of manganese, iodine, cobalt and copper, stimulate the formation of compounds connected with cardio-vascular and sedative activities in Motherwort. Dranitsyna et al, *Biol Aktivn* 1975.

Motherwort has been investigated for veterinary use. Work by Nikolaenko, *Veterinariya Moskva* 1990 4 looked at the protective effect of plant infusions during vaccination of chicken broilers.

MEDICINAL

CONSTITUENTS- *L. cardiaca-* a number of alkaloids including leonurine (0.0068%), leonurinine, leonurine A&B, stachydrine (a pyrrolidine type alkaloid), betaine, betonicine and turicin, iridoid monoterpenes like leonuride (ajugoside and ajugol), galiridoside, and reptoside; various bitter glycosides ; alpha humulene, furanic labdane diterpenes (20-70 mcg/g fresh wt) leocardin, leosibirin, preleosibirin, and isoballotenol acetate; bufenolide glycosides, tannins (9.5-10%), leonurin, stachyose, choline, lavandulifolioside, malic acid, calcium chloride, trace minerals, resins, essential oils, lauric acid, citric acid, malic acid, oleic acid, ursolic acid, caffeic acid 4-rutinoside.
Also contains a number of flavonoids including rutin, quinqueloside, genkwanin, quercitin, quercetrin, isoquercitrin, hyperoside; as well as apigenin and kaempferol glucosides.
seeds- a Cad-specific lectin; 22% protein; 30% fat; root- stachyose
L. sibiricus- sibiricinones, three diterpenes, leosibiricine, leosibirine, and isoleosibiricine, 15-epi-sibiricinones, genkwanin (flavone), rutin, four quanidine derivatives (4-guanidinobutanol, arginine, 4-guanidine butyric acid and leonurine), l-stachydrine, syringic acid, rosmarinic acid, caffeic acid depsides, various alkaloids including stachydrine, leonuridine, leonurinine, and leonurine; various acids, including benzoic, lauric, linoleic and oleic; phytosterols, arginine, 4-guanidino-1-butanol, 4-guanidinobutyric acid, stachyose, flavonoids, bitter glycosides, tannins, stachyose, potassium chloride, trace minerals, vitamin A, and a variety of flavonoids

including rutin, kaempferol, hyperoside, quercitrin and quercitin.
seed- leonurine
plant- 0.01-0.04% leonurine, stachydrine, prehispanolone, apigenin, genkwanin, isoquercitrin.

Motherwort is used worldwide for treating the heart and uterus. The herb is most reliable in cases of PMS associated with frustration, irritability, depression, heart palpitations and insomnia. Delayed or suppressed menstruation, associated with anxiety, tension, or cold is relieved, combining well with vervain as a relaxing nervine. It helps relieve smooth muscle parasympathetic cramping. In China, it is used to relax muscle tension associated with painful and frustrating vaginismus.

It is a mint with bitter acrid taste, calming to the sympathetic nervous system.

Menstrual cramps with little or no bleeding are relieved. Taken over time, motherwort encourages strong uterine contractions, by strengthening tissue. As the uterus is more toned, less cramping occurs in the future.

Motherwort may reduce endogenous inflammatory mediators by enhancing the synthesis of prostaglandins via prostaglandin E9-ketoreductase that is important in synthesis of useful PGE2 prostaglandins. Hsieh et al, *Proc Nat Sci Council Repub China* 1985 9:3.

The herb brings more blood to the pelvic region and thickens the bladder, uterus and vaginal tissue, increasing tone and elasticity. It possesses beta-blocking activity with specific affinity to the uterus and vascular tissue.

It contains some of the same constituents as wood betony, and shares both nervine and uterine stimulating properties. The plant is warming in nature, with a bitter or acrid bent, similar to valerian root.

Clymer suggests small amounts can be taken prenatally for preventing toxemia. I have no experience with using the herb in this way, but I would exercise caution, due to the oxytocic effects. For painful dysmenorrhea, delayed labour and as a hemostat for postpartum hemorrhage, the herb is most effective.

Stachydrine, for example, possesses oxytocic activity. Dosage is important, as too much of the herb before the uterus has clamped down, may precipitate bleeding. Small amounts assist the uterus in contract after delivery, in a manner more effective than ergot.

Leonurine induces uterine contractions at low concentrations, but inhibits at higher, in test tube studies. These seemingly opposite results may explain how motherwort can induce labour and menstruation, as well as relax the uterus after childbirth. Yeung et al, *Planta Medica* 1977 31; Kong et al, *Am J Chin Med* 1976 4.

Taken once or twice daily for a week, beginning the day after giving birth, can help ease tension in the new mother, and prevent uterine infection. Sitz baths with uva ursi will also help. If it causes increased flooding, replace the herb with bugleweed, according to Michael Moore.

Taken immediately after birth may increase bleeding so use caution, but it will stimulate suppressed lochia and help promote postpartum uterine drainage. It will not increase post birthing uterine contractions induced by nursing.

Ellingwood writes, "Professor John King regarded motherwort as superior to all other remedies in suppression of the lochia, giving it internally and applying a fomentation of the herb over the lower abdominal region."

For fibroids, it combines well with black cohosh. Add cramp bark to these two herbs as a combination for painful dysmenorrhea, but do not use when bleeding is heavy. For amenorrhea, combine with thuja or yarrow to promote menstruation.

Lectins from seeds affect red blood cell agglutination and believed part of blood flow enhancement. Bird et al, *Clin Lab Haematol* 1979 1:1.

Motherwort helps relieve stress affecting the heart, such as in hyperthyroid conditions; combining well with bugleweed.

Various glycosides are cardiotonic and anti-spasmodic, which are of cumulative benefit over time, helping ease palpitations and tachycardia.

Motherwort, combined with hawthorn, will slow the heartbeat, lower blood pressure, and give a steady, strengthened pulse. Both contain organic sources of calcium chloride that supports and nourishes cardiac muscle.

Work by Ritter et al, *Planta Medica* 2010 76:6 572-82 suggests various pathways related to improving cardiac function.

It exerts calcium antagonistic activity by $I_{ca.L}$ blockade, reduces the repolarising current $I_{k.r}$, and prolongs AP duration. I_{na} is not affected. It therefore works on multiple electrophysiological targets at whole organ and single cell levels.

Michael Moore put it well. "I am not referring to thyroid disease here but the tendency for a certain subset of folks to increase thyroid levels under stress (and decrease them under depression), rather than the more common use of flight or fright responses (adrenergic stress) or increasing blood mass from anabolic stress (the hibernating bear syndrome). If the primary symptoms of thyroid stress (not disease) are sweating, rapid gut transit time, and nervous lethargy, Bugleweed is the preferred herbal approach. If the primary symptoms are tachycardia and palpitations, Motherwort is better. If in doubt, use both; they are complementary."

It is a hypotensive nervine that will help headache, insomnia and vertigo.

For intermittent claudication, relaxing the smooth muscles will help improve blood flow. For this combine motherwort with cramp bark, scullcap and valerian. To slowly dissolve the arterial plaque, add linden blossom.

Work by Milkowska et al, *J Ethnopharm* 2002 80 identified lavandulifolioside, and found it reduced the heart rate and blood flow in rats. It induced widening of the QRS and prolonged Q-T interval. The authors suggest the compound is akin to quinidine, and has different activity than various cardiac glycosides in the herb.

This makes it a good choice for women suffering night sweats and hot flashes associated with the menopausal transition. Motherwort helps lessen the severity, frequency and duration of hot flashes, even after they have begun.

It alleviates the shortness of breath and respiratory congestion associated with menopause. Insomnia and night sweats, as well as disturbed dreams and nightmares suffered by some women, are likewise relieved.

Women who are nervous, and quick in thoughts and actions can benefit.

As well, it helps relieve muscle twitching and spasms, especially in cases of restlessness and nervous debility. It will relieve the irritation of herpes and shingle pain.

It combines well with elecampane in the treatment of tachycardia associated with symptoms of Grave's disease.

Taken hot, motherwort tea promotes diaphoretic activity, and can be used in fevers, colds, and even chronic bronchitis, relaxing spasms and removing toxins via the skin. As a calming expectorant for bronchitis, it is similar in activity to ground ivy.

Dr. Christopher mentions that motherwort can be used "as a healing tonic in recovery from debilitating fever where other tonics are inadmissible."

At body temperature, the herb has more direct action on the kidneys, and may be useful in both acute or chronic nephritis, water retention and edema of the lower limbs associated with kidney stagnation, cardiac weakness, and scanty urination. Motherwort appears to help clear protein and blood from the urine, including that caused by renal calculi.

Motherwort may be useful in early stages of prostate enlargement, combining well with nettle root.

Likewise, skin conditions, such as eczema respond, if taken over time at a cooler temperature, and combined with goldenrod, nettle leaf and such.

Herpes and shingle irritation may be somewhat relieved, and well as neuralgia, according to Michael Moore. Motherwort helps relieve headaches, vertigo and peripheral circulatory deficiencies. In clinical trials, it showed impressive results for treating numbness of the limbs, dizziness, and insomnia.

Motherwort can be useful in exhaustion and cardiac stress associated with chronic fatigue syndrome, fibromyalgia, panic attacks, anxiety and bipolar disorders.

Matthew Wood reports on an unusual constitutional indication given by William LeSassier. "He associated it with a hollow, caved-in chest, odd shapes in the sternum, and scoliosis."

Small doses of the herb help relieve gas and flatulence, as well as improve digestion and encourage regular bowel elimination.

A small amount may be useful for children on their first day to school, or when introduced to new school environment.

Motherwort taken within 10 days of a tick bite may help to prevent secondary viral infections, such as Lyme disease.

Water extracts of motherwort were tested against tick borne encephalitis virus, in vitro, and almost completely inactivated the virus. Other herbs with similar activity, in this study by Fokina et al, *Voprosy Virusologii* 1991 36:1, were labrador tea (*R. palustre*), greater celandine (*Chelidonium majus*), bog cranberry (*V. vitis-idaea*), bilberry (*V. myrtillus*) and black currant (*Ribes nigrum*).

Ursolic acid is anti-viral, and inhibits the Epstein Barr virus in vitro. Ursolic acid, in vitro, is cytotoxic to lymphatic leukemia P388 and L-1210, human lung carcinoma A-549, KB cells, human colon HCT-8, and mammary tumour MCF-7. Li et al, *World J Gastroenterology* 2002 8:3.

Ursolic acid inhibits tumour production in a manner comparable to retinoic acid.

The herb possesses significant anti-oxidant activity in work by Matkowski et al, *J Med Plants Res* 2:11. This was confirmed by Bernatoniene et al, *Acta Pol Pharm* 2009 66:4 415-9. He noted the anti-oxidant benefit was higher than ginkgo biloba or hawthorn.

Motherwort could be useful remedyto protect cardiac muscles from pathogenic process, due to partial uncoupling of mitochondria, respiratory inhibition and decreased ROS production.

A review of its phytochemistry and pharmacology was published by Wojtyniak K et al, *Phytother Res* 2013 27:8 1115-20.

The closely related Asian Motherwort *(L. artemisia)* is nearly identical in action, and is widely used in China after delivery to help the uterus contract, reduce pain and stop bleeding.

Studies have shown decoctions of the herb as effective as the drug ergotamine in contracting the uterus after delivery.

Modern research suggests it is similar in effect to posterior pituitary hormone.

For dysmenorrhea, retention of lochia, and placenta, the wine mix-fried herb is preferred.

For amenorrhea it combines with red peony root.

The uncooked herb is often combined with dandelion root, violet leaves, and forsythia fruit for skin inflammations and erysipelas due to heat toxins. For edema and water retention it is combined with plantain seed that is salt-processed.

Experiments on this species have found it decreases blood viscosity and reduces platelet aggregation rates. Intravenous drips of asian motherwort herb have been used in China since 1978 for treatment of coronary myocardial ischemia in several hospitals.

One recent clinical study from Shanghai looked at 100 patients with heart disease. All had symptoms of angina pectoris, palpitations, shortness of breath, and chest tightness.

The patients were divided into the five Traditional Chinese Medicine syndromes including 41 cases of chest yang, 22 cases of heart blood qi and yin deficiency, 9 cases of kidney yang deficiency, and 17 with lung/phlegm congestion.

The latter two divisions did not respond well to Asian Motherwort. The first two had great success with 45% showing marked improvement, 39% moderate improvement, for total of 84% efficacy.

Other studies have shown Motherwort extracts help activate blood circulation and remove blood stagnation, relieve chest pain and palpitations. Increased blood flow in the coronary artery and PAF, platelet activating factor, inhibition was noted.

Work by Pang et al, *Japan J Pharmacology* 2001 86:2 found an un-named compound showed vaso-constrictive activity similar to nitro-L-arginine methy-ester, an inhibitor of nitric oxide synthase.

Early work by Zou et al, *Am J Chinese Med* 1989 17:1-2 examined blood hyper-viscosity in 105 patients.

Given intravenously, over a 15 day period, produced clinical benefit in reduced blood mammary viscosity, fibrinogen volume, as well as increases in deformability of RBC, and enhanced anti-platelet aggregation.

It may have therapeutic possibilities with stroke. Loh et al, *J Ethnopharm* 2009 June 1.

Stephen Buhner mentions the use of Asian motherwort for mitochondrial protection and support. He is much better writer than me, so let us read what he has to share in his new book on Healing Lyme Disease Coinfections.

"Motherwort has been found to be strongly neuroprotective, especially in ischemia-reperfusion-induced mitochondrial dysfunctions in the brain, including the cerebral cortex. It significantly improves neurological outcomes and reduces ischemia-reperfusion impacts in the brain.

It decreases reactive oxygen species (ROS) levels in the brain mitochondria and, importantly, reduces mitochondrial swelling and restores mitochondrial membrane potential. Motherwort decreases the expression of a protein, B-cell lymphoma 2 (Bcl-2), in the brain.

Increased Bcl-2 levels in the body have been implicated in the generation of various cancers including prostate, as well as various psychiatric disorders of the CNS and autoimmunity problems, all part of the mycoplasma symptom range. Part of the function of the protein is interfering with apoptosis, that is, cell death."

He continues. "Motherwort decreases its expression and increases the levels of Bax. Bax is a protein, closely related to Bcl-2, that acts to increase apoptosis in cells. Bcl-2 and Bax normally exist in a modulated balance and their expression is controlled by a protein, p53.

This protein is intimately involved in controlling the emergence of cancers in the body as well as protecting the genome from damage." Reishi mushroom regulates this gateway as well.

Leonurus sibiricus contains diterpenoids which show strong inhibition of estrogen sulfotransferase comparable to meclofenamic acid. Narukawa et al, *J Nat Med* 2014 68:1.

In China, it is being tested experimentally, as a morning after contraceptive. It is an energetic uterine stimulant, and the fresh herb juice is often used in difficult childbirth situation. For poor blood circulation in the mother after childbirth, a cup of the fresh juice is often prescribed.

Tao et al, *J Ethnopharm* 122:2 found water extracts of chinese motherwort inhibit proliferation of breast cancer cells through cytotoxicity and cell cycle arrest. It was non-apoptotic and ER independent.

Chinwala et al, *J Altern Comp Med* 2003 9 identified activity via apoptosis against several cancer cell lines.

Asian Motherwort is used alone for treating acute nephritis, a derivation from the often complex combinations used in TCM. Clinical studies show the herb useful in treating acute glomerulonephritis, and edema associated with acute or chronic nephritis. Lin P S, *J Trad Chin Med* 1959 6:18.

In another study of acute nephritis, the fresh herb decoction was more effective than dried, but both reduced edema. *Yunan J Chin Med* 1984 2:48.

Isoquercitrin, isolated from *L. heterophyllus*, shows activity against leukemia K562 cancer cell lines. Cong et al, *Zhong guo Zhong Yao Za Zhi* 2009 34:14.

Work by Nagasawa et al, *Anticancer Research* 1992 12:1 found both absorbed and un-absorbed motherwort fractions suppressed the incidence and growth of mammary tumours in mice. An earlier study by the same author found adding just 0.5% methanol extract of the herb to drinking water suppressed mammary cancers.

Siberian Motherwort is known as a heart herb, in that part of the world, and used for cardiac neurosis, epilepsy, insomnia and various menstrual conditions.

Extracts enhance insulin secretion and/or foster cell proliferation, suggesting one mechanism for the traditional use in diabetes mellitus. Schmidt S et al, *J Ethnopharm* 2013 150:1 85-94.

Asian Motherwort seeds, **CHONG WEI ZI**, are hypotensive. They are traditionally used to increase sperm count, vitality, enhance vision problems including nebula, due in part, to their large vitamin A content.

The seeds are sweet and mildly cold, and used especially for menorrhagia and continuous hemorrhage conditions.

They help break up congealed blood, astringe and tone the uterus. The seeds cool the liver, and are used in heat conditions with red, painful, swollen eyes.

Both water and alcohol extracts help decrease blood pressure, according to pharmacological studies.

The stalks are used to treat addictive itching papules, or to bathe newborns and prevent skin irritation. Another name is **YI MU**, meaning Mother Booster, or **YI MING**, meaning Brightness Booster.

HOMEOPATHY

Motherwort influences pelvic organs, allays spasms and nervous irritability, promotes secretion and reduces febrile excitement. Valuable in suppressed menses and lochia, dysentery, vomiting, frightful pain in abdomen, violent thirst, tongue dry and cracked.

Tinnitus, ringing in ears, and teeth sensitive to sugar are symptoms to observe. Burning in urethra during urination. Loss of ambition, indifference, dissatisfied with everything, needs a change. Disconnected, need stimulation. Irritable, annoyed by needs of others, with feelings of contempt, yelling, cursing.

DOSE- Tincture and lower potencies. The mother tincture is prepared from the fresh plant above ground as it comes into flower. This was based on an involuntary proving by Clarence Bartlett in 1888.

A more recent proving by Joy Lucas on 8 females and 2 males at LM1, 6c, 12c, 30c, and 200c in 2006, showed many mental and emotional patterns.

ESSENTIAL OIL

The essential oil of *L. cardiaca* is diuretic and relaxant, according to Bezanger-Beauquesne et al, *Plantes Medicinales des Regions Temperees*, 2nd Edition, Paris: Maloine 1990. It is lemon scented and may create photosensitivity or dermatitis is sensitive individuals.

It is composed of 49 compounds that comprise 84% of the oil; 26-35% germacrene D.

The essential oil of *L. sibiricus* contains three diterpenes with psychoactive properties.

PLANT OIL

The plant oil was used in a trial of patients with arterial hypertension, accompanied by anxiety and sleep disorders. Fifty patients were treated for 28 days with 1200 mg of oil extract per day. Significant improvement was observed in 32%, moderate improvement in 48% and weak effect in 8%. The authors conclude that the oil extract may have potential in treating patients with arterial hypertension with concurrent psycho-neurological disorders. Shikov AN et al, *Phytother Res* 2011 25:4 540-3.

HYDROSOL

Motherwort water is distilled from all parts of the plant. It can be put into wine that is unclean and turbulent for clarifying.

Motherwort water is for sharp wit, good understanding and good memory. It helps promote good minds and amiable color, and dissipates anger. It prevents grey hair, taken both internally and applied to head. It helps trembling and palsy, mouth abscess including gum and tooth pain, and bad breath. It improves appetite and digestive power, and relieves dropsy, melancholy, comforts the heart, and thoughts of fear.

It is used for scrofula, quarternary fevers, melancholic and phlegmatic temperaments, scabs and abscesses of skin. It is also an effective spray for flies. **BRUNSCHWIG**

FLOWER ESSENCES

Motherwort flower essence improves the communication with all devic spirits, particularly of the water. A greater understanding of relationships to plants, animals and the land is enhanced. Finer attunements to geopathic zones are noticed.

It improves ability in landscaping, and for those who work with numbers it will be balancing. The flower essence is for accountants.

PEGASUS

Motherwort essence helps heal energies that surround auto-immune illness such as Lou Gehrig's and Parkinson's Disease. It heals the energies surrounding brain aneurysms, scar tissue, heart murmur and muscle apathy. **AVENSARO**

Motherwort flower essence teaches about and heals an aspect of the psyche that deals with hardness and softness. A person needing Motherwort can also have difficulty setting boundaries in some situations, allowing themselves to be used or mistreated, especially by people they have developed some trust with.

Use Motherwort in many stages of psychotherapy where the individual is learning constructive, assertive behavior to set appropriate boundaries. **DALTON**

Motherwort essence is female (yin) energy and works on the intuitive crown to heart charkas, helping to eliminate negative cords and behavior taught by your mother. Perfect for those with mothering issues, the essence brings a better balance in relationships, especially for an overprotective mother. It rebalances mind and body, creating peace and understanding. It may also help with hormonal imbalances, PMS, and birthing issues. **OLIVE**

Motherwort flower essence works on family patterns. Helps those who don't feel at home in their family and on the earth. For lack of warmth and love in the family, resulting in becoming hardened, rigid and feeling like a stranger on the earth. **BLOESEM**

Motherwort essence helps you reconnect to your heart's life force, and helps us remember that we are integral to the web of Life.

TREE FROG

Motherwort helps re-integrate a wobbly energy in body. It is for the mothering figure who clings rather than lets go.   **ILMINSTER**

SPIRITUAL PROPERTIES

In calling on the spirit of the plant, a vision appears of many spirits playing their trumpets as they await for a special being to join them. They announce her entrance with the songs of the heavens and upon their last note, a regal being appears with all her glory. She is a queen in the spirit world. She know exactly what her purpose and mission is and is ready and willing to perform her duties…When one uses the plant for medicinal purposes, know that you are receiving the energy of the miracle that was performed by this noble spirit.   **AVENSARO**

In the first period after the influx of *Leonurus sibiricus* smoked, little happened apart from the fact that I got into a basic meditative state in which all material things appeared to increase in depth and importance.

FELIX HASLER

Motherwort helps us to enjoy freedom in new thought. Motherwort is in the realm of communication. It allows the transmission of knowledge, of ancient wisdom, of the joining of the intuitive with the scientific.   **EVELYN MULDERS**

PERSONALITY TRAITS

Motherwort…best fits women who are underweight and emotionally unbalanced largely because of external life stresses.

If sleep is problematic, and there is anxiety and restless, particularly in the days preceding the onset of menses, Motherwort will prove relaxing. If is specific for women with long cycles, who have breast tenderness, painful or sluggish onset of menses, and possible heart palpitations during this time of month.   **CHARLES W. KANE**

Unlike other members of the mint family, which are usually more soft and inviting, Leonurus presents as a bit more tough and prickly, perhaps a good doctrine of signatures to encourage women to be a bit prickly if that is what it takes to get their need met before getting frazzled. **DEBORAH FRANCES RN ND**

This European and Asiatic plant…intermingles leaf and flower formation, drawing the inflorescence down into the region of leaf rhythm; it is divided and arranged in triangular lappets.

The plant is only faintly aromatic, with a musty and a slightly repellent scents, and the taste is very bitter. Corresponding to the nature thus expressed, the medicinal action has largely shifted from the metabolic to the rhythmic action.

Amenorrhea, dysmenorrheal, sterility and climacteric symptoms do also benefit, but the accent lies on the help this plant gives with palpitations, anxiety, dyspnoea, weak cardiac function with intermittent pulse, angina pectoris; oppression of the heart from the metabolism, Roemheld's syndrome. **WILHELM PELIKAN**

MYTHS AND LEGENDS

A mother was living with her ten-year old son. She had been ill since giving birth with abdominal pain, and menstrual irregularity.

The son wanted to help her and so went to an herbalist. He bought an herb and decocted it for his mother. She took it and felt better. The son went back to herbalist and asked if he could cure his mother. He said yes, but it would cost him 500 pounds of rice.

He could not afford this, but suddenly had an idea and asked if he could pay after his mother was cured. The herbalist agreed.

At midnight, the son followed the herbalist into the mountains and watched him dig herbs. He waited for the herbalist to leave and then picked them himself.

The next day, the herbalist came to the house, but the son said he could not come up with the rice and was sorry. The herbalist left. The mother was cured by the herb and has been called "good-for-mother" ever since. **HENRY LU**

BOTANICA POETICA

If your heart is ticking fast
You tend to be the nervous sort
Your friends describe you as high strung
You just might need some Motherwort
Leaves and flowers, not the stem
A tonic for a nervous heart
And if menstruation is delayed
This herb can help your cycle start
Stimulates the uterus
Helps promote the circulation
Leonurus Cardiaca, a bitter mint
Take it for your palpitation
Ease a spasm or a cramp
Or if you can not sleep at night
Menopause has set you off
Motherwort might set you right.

SYLVIA CHATROUX

RECIPES

INFUSION- 20-40 grams

TINCTURE- 30-60 drops as needed. The recently dried plant is tinctured 1:5 at 45%; the fresh plant at 1:2 and 60% alcohol.

A Russian recipe is two parts fresh plant juice to three parts vodka (strength not mentioned, maybe 40%).

POWDER- dry powder, according to the European Pharmacopoeia 7th ed, should have a minimum of 0.2% flavonoids, expressed as hyperoside. Odd.

SEED DECOCTION- 4-10 grams for less than five minutes.

CONVACARD- enteric coated tablet available in Europe.

CAUTION- Do not use in patients with pupil dilation.

ASIAN MOTHERWORT DECOCTION FOR ACUTE NEPRHITIS- Take 250 grams of fresh herb or one half of dried and decoct in 700 ml of water down to 200 ml. Divide and drink throughout day.

CAUTION- Motherwort is a uterine stimulant and in contraindicated during pregnancy, or Blood or Yin deficiency except where noted. It may be used in the third trimester, but not in first three months of pregnancy. May interfere with blood thinners. It probably should not be taken with beta-blockers like Inderal or Tenormin.

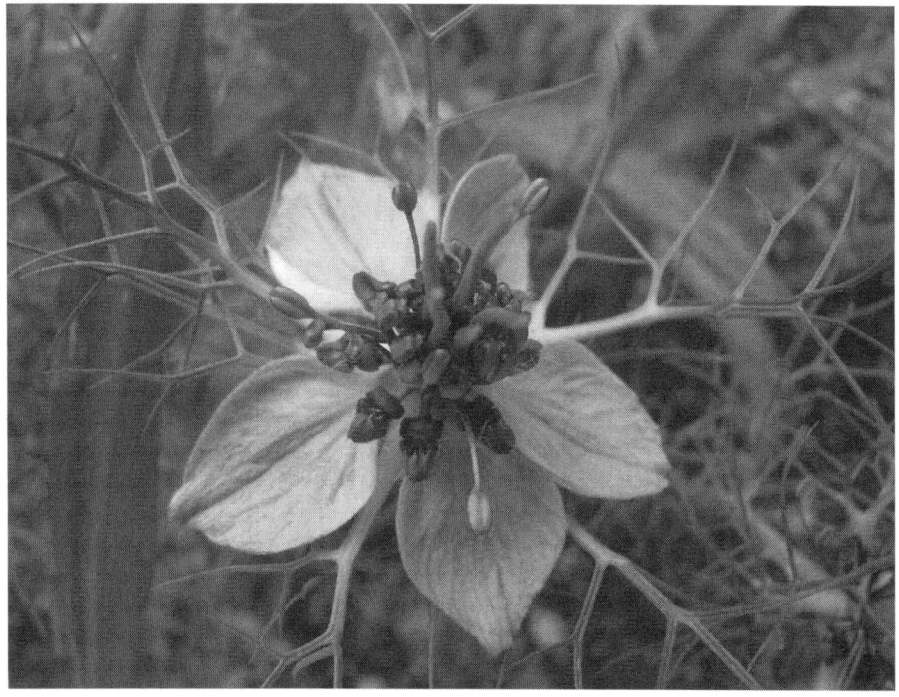

Love in a Mist

NIGELLA
BLACK CUMIN
FENNEL FLOWER
BARAKA
(*Nigella vulgaris*)
(*N. sativa* L.)
(*N. indica* Roxb. ex Flem.)
LOVE IN A MIST
VIRGIN IN THE GREEN
STRAWBERRY CUMIN
(*N. damascena* L.)

Their names were nymphs, and they were nymphs indeed
A whole mythology from pinch of seed,
Nemesia and Viscaria, and that
Blue as the butterfly, Phacelia;
Love in mist Nigella whose shining brat
Appears unwanted like a very weed.   **V. SACKVILLE-WEST**

Black cumin is good for all ailments except death.   **MOHAMMED**

Curative black cumin.   **ISAIAH 28:25**

Nigella is the diminutive of Latin **NIGER**, meaning small black, referring to seed colour and size. Damascena refers the city of Damascus where the plant was believed to originate.

Both Nigella species are annuals that will complete to seed on the prairies if they get enough heat. They require minimal moisture and love porous, sandy soil.

Love in a Mist refers to the fine hair-like leaves surrounding the flowers. The fine hairs must have been suggestive, the French calling them "Chevaux de Venus", the Germans "Venushaar", meaning Venus Hair. Up until the 18th century, brides wore long hair decorations to demonstrate virginity. Another name was Capuchin's Beard.

In the Middle East, Love in a Mist seeds are put into cakes and breads. The Syrian Book of Medicine suggests its main use is for headaches.

The German nickname, strawberry cumin, or **ERDBEERKUMMEL** does not really explain the flavour, which is more pineapple-like when the seeds are crushed.

Gerard wrote the seed drunk with wine is a remedy for shortness of breath. He suggested that Love in a Mist would "bringeth down the menses".

Egyptian ladies were said to eat them to produce stoutness.

Medicinally, it was combined with *Plumbago* root for digestive complaints and intermittent fevers. It was a favoured medicine in India, to give to new mothers after childbirth.

The seeds are often used to adulterate the more valuable black cumin, but the oil, which can be obtained in larger amounts, is lower in active constituents.

194

The seed of *N. damascena* smells like grape soft drink when rubbed between the fingers.

An early Latin name was *Papaver nigrum*, meaning Black Poppy, due to the narcotic effect of the alkaloid damascene.

It is dedicated to St. Catherine, and the patron of spinsters. She was successful at converting folks to Christianity, and ordered to death by Emperor Maxentius.

She met her death via a wheel stuck with spikes; and then beheaded. The linear foliage bears some resemblance to a wheel.

It has another side. If a young girl handed the flower to an admirer, it meant to leave her alone. It was used to send someone packing by placing it in a covered basket. In Victorian flower symbolism it stands for perplexity and "you puzzle me".

The flower is used in bread dough as a topping for decoration.

At one time, the seeds were burned to protect against fleas, gnats and other insects.

The flower has an ingenious hinged-lid that keeps unwanted insects from stealing nectar.

Black Cumin is a popular spice in India, Turkey, Greece, and all over the Middle East, including Tunisia, and Egypt.

The seeds have a spicy, fruity taste, but were supplanted with the more recent popularity of pepper.

They smell aromatic, more like fennel than cumin with a touch of nutmeg or camphor. Others describe the aroma like lemony carrots with hint of nutmeg. Some authors say oregano-like with a peppery nutmeg taste.

It is popular in spreads and soft cheeses. A popular hot dog-shaped croquette in the Middle East made with bulgar and lamb is spiced with the ground seed.

Dioscorides called the pale white-flowered, black-seeded plant, **MELANTHION**, meaning Black Leaf. He recommended the seed for headache, toothache, nasal congestion and intestinal worms. The seeds were found buried with King Tut, suggestive of their value.

Greek physicians classified the herb as hot and dry to the third degree, meaning it warmed up the center and opens the skin to release toxins.

In ancient Latin, the seed was called **PANACEA**, meaning cure-all. See Ginseng.

Arabic, Persian and Hindu physicians know Nigella as **HABBATOUSSOUDA, SIYAN-DANAH,** or **KALA-DANAH**, meaning Black Seed in all three languages. **HABBAT EL BARAKA** is an Arabic word meaning "seeds of blessing".

An ancient Syrian herb book calls it Black Tin-tir.

In the Old Testament of the Bible, it is called **FITCHES** from the Hebrew for vetch, **KETZAH**.

Kala-Danah is a common Asian name associated with pre-European medicinal and religious plants. Pliny called it Git, similar to the Arabic Gith.

Black cumin use medicinally goes back at least 3600 years. A recent archeological find in north-central Turkey was a flask containing the seed mixed with propolis and beeswax.

Hildegard de Bingen, under the name **GITHERUM RATDE**, suggested crushing the seeds and combining with honey. This is smeared on the wall to attract flies that will taste it, sicken and fall dead.

The Romans used it for flavouring food; the French as a substitute for pepper, calling it **QUATRE EPICES**, or **TOUTE EPICE**.

The seed is spicy, and pungent, and is commonly used all over the Middle East and into India for flavouring curries and a sprinkle on cakes and breads.

In Ethiopia, it is a spice in alcoholic beverages, like adding celery salt to rim of Bloody Mary cocktail on this continent.

It was added to breads in Poland, known as **CZARNUSZKA SIEWNA**. The seeds were added to wine to remove phlegm from the lungs and increase mother's milk. It was combined with wormwood as a summertime mosquito deterrent.

At one time, the warm, ground seed was used in sweet powders and sniffed to restore a lost sense of smell.

The seeds were put among linen to keep away insects, and used by veterinary doctors to strengthen the immune systems of animals (two pounds of seeds per ton of animal feed). It has been shown to reduce allergic symptoms such as asthma and eczema in horses, and prevent mastitis in cows.

When added to diet of broiler chickens, it proved to be both an economic and efficient growth promoter. Mahmood et al, *Int J Ag Bio* 11:6.

Akhtar and Javed, *Indian Veterinary Journal* 1991 68:8 found powdered seeds (suspended in 2% tragacanth gum) were as effective as Niclosamide in treating *Moniezia* infections in sheep. Essential oil activity against tapeworm was found comparable to piperazine.

Other veterinary uses include increasing milk production in ruminants, and anti-oxytocic during pregnancy and birthing to retain placenta. Lab studies suggest it is a more potent galactagogue than cumin seed.

The seed alone, or combined with *Thymus vulgaris*, appears useful in raising healthy rabbits, with a high level of safety. Tousson et al, *Toxicol & Health* 2011 27:2.

It was traditionally used in medicine for dropsy and kidney complaints. In fact, the hard small black seeds look like kidneys in the doctrine of signatures, even the kidney stones they help eliminate.

Readers interested in a more intensive history are referred to *The Healing Power of Black Cumin* by Sylvia Luetjohann.

The seeds were one of the first in space, travelling on Sputnik III in 1958.

MEDICINAL

CONSTITUENTS- *N. sativa* seed- 21% protein, 38% carbohydrates, and 35% oil. High levels of linoleic acid, alkaloids such as nigelline, nigellone, nigellimine, nigellidine, nigellicine, nigellamine A-C, and the glycoside melanthin, volatile oils, alpha hederin, kalopanaxsaponin I, thymoquinone,
Shoot, root- vanillic acid*N. damascena* seed- 1-0-(2,4-dihydroxy) benzoyl-glycerol (phenolic ester); and three other phenolic compounds, 3,4-dihydroxy-beta-phenethyl alcohol; 2,4-dihydroxyphenylacetic acid, and 2,4-dihydroxyphenylacetic acid methyl ester; alkaloids, flavonoids, sesquiterpenes germacrene; damascenine, and elemene, sterols, saponins, polyols, and fatty acids.

Black cumin has a long history of medicinal use in Islamic countries, exported to Malaysia; and widely used by Unani physicians of Pakistan and region.

The seed is laxative, stimulates the uterus, increases lactation, reduces inflammation and improves digestion due to the bitter compounds.

The seed infusion reduces painful menstruation, and postpartum contractions. It combines well with demulcent herbs for various bronchial complaints, including asthma.

Combine black cumin seeds (3 parts) with licorice root (2 parts) for a great cold and flu tea.

Nigellone, in low concentrations, inhibits the release of histamine from mast cells. Chakravarty et al, *Ann Allergy* 1993 70.

Decoctions of ground seed help relieve airway constriction, but are less powerful than theophylline. Boskabady et al, *Phytomed* 17:10.

Work by Weinkotter et al, *Planta Medica* 2008 74:2 confirmed the anti-spasmodic and muco-ciliary clearance of nigellone.

Nigelline (damascenine) reduces edema and is anti-pyretic in activity.

Salem et al, *International Journal of Immunopharmacology* 2000 22:9 looked at the anti-viral effects of black cumin seed. It showed a striking ant-iviral effect against murine cytomegalovirus infection that may be mediated by increasing the Mphi number and function, as well as IFN gamma, or interferon production.

Black Cumin seed supports metabolism, digestion, and helps lower blood sugar levels. Al-Awadi et al, *Diabetes Research* 1991 18:4.

Meral et al, *J Vet Med A Physiol Pathol Clin Med* 2001 48:10 found Nigella may be useful in diabetic patients, to prevent lipid peroxidation, increase anti-oxidant activity and prevent liver damage.

Ethanol extracts are agonist to PPAR gamma and produce insulin-like stimulation of glucose uptake in skeletal muscles. Benhaddou-Amdaloussi et al, *Diab Obes Metab* 2009 September 25.

Studies conducted by Nabil et al, *Pharmaceutical Biology Journal* 1998 used various fractions of black cumin, tested on rats vaccinated with *Brucella* vaccine (Rev 1).

Examination of lymph nodes revealed a remarkably consistent reactive lymph hyperplasia; and infiltration of the medullary sinuses with plasma cells, lymphocytes and macrophages.

One study, on cisplatin-induced toxicity in mice, found black cumin offered protection, and increased life span from 150-200%. Reductions in leukocytes and hemoglobin count were prevented. Cisplatin is a widely used, extremely toxic, cancer therapeutic drug with devastating side effects in most patients.

If lab studies can be extrapolated, it appears that the toxic principles are somehow neutralized and not present in excreted urine.

Various *in vitro* and *in vivo* studies indicate some selective toxicity to certain cancer cells. Abuharfeil et al, *J of Ethnopharmacology* 2000 71:1-2, found fresh plant water extractions exhibit maximum natural killer activity (62.3%) against tumour cells at a 1:50 dilution.

Black Cumin contains 23 different plant sterols that fit hormone receptors in the human body. This may be one of the reasons relief from menopausal symptoms, prostate inflammation, and other hormone-related conditions is experienced by many individuals.

In one study, an ether extract of the seed at 1.8% concentration shows a more powerful galactagogue effect than 0.5 mcg of estrogen.

Various fractions including the volatile oil, ethanol extracts and polysaccharide compounds were effective; with the latter the most effective fraction of all. Alcohol extracts of the seed inhibit growth of *E. coli* and *Staphylococcus aureus*.

Work by Hannan et al, *J Ajub Med Coll Abbottabad* 2008 20:3 found ethanol extracts inhibit methicillin-resistant strains of latter.

Petroleum extracts are effective against *B. subtilis, Micrococcus pyogenes* var. *aureus, Diplococcus pneumoniae* and *Streptococcus pyogenes.*

A combination of six parts nigella and one part *Phyllanthus niruri* showed significant improvement in the treatment of tonsil pharyngitis over seven days compared to placebo. Dirjomuljono et al, *Int J Clin Pharmacol Ther* 2008 46:6.

Work by Gilani et al, *Journal of the Pakistan Medical Association* 2001 51:3 confirmed the anti-spasmodic and broncho-dilating effect of nigella seed, or **KALONGI** as it is more well known. The mechanism is believed to involve calcium-channel blockade.

Boskabady et al, *Fund Clin Pharm* 2007 21:5 suggests benefit in treating asthma.

Efficacy against allergic rhinitis was noted. Nikakhlagh et al, *Am J Otolarynol* 2010 October 12.

Nestle scientists have found thymoquinone useful in food allergies and have registered a patent on a compound to treat and prevent. A huge cry went out across the web when some people speculated the company was trying to patent the plant. Not true. You cannot patent a plant.

Work published in *Biol Trace Elem Res* 116:3 found parathyroid hormone and nigella seed taken together were more effective in treating induced diabetic osteopenia.

A US patent was issued in 1996 for the use of *N. sativa* to stimulate immune competent cells in humans. However, as the patent has no specific proprietary processing method, the patent offers rather weak protection to the "inventor". One study found nigella seed enhances production of certain human interleukins and alters macrophages, suggesting changes in immune response. Haq et al, *Immunopharmacology* 1995 30:2.

In fact, black cumin is an immune modulator, helping to balance the body's response to under or over-active conditions. One study found people treated with the herb had a 30% increase in natural killer cell activity.

Rheumatoid arthritis, for example, is an auto-immune condition. Sajad et al, *J Comp Integr Med* 2010 7:1 found water and alcohol extracts reduced inflammation in patients.

Cancer cells are controlled in four different ways, through stopping proliferation, stopping metastases, initiating apoptosis and enhancing effectiveness of chemotherapy.

The seed appears to induce apoptosis in HepG2 cancer cell lines. Hassan et al, *Integr Cancer Ther* 2012 11:4 354-63.

The seed extract induces apoptosis in SiHa human cervical cancer cells through both p53 and caspases activation. Hasan et al, *Nat Prod Commun* 2013 8:2 213-6.

It appears people of African descent are more sensitive to the anti-tumor compounds alpha-hederin and its derivative kalopanaxsaponin I. Feller et al, *Planta Medica* 2010 76:16 1847-51.

Matthew Wood puts it well. "Thus, it balances the inflammatory suppressant side of the adrenal cortex associated with high cortisone (high blood sugar, digestive heat, impotence) and on the other it controls excessive immune reaction associated with high aldosterone and androgens (hyperactivity, allergies, asthma, gum disease, food allergies, inflammatory and degenerative arthritis, skin eruptions)."

By blocking cell receptors for androgen, it may be effective in preventing or treating prostate cancer.

The seeds increased splenocyte proliferation, decreased Th1 cytokines, increased Th2 cytokines, decreased macrophage inflammation, and increased NK (natural killer) cytotoxicity. *Journal of Ethnopharmacology* 131:2.

The seeds reduce toxicity of drugs used to treat pancreatic cancer, and increase tumor inhibition by 60-80% according to article in *Cancer Research*.

Cervical cancer cells are killed by powdered seeds, in work published in *Cancer Cell International*.

Work by Meddah et al, *J Ethnopharm* 121:3 found water extracts of the seed inhibit intestinal absorption of glucose.

Khan et al, *Hamdard Medicus* 1998 41:3 found female patients with urinary tract infection had decreased pus cells in urine after taking *N. sativa* seeds.

Ethanol extracts appear to lower calcium oxalate levels and reduce their deposition, suggesting benefit in treating kidney stones. Hadjzadeh et al, *Urol Journal* 2007 4:2.

The same study found that men with normal blood pressure, showed decreased systolic and diastolic readings after taking the seed. Systolic pressure was depressed after one hour and continued for four hours.

Diastolic was significantly depressed for two hours from ingestion onwards.

This may be due, in part, to thymoquinone that decreases heart rate.

A two-month randomized, double-blind, placebo-controlled trial found seed extract lowered systolic and diastolic blood pressure in hypertensive subjects and decreased LDL cholesterol. Dehkodri et al, *Fundament Clin Pharmacol* 2008 22:4.

Work by Kocyigit et al, *Saudi Med J* 2009 30:7 found seeds supplemented in diet increased good HDL and lowered LDL cholesterol and triglyceride levels.

A study of 123 patients taking nigella seed found serum lipid levels, blood sugar and pressure and obesity favorable over placebo. The small sample size did not make the difference statistically significant. Qidwa et al, *J Altern Complem Medicine* 2009 15:6.

Work by Leong et al, *Evid Based Compl Altern Med* 2013:20732 confirmed lowering of blood pressure and cholesterol in a human study.

A randomized, placebo-controlled trial of hyperlipidemic menopausal women showed a significant improvement in lipid profiles after two months. Ibrahim RM et al, *J Transl Med* 2014 12:1 82; *Adv Pharm Bull* 2014 4:1 29-33.

Parvadeh et al, *J Med Plants* 5 found thymoquinone as effective as anti-seizure compounds due to activity on benzodiazapine receptors.

Akhondian et al, *Med Sci Monit* 2007 13:12 found water extraction from seeds exhibit anti-epileptic activity in children with refractory seizures, in a double-blind, crossover study involving 23 patients.

Sayeed MSB et al, *J Ethnopharm* 148 780-6 conducted a study on memory, attention span and cognition in 40 elderly volunteers, and found significant benefit in nine week trial.

The seeds modulate mood, anxiety and cognition in healthy adolescent males in a four week trial, compared to placebo. Bin Sayeed MS et al, *J Ethnopharm* 2014 152:1 156-62.

Animal studies suggest it may be useful in treating multiple sclerosis.

The seed shows activity against *Helicobacter pylori*, associated with peptic and duodenal ulcers. Salem et al, *Saudi J Gastroenterol* 2010 16:3.

A review of the seed's medicinal properties, from 1960 to 1998, was published by Khan et al, *Inflammopharm* 1999 7:1.

Both the root and shoots contain vanillic acid, the former more anti-mutagenic and the latter more anti-oxidant in nature. Bourger et al, *CR Biol* 2008 331:1.

One mouse study by Vahdati-Mashhadian et al, *Pharmazie* 60:7 found water extracts toxic to liver cells. Do not feed your pet mice seed water until further useless studies are conducted.

The seeds of *N. damascena* possess analgesic and diuretic activity. Work by Agradi et al, *Phyto Res* 16:5 found seeds possess low estrogenic influence.

Work by Toma et al, *Rev Med Chir Soc Med Nat Instit* 111:1 found seed and leaf extracts active against *Leishmania promastigotes*. They may be a natural alternative to pentamidine and amphotericin B.

The seed is used in treatment of fevers and inflammation, to regulate menstruation and to expel tapeworms.

The compound damascenine lowers body temperature and reduces inflammation.

Love in a Mist is used in the commercial production of a hypertensive pharmaceutical.

HOMEOPATHY

Nigella sativa symptoms include nervousness, anxious fearful-ness, fear of death, discouragement, tendency to start and out of humor. The voice is anxious, hurried and interrupted.

Violent, darting stitches in occiput and vertex. Intolerable pressure and digging in frontal eminences. Cutting in the middle of brain, with continual throbbing. Dullness of eyes with frequent obscuration of sight. Twitching of right upper eyelid. Tip of nose cold as ice, dryness of nose, face pale and bluish with pale lips. Scanty urine, soreness in vagina, with heat and dryness. Violent tearing pain in back. Legs feel paralyzed.

DOSE- 6x potency. Ruckert reported three cases cured with this potency. All cases concern inflammatory conditions brought on by cold. It was given after inflammatory symptoms were subdued by Aconitum.

ESSENTIAL OIL

CONSTITUENTS- *N. sativa* seed- 0.5 to 1.5% consisting of 15% p-cymene, 20% trans-anethole, alpha thujene, alpha and beta pinenes, sabines, sabinen hydrates, thymol, carvacrol, 1,8 cineol, borneol, carvone (4%), d-limonene (4.3%), linalool, nigellone semohiprepinon, thymochinon, thymoquinone 37%, (+) citronellol, *N. damascena* seed- damascenine (8-10%), sesquiterpenes including beta elemene 59%, beta (12.8%) and alpha selinene (12%), beta caryophyllene and alpha humulene, as well as methoxy anthranylate of methyl esters 30% and 47 other compounds.

The essential oil of black cumin decreases blood pressure and increases respiration. It is used topically for hemorrhoids and skin conditions such as eczema and infections, diluted of course.

Chowdhury et al, *Phytotherapy Research* 1998 found essential oil of *N. sativa* exhibited activity against various drug-resistant strains of *Shigella in vitro.*

Synergistic activity with streptomycin and gentamicin. Ferdous et al, *Phytotherapy Research* 1992 6:137.

Various bacterial and fungal conditions, including *Candida albicans* overgrowth, are inhibited by the volatile oils. Dental plaque is prevented.

Staphylococcus aureus, Vibrio cholerae, Streptococcus pyogenes and *S. viridans* are most susceptible, with *in vitro* studies indicating activity comparable to ampicillin. The essential oil inhibits *Bacillus subtilis, B. anthracis, B. pumilis, Staphylococcus luteus, E. coli, Salmonella typhi,* and *Pseudomonas aeruginosa.*

Methicillin and drug resistant strains of *S. aureus* and *P. aeruginosa* succumb to essential oil. Salman et al, *Nat Prod Rad* 2008 7:1.

The oil inhibits various fungi, including *Candida albicans, Aspergillus niger, A. flavus, M. gypseum, Trichoderma viride* and *Curvularia lunata.*

In vivo activity against *S. flexneri*; fully curing infected monkeys within three days.

Nigellone semohiprepinon, when inhaled or rubbed on chest, enlarges the bronchi, reduces cramps and raises the temperature, to quickly alleviate bronchial asthma, whooping cough.

Nigellone inhibits release of histamine from mast cells. Thymochinon inhibits infection, is anodyne, anti-oxidant and stimulates gall bladder function.

Aqel and Shaheen, *Journal of Ethnopharmacology* May 1996 tested the effects of black cumin essential oil on uterine tissue. Their results suggest anti-oxytocic potential.

Badary et al, *Drug Development Research* 1998 44:2-3 showed thymoquinone induced significant decreases in fasting plasma glucose concentration.

Thymoquinone is very potent, with approximate IC50 values against 5-lipoxygenase and cyclooxygenase of <1 and 3.5 ug/ml, respectively.

Thymoquinone possesses hepato-protective activity. Daba et al, *Tox Letters* 1998 95:1.

The essential is active against Jurkat T-cell leukemia cells, *in vitro. Int Journal Pharmacognosy* 1995 33.

The essential oil suppressed cancer cell proliferation in colon mucosa. Salim and Fukushima, *Nutr Cancer* 2003 45:2.

Administration of the essential oils into tumor sites inhibits liver metastasis development and improved mice survival. Ait et al, *Braz J Med Biol Res* 2007 40:6.

Thymoquinone, and alpha pinene affect benzodiazepine receptors associated with anti-anxiety. Raza et al, *J Herb Spice Med Plant* 12:1-2.

Oral ingestion increases levels of 5-HT and tryptophan in both blood plasma and brain, suggesting a mechanism for reduced anxiety.

Toxicology testing on mice, at significant doses for up to ninety days showed no signs of toxicity. Acute oral administration gave an LD50 of 2.4 g/kg.

Water stress increases the content of both seed and essential oil. Water stress produced by irrigating every 12th day increases thymoquinone content.

The seeds of *N. damascena* are distilled to produce an essential oil of quite unique and interesting aromatic potential.

This oil is not medicinal, like its more famous cousin, but mostly used for the perfume and cosmetic industry. Elemenes are the most abundant volatiles (22-29%), as well as up to 30% methyl-3-methoxy-N-methyl anthanilate. Beta elemene and beta selinine make up nearly 70% of composition.

The oil is yellowish and intensely sweet and fruity with a somewhat unpleasant odour when first distilled. This dissipates rather quickly, and on blotter paper shows a great tenacity, and very pleasant wine or brandy-like character similar to ambrette seed oil.

The citrus, peach-like notes have been compared to the scent of wild strawberries. Sweet and fruity, the oil must be used in small amounts 0.2-0.5% to avoid a perfumery scent.

The oil, when diluted, has a blue fluorescence due to content of damascenine.

Butanol extracts show activity against *Staphylococcus aureus* and *Pseudomonas aeruginosa. Phyto Res* 18:6

The oil cannot be used in food flavour work, as it loses its flavour in an acid medium, and grape and peach are usually presented as acidic flavors.

However, the oil can be used in lipsticks as well as fruity and floral perfumes, combining well with gardenia, jasmine, bergamot, neroli, etc.

It has a few medicinal applications, especially as a powerful anti-histamine and anti-allergenic for treating bronchial asthma. Its cousin is a better medicinal, however.

SEED OIL

CONSTITUENTS- *N. sativa-* thymoquinone, 23-49% oleic, 38-55% linoleic, 12% palmitic and 2% linolenic acid; Total sterol content is 0.51% consisting of 63% beta sitosterol, 17% stigmasterol, and 15% campesterol.
N. damascena- linoleic acid (43-50%), oleic (14-23%), stearic (15-23%), and palmitic (10-12%) acids. Beta elemene is 73.2% of oils.

The fixed oil of *Nigella sativa*, like essential oil, contains thymoquinone, a potent anti-inflammatory and anti-oxidant constituent. It contains an unusual C20:2 unsaturated fatty acid that may play a role in these functions.

One of black cumin's strengths is anti-allergenic and anti-histamine activity. One study from Munich on 600 allergy patients found that 500 mg of black cumin oil twice a day for three months showed clear improvement in 85% of patients.

Seed oil was compared with control in 84 patients with asthma wheeze. Statistically significant difference was found by day three in a 14 day study. Ahmad et al, *Afr J Pharm Pharmacol* 2009 3:5.

The fixed oil obtained from the seeds should be processed with the same care afforded organic flax and hemp seeds oils in this country. One of the great disadvantages at the present time is uncertainty of oil products from Middle East and Egypt. The seeds do produce from 30-35% oil, with over 60% linoleic acid.

Small amounts, up to 10% of the fixed oil, may be added to other carrier oils, for conditions related to inflammation, such as arthritis, bursitis, and other conditions both acute and chronic. The seed oil is used externally for abscesses, hemorrhoids and orchitis.

A randomized PC, DB clinical trial of infertile males found the intake of 2.5 ml daily improved abnormal semen quality without adverse effects. Kolahdooz M et al, *Phytomedicine* 2014 March 25.

The seed oil combined with exercise in sedentary overweight females for eight weeks showed improved lipid profiles. Farzaneh E et al, *Int J Prev Med* 2014 5:2 210-6.

The fixed oil and unsaponified portions show anti-fungal activity against *Fusarium solani, F. moniliforme, Helminthosporium turcicum, H. oryzae, Alternaria helianthi, Colletotrichum capsici* and *Pyricularia setariae.*

Recent work by Enomoto et al, *Biological and Pharmaceutical Bulletin* 2001 24:3 found methanol soluble portions of the fixed oil show inhibitory effect on arachadonic acid- induced platelet aggregation and blood coagulation. In a randomized, DB PC trial of 70 volunteers, the seed oil (5ml daily) lowered systolic and diastolic blood pressure without side effects. Fallah Huseini H et al, *Phytother Res* 2013 27(12): 1849-53.

Compounds in the oil possessing aromatic hydroxyl and acetoxyl groups had more potent activity than aspirin as anti-thrombotic agent.

A study at the Amala Nagar Cancer Research Centre found evidence that long chain fatty acid in oil has potent anti-tumour activity. Salomi et al, *Cancer Letters* 1992 63:41.

The fixed oil has been shown to prevent chronic cyclosporine nephrotoxicity. Uz et al, *Am J Nephrol* 2008 28:3.

The seed oil appears to alleviate the deleterious effects of highly active anti-retroviral drugs, reducing insulin-resistance by stabilizing beta cells and insulin activity at periphery of body. Chandra et al, *Can J Physio Pharmacol* 2009 87:4.

Thymoquinone reduces release of inflammatory mediators in pancreatic cancer cells. Arafat et al, *Am Assoc Cancer Research* Denver April 2009.

Previous studies found nigella possesses anti-cancer effects on prostate and colon cancers. Afarat and colleagues compared thymoquinone, with trichostatin A, an HDAC inhibitor that has been shown to ameliorate inflammatory-associated cancers.

Seed oil reduces viability of human lung cancer cell lines. Al-Sheddi ES et al, *Asian Pac Journal Cancer Prev* 2014 15:2 983-7.

Inhibition of NFkappaB was noted. When animal models with pancreatic cancer were treated with thymoquinone, tumors shrank 67% and pro-inflammatory cytokines were reduced.

FLOWER ESSENCES

Love in a Mist (*N. damascena*) flower essence assists in allowing free association of thoughts, feelings and ideas. It can be very useful in hypnosis or other trance work. For individuals who have difficulty with the Air elements, this essence helps one to achieve oneness with one's soul family.   **PEGASUS**

Love in a Mist flower essence helps purify the aura, clarifies issues of etheric and auric boundaries, clearing out distracting energies. Use it as a ritual ablution or cleansing before prayer; it sets the intention of purity.   **HUMMINGBIRD**

Love in a Mist, a very gentle flower essence, works on the strands between the heart chakra and other, smaller charkas of the body and encourages you to be both strong and courageous. A physical cleanser, Love in a Mist also clarifies your emotional motivations, helping to ease frustrations and allow clear choices to be made.   **OLIVE**

ASTROLOGY

The flowers of the love-in-a-mist are surrounded by a group of pinnate leaves, so that they are hardly noticeable. Their petals are pointed as though in an intermediate form between the simple leaf and the sepal; they are like an early stage of the metamorphosis ending in the perfect petal…the development of the flowers is deeply rooted in the vegetative processes. Even the green stamens remind us of vegetative life…in the love-in-a-mist, the carpels grow together into one common ovary. A very strong influence from the moon manifests itself in this organ, which isolates itself uniformly from its surroundings and dominates the entire flower.   **KRANICH**

SPIRITUAL PROPERTIES

The flower spirit of Nigella, also known as Love-in-a-Mist, reminds you to pause and breathe. Close your eyes and slowly fill your lungs with cool, blue celestial light. Imagine the soft, hazy blue of the Nigella flower flowing into the crown of your head from above, filling first your stomach and then your lungs.   **ECLARE**

PERSONALITY TRAITS

Love-in-a-mist, *Nigella damascena*, is one of the frothiest of plants. Mingling into surrounding greenery, it makes the planting float. Its relatively large flowers add to the impression as they hover above the fuzzy leaves.   **CAROL KLEIN**

RECIPES

GROUND SEED- Two grams daily for up to four weeks to improve immune system.

Do not use *N. sativa*, in any form, during pregnancy.

TINCTURE- Make a 1:5 tincture with freshly ground black cumin seeds in 60% alcohol. Use 10-30 drops as needed.

NODDING ONION
HOOKER'S ONION
LADY'S LEEK
(*Allium cernuum* Roth.)
(*A. recurvatum* Rydb.)
PRAIRIE ONION
(*A. textile* Nels. & Macbr.)
(*A. aridum*)
GEYER'S ONION
(*A. geyerii* S. Wats.)
WELSH ONION
JAPANESE BUNCHING ONION
CIBOULE
SPRING ONION
(*A. fistulosum* L.)
SHALLOT
(*A. ascalonicum* Hort.)
(*A. cepa* var. *aggregatum*)
CULTIVATED ONION
RED ONION
GREEN ONION
SCALLION
(*A. cepa* L.)
GARLIC
(*A. sativum* L.)
GARLIC CHIVES
CHINESE CHIVES
ASIAN LEEK
(*A. tuberosum* Rottler ex Spreng.)
(*A. uliginosum* G. Don)
WILD CHIVES
CULTIVATED CHIVES
RUSH LEEK
(*A. schoenoprasum* L.)
(*A. tenufolium*)
SIBERIAN CHIVES
(*A. schoenoprasum ssp. sibiricum* [L.] Hartman)

(*A. sibiricum*)
ELEPHANT GARLIC
(*A. ampeloprasum* L.)
LEEK
(*A. porrum* L.)
EGYPTIAN ONION
WALKING ONION
CATAWISSA ONION
(*A. cepa var. proliferum*)
(*A. x proliferum*)
(*A. cepa var. viviparum*)
RAMPS
(*A. tricoccum* Ait.)
PARTS USED- bulbs, seeds

Mine eyes smell Onions;
I shall weep anon.   **SHAKESPEARE**

He who bears chives on his breath
Is safe from being kissed to death.
                      MARCUS V MARTIALIS 100 AD

"The onion and its satin wrappings is among the most beautiful of
vegetables, and is the only one that represents the essence of things. It
can almost be said to have a soul.   **C. D. WARNER 1870**

An Onion a day keeps arteriosclerosis at bay.
                              DR VICTOR GUREWICH

Life is like an onion; you peel it off one layer at a time, and sometimes
you weep.   **CARL SANDBURG**

An onion can make people cry, but there's never been a vegetable that
can make them laugh.   **WILL ROGERS**

Eat Leeks in March and Ramsons in May,
Then all the year after physicians can play.   **OLD ENGLISH**

I stand erect and tall, well-rooted
I stand proud in bed
I am hairy below, sometimes the fair peasant's daughter grips my body
and holds me hard…
I will bring tears to her eyes.   **ANGLO SAXON RIDDLE 1066 AD**

Onion is derived from the Latin, **UNUS**, meaning the numeral one. This evolved into **UNIO**, or **UNIONIS**, meaning a unity, one large pearl, or a oneness of note; and then into the French **OIGNON**.

In 42 AD, Columella introduced the word **UNIONEM**.

It was called **YN-LEAC** in Saxon, and oinnum, onyoun and onyoun in 10th century leech books.

Allium is from the Greek meaning Garlic. This, in turn is related to the Celtic **ALL**, (hot, pungent or burning), and the French **AIL**, and Italian **AGLIO**. Cernuum means nodding, in reference to the slant of the flower stem.

Cernua means a shepherd's crook, and refers to the manner in which the flowers gently bend over like the top of a cane.

Geyerii is named after the botanist, Carl Geyer, who identified it in Washington State in 1844.

Cepa is from **CEP**, a head, referring to the bunched florets. One Chinese name for Onion is "jewel among vegetables".

Caepula was the Roman name for onion. From Cepa came the French **CIVE**, and hence Chive. Schoenoprasum is from the Greek **SCHOINOS**, meaning rush or reed, and **PRASON**, for leek; hence Rush Leek.

Garlic is from the Anglo-Saxon **GAR-LEAC** or Spear Plant.

Welsh Onion has nothing to do with Wales, but is derived from the German, **WELSCHE**, meaning foreign.

Scallion is from the Late Latin **SCALONIA**, the same root as Shallots, which take their botanical name from the city of Ashkelon in Palestine, or less likely, from the French name Echalogne.

The Emperor Nero was contemptuously nicknamed Porrophagus, or leek eater, for his use of the vegetable to improve his singing voice. The Romans called them Porrum, and the Greeks, Prasa. Leek is corrupted from the Anglo Saxon **PORLEAC**.

Nodding Onion is found in dry, open areas on the plains and into the foothills, from Alberta down to New Mexico.

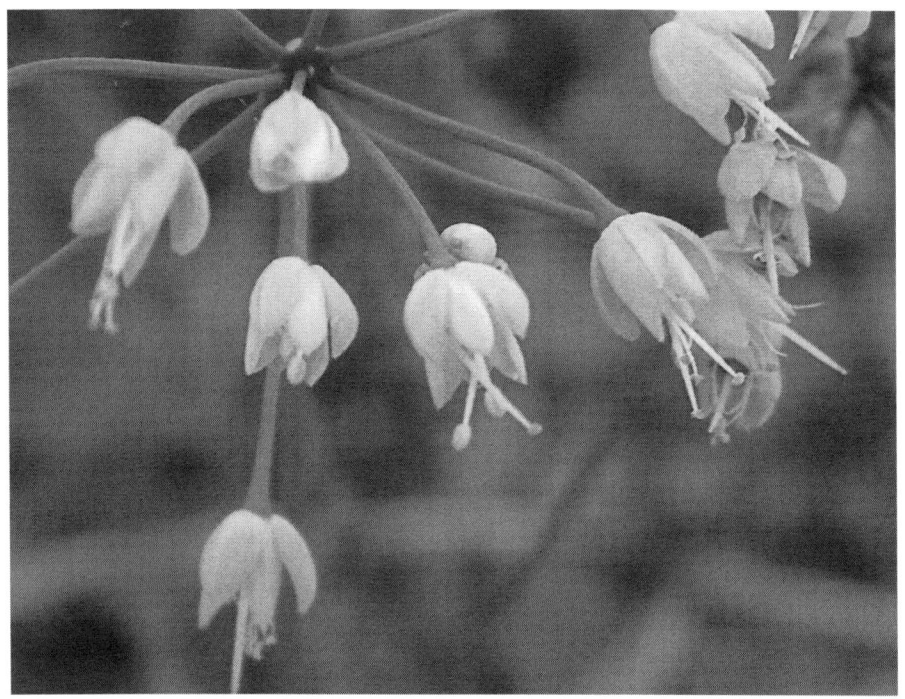
Nodding onion

The bulb is edible and can be eaten raw, baked, boiled, or dried for use in winter.

The cooking removes some of the strong smell and flavour, and converts the carbohydrate inulin into the more digestible, and sweeter fructose.

Native tribes harvested the bulbs and leaves before flowering, for steaming pits, or boiled or roasted in stews. They were bundled or woven together, and used to flavour meat or fish, or improve the blandness of Black Tree Lichen.

After cooking, they can be eaten immediately, or dried, and pressed into thin cakes for winter.

Because Nodding Onion, Geyer's Onion and other onions resemble and grow in areas of Mountain Death Camas, you must be certain of identification. One of these is that Death Camas does not smell like an onion.

The Northern Cree call it Stinking Grass, or **WECHEKASKOSE**. Other Cree call both Nodding and Prairie Onion, and even Wild Chives by the same name or **PIKWACIWICIKASKOSI**.

The Cheyenne call it **KHA-A-MOT-OT-KEWAT**, or "Skunk Testicles". The Chipewyan call the wild onion, **TLH' OGH TS IAZE**, meaning "little beaver grass". The Blackfoot call it **PIS SATS'E MI KIM**, or **PESAT SE NEKIM**. They used the entire plant as a sore throat remedy, and the whole plant with flower as a tea for abdominal pain. An alternate name is **SAOKIIPISATSIINIKIMM**.

The neighboring Blood tribe used the nodding onion as a nasal decongestant, to treat a swollen penis in an unspecified manner, and decocted the dried plant for pains in the waist area. They refer to the plant as Prairie Funny Vine, according to Joan Kerik, who compiled Living with the Land.

The Gitxsan of British Columbia call it **TS'ANKSA GAAK**, meaning roughly "raven's underarm odour" or "armpit".

Prairie Onion, which is more common and used in a similar manner, is often called Wild Garlic, due to stronger garlic flavour. Nodding onion is much milder.

Geyer's Onion has tiny pink flowers that point upwards, and form tiny bulbs that form the next year's seed.

Wild Chives are a hardy perennial, originally from Siberia, that spread to Alaska and eventually everywhere.

When Alexander the Great, 300 BC married Princess Roxana, the Siberians sent Wild Chives as a wedding gift. This was considered appropriate due to its reputation as an aphrodisiac. Romanian gypsies use chives in their fortune telling rituals.

Wild Chives are added to boiled fish for flavour by the Woods Cree of Saskatchewan. They sometimes call it **PIKWACIWICKASKOSI**, the same name as Nodding or Prairie Onion.

Wild Chives are boiled down to thick syrup for coughs and colds.

The dried bulbs were burned traditionally in smudges to fumigate patients, or the dried powder was inhaled as a snuff for congested sinuses.

Wild Chives were crushed and soaked in water overnight. This was taken on an empty stomach by patients suffering from worms and parasites.

You can make tasty and beautiful pink vinegar from chive flowers. Or pick off the petals, and put them into potato salad, green salad, soups, and marinated vegetable dishes.

In Norway, the leaves were salted and stored in wooden barrels during the winter. Today, they are still collected and used in fish and meat dishes.

In Newfoundland, wild chives are sometimes known as Chibbles.

In Japan, there are two recognized varieties of Wild Chive. The "orientale" form is known as **SHIROUMA-ASATSUKI**; and "yezomonticola" is called **HIME-EZO-NEGI**.

Chives make a good companion plant for carrot, as they deter the carrot root fly. Made into a tea, the herb is especially useful against the gray mold that affects roses, and good companions to tomatoes. The same cooled liquid is also used for gooseberry mildew and apple scab. Chives are said to inhibit the growth of beans and peas, however.

Cultivated Chives are easy to grow inside as a winter kitchen herb. The root bulbs should be dug up, divided and replanted every three years; about six bulbs to a cluster. Chives make a nice addition to sour cream for potatoes, with fresh tomatoes in salads, or in soups and egg omelet. The secret to chives is never to cook them, but to add at the last minute. Chives have been found to hyper-accumulate cadmium, in work by Khadka et al in Israel.

Most chives bloom in the spring, with purple blossoms, while Chinese Chives bloom in the fall with white blossoms. Also known as Lazy Fellow's vegetable, it is a favourite kitchen vegetable in Chinese cuisine.

Chinese Chive (*A. tuberosum*) seed oil is used in China and the Philippines for flavouring foods like fish. The leaves have been used in TCM for treating abdominal pain, diarrhea, hematemesis, snakebite and asthma, while the seeds are used as a tonic and aphrodisiac.

The herb goes by several names including Flat Vegetable **(BAIN CAI)** and Rising Sun Grass **(QI YANG CAO), GOW CHOY**, and **JIOU CAI**. A yellow, blanched cultivar, even more tender and delicious, is grown in the dark and known as **JIOU HWANG**.

The star shaped white flowers smell like roses, and are often planted on kitchen windowsills. The leaves are more garlicy than onion.

Chinese herbals suggest this species as an antidote for poison and to control excessive bleeding.

The Japanese call it **NIRA**.

In Ayurvedic medicine, the onion is said to balance both Vata and Kapha, but may moderately aggravate Pita.

Onions have been eaten for more than 6000 years by humans as a universal flavouring and medicinal agent.

The Onion motif is a symbol of growth and evolution and the shape is found on Egyptian pillars, East Indian and Chinese ornaments, Arabic frescoes, Byzantine domes, and Greek Orthodox Church steeples.

Ancient Egyptians used onions in mummification, one or two placed in the thorax or pelvis, or in the ear or near the eyes. It is said that during the building of the pyramids, nine tons of gold were spent to buy onions for the workers.

Another author states that the Giant Pyramid of Cheops built around 3700 BC, contains an inscription that 1600 talents of silver ($3.5 million) were paid out to provide workers with onions, garlic and radishes.

Egyptians saw onions as symbols of the universe, as their cosmogony saw the spheres of earth, heaven and hell as concentric, like the layers of an onion. It was also an emblem of the moon as the various phases were seen when the bulb was cut. Thus it was dedicated to Isis, the goddess of the moon. Oaths of office were sworn over an onion in ancient Egypt.

The importance of Onions in our day-to- day lives was brought home recently with reports of onion riots in India. Residents of Turkey are the biggest consumers in the world with a per capita annual use of 36 kilograms. Jainism, a religious sect of India, eat no onions.

The largest onion in the Guinness Book of World Records was grown in England, and weighed in at 4.9 kilograms.

For protection in the home, take a small white onion and stick it full of black- headed pins and place in a window. The flowers can be dried and placed in the home as a protective amulet.

Onion skins should never be thrown onto the ground, but burned in a fire to attract riches. A large red onion tied to the bedpost was believed to protect from sickness. The relationship of onions and protection from evil forces may originate in the name **HEDJW**, for onion, and its being punned with **HEDJET** meaning damage, as in to evil forces.

To dream of peeling onions suggests domestic strife and illness, but to dream of eating them suggests finding treasure.

A Muslim legend says that when Satan left the Garden of Eden after the fall, garlic sprang from his left footstep, and onion from his right.

The Perfumed Garden, a 16th century book mentions that the hero's member, after eating onions, stayed erect for 30 un-interrupted days.

Lewis and Clark, on their famous expedition in 1805, related the following story about an island on the upper Missouri: "Here were found great quantities of a small onion about the size of a musket-ball, though some were larger; it is white, crisp and as well flavored as any of our garden onions; the seed is just ripening, and as the plant bears a large quantity to the square foot, and stands the vigors of the climate, it will no doubt be an acquisition to settlers. From this production we called it 'Onion Island'."

Early settlers used onions to help preserve bacon and other fat on long trips. Without knowing it, they were taking advantage of quercitin, or flavone polyphenols, and their lipid stabilizing property. More recent work indicates that adding an onion, when cooking ground beef, helps reduce the mutagenicity associated with the meat. Kato et al, 1998.

Some authors believe that Chicago is derived from the native **CHECAGOU**, which refers to the pungent smell of onions (*A. cernuum*), or ramps (*A. tricoccum*) growing wild along the south shore of Lake Michigan.

The Menomini of the Great Lakes called wild leek **SKAKU** meaning skunk, and **SKIKA'KO'** was skunk place.

Others say this was a fraudulent translation by the French explorer Marquette, as the Chippewa word for wild leek is **SHE GAU GAWINSHE**.

While full of flavour, these small native onions never grow to any great size.

Green onions are believed to be immature *A. cepa* by most authors. One farmer in Ohio is the Green Onion King, growing over 96 million on only 100 acres in a single season.

As mentioned, the seeds are numerous, and can be collected for transplant, or to sprout in the middle of winter.

An old folk remedy for dissolving kidney stones involves burning onion in a fire to a white ash. One teaspoon was taken in white wine morning and evening.

Commercial onion growers can take advantage of a discovery by R. Vernon of the Ag Research Station in Vancouver. Vernon found that the adult flies of onion maggots fly at less than four feet, so that most could be prevented from reaching plants by a simple nylon window screen fence, three feet high, with the top edge bent outwards.

China is the largest grower of onions, producing ten million tons in 1998. Full of heavy metals!

Onion juice makes a perfect invisible ink that magically appears on paper after exposure to a fire or clothing iron.

Decoctions of dry onions are gargled by conjurers that place fire and lit candles in their mouth.

Research from India and Russia, indicates that onions may also create electrical fields with healing energy.

Dr. S. S. Nehru, president of *Agriculture in India Science Congress* isolated mashed onion in cellophane and quartz containers so no actual contact with human skin occurred. He found treatment of inflamed throat and sinuses still happened but were blocked when the onions were put into lead, iron, glass or aluminum containers. This indicates that some unusual electrical energy rays are at work.

Dr. Gurwitsch, an electrobiologist from Russia, also investigated this unusual property of onions. He found they emit a form of ultraviolet radiation he termed "mitogenetic". He found that pointing the growing end of an onion toward another began cell division in three hours.

When quartz crystal was placed between it still occurred, but stopped when glass was used, as it does not transmit ultraviolet light.

He found that this energy appears to stimulate general cell activity and produce rejuvenating effect. This same energy has been observed in garlic, ginseng and penicillin; and although dismissed by some scientists, the observed effects have never been fully explained.

Dr. Fritz Popp, a German biophysicist, is a proponent of his work and calls it biophotons. This light carries intelligence and may be the foundation of why plants and humans can communicate with each other.

Garlic is a well-known vegetable. Long term use for prevention of atherosclerosis, as well as stomach and intestinal cancer is well-known. Organic garlic is highly recommended, due to the flood of cheap Chinese garlic contaminated with heavy metals. The fatty oils in garlic bulbs allow for increased metal absorption of lead, mercury and other undesirable contaminants.

Over 3000 scientific papers on activity of garlic have been published. Traditional usage for coughs, colds, rhinitis and sinusitis are not supported by clinical trials, but are effective. Many of the attributes of onion listed below apply as well to garlic, the more powerful cousin.

Two compounds in garlic need to react in order to produce an effective medicinal product. Crushing the clove and waiting ten minutes will accomplish this, and then use fresh, infused or make a tincture.

Shallots are mild aromatic bulbs that grow in clusters of two to six, like garlic.

The green tops are sometimes harvested in early summer and sold as scallions (hence the confusion with names), and the dried bulbs harvested in fall like onions.

Shallots are hardy, mature rapidly, and are good for cold climates. I prefer them to onions for some recipes!

Pliny, the Elder described six different types of onions with therapeutic value, and indicated that shallot was the most important one.

In the 9th century, shallots were one of the 18 herbs grown in the Monastery Gardens of St. Gall in Switzerland; in its time one of the great centers of civilization.

They probably came to the New World by De Soto to Louisiana. French Huguenots were growing them in North Carolina around 1710.

Shallots are considered essential to fine French cuisine, as they are neither onions nor garlic, and their mildness makes them perfect for delicate sauces as they emulsify more easily than onions.

Shallots are sweeter, milder and more subtle than other onions. They are indispensable for Bernaise sauce, cooking down to a thick, creamy consistency.

The red-brown skins are used to dye Easter eggs.

Japanese bunching onion, or Welsh onion (*A. fistulosum*) is actually native to Siberia, not Wales.

Welsh is a corruption of the German **WELSCHE**, meaning foreign, and comes from the introduction of the onion into Europe towards the end of the Middle Ages. It is descended from *A. altaicum*, a wild plant from eastern Kazakhstan.

The plant is known as **CHANG FA** in China, and **NEBUKA** or **NEGI** in Japan. The seed is known as **CONG SHI**, and widely used in older texts, but rarely in modern prescriptions.

Welsh Onion or Ciboule growing naturally is said to be a geo-botanical sign of precious metals.

About 800 AD, Tuan Ch'eng-Shih wrote, "when in the mountains there is a ciboule onion, then below silver will be found. When...there is Hsiai (a type of shallot), then below gold will be found."

Elephant Garlic is a giant, milder version of regular garlic. It cannot tolerate very cold winter temperatures, but requires fall planting to mature fully. Elephant Garlic is included for general interest, but has no real commercial future on the Canadian prairies.

The Romans brought leeks to Britain, via Egypt. They are frost hardy, and well adapted to northern climates, but require transplantation in our short season.

The Romans believed it prolific of virtue, because Latona, mother of Apollo, longed after leeks.

Ancient Greek translators used the word **PRASIA** for leek bed, literally meaning garden plot. The ancient Egyptian name for leek also means "vegetables" in general.

Leek is the national emblem of Wales, to commemorate victory over the Saxon invaders by St. David, the patron saint of Wales, in the sixth century; or that the Welsh soldiers wore leeks to distinguish themselves from the enemy.

On St. David's Day (March 1), the Welsh will wear the leek in their hats.

There is a legend that St. David lived on leeks and water during his retirement in the Vale of Ewias.

It is now believed that no such person existed, and his "life" was composed of an 11th century bishop of St. David's, to canonize Dewi, the sea spirit that also became the Red Dragon of Wales.

The European community produces over 7 million tonnes annually to meet demand. It grows well with celery

In Traditional Chinese Medicine, the leek is known as **SUAN**, and used for its warm and acrid taste.

Leeks are often recommended for expectant mothers, supplying a wealth of nutrients to the growing fetus.

Egyptian Onion is a hardy perennial and was one of my first transplants when I lived near Lesser Slave Lake in the early 1970s. It has been recently found to be a hybrid between *A. cepa* and *A. fistulosum,* but has been noted in Europe since the 16th century.

It is unusual, in that it develops little bulblets, or bulbils that grow to the size of hazelnuts or larger. They may start sprouting and can be removed and planted to increase your production. The weight of the bulblets, if left unattended, find their way to the ground and do the job for you. They are one of the first fresh greens of spring.

In the US, they are called walking onion due to their unusual habit. In Japan, it is known as Kitsune Negi, meaning foxy or mysterious onion.

Ramps are delicious but endangered wild plant in Canada. Some parts of the continent celebrate Ramp Festivals, in areas of plenty.

MEDICINAL

CONSTITUENTS- *A. cernuum*-sugars, Vitamins A, B and C, minerals, adenosine, organic acids, propenethial-s-oxide, and enzymes. Diosgenin, a steroid is also present 0.3-0.5% in flowers, and 0.1-0.2% in roots.

A. cepa bulb- alliins (alkylcysteine sulphoxides): in particular allyl alliin and its gamma-glutamyl conjugates that in the course of cutting are transformed into so-called alliaceous oils; allithiamines (benfotiamine), disulphides, trisulphides, zwiebelanes, methylalliin, proplylalliin, fructans (35-40% dry wt), saccharose, saponins (0.095%) sterols, fatty acids, vitamins, prostaglandins, flavonoids including four cyanidin bssed anthocyanins; pectin and other sugars. Bulb contains 48,100 ppm of quercitin.

When crushed the cysteine sulphoxides contact allinase in adjacent cells forming the odorous thiosulphonates.

Red Onions are similar, and contain ascalonicosides, and tropeosides.

leaves- 8 querctin glucosides and 8 anthocyanins; 2.7% free sterols and sterol esters, 1.7% sterol glycosides, and 0.8% acetyl sterol glycosides.

skin- quercitin

A. fistulosum bulb- essential oil, allicin, allyl sulphide, pectin, malic/palmitic/stearic/arachidic/oleic/
linoleic acids, Vit A, thiamine, riboflavin, Vit C, Vit E (74.6 mg/kg), iron salts, S-(prop-1-enyl)-cystein-sulfoxide, cycolalliin; fistulosides (yuccagenin glycosides), two diosgenin glycosides, dioscin and saponin P-d.

A. tuberosum seed- essential oil, sulphates, gycosides, vit C.
leaf- N-p-coumaroyl tyramine, and bis (p-hydroxyphenyl) ether.

A. schoenoprasum- methyl alliin and pentyl alliin, as well as gamma-glutamyl conjugates. When cut, or the dried chives are re-wet, these compounds transform into alliaceous oils such as diakyl-disulphide-mono-S-oxides and diallyl-di and trisulphides. The fresh leaves contain 52 mg/100 grams of Vit C; and 0.2% phosphorous pentoxide.

A. ascalonicum- bulb- furostanol saponins called ascalonicosides; quercitin, isorhamnetin, and their glycosides.

Onions are diuretic, stimulating, expectorant, antiseptic, hypotensive, anti-spasmodic, and help reduce blood sugar levels. The juice is the most valued and combines well with honey, or carrot juice as a reliable cough syrup (see recipes below).

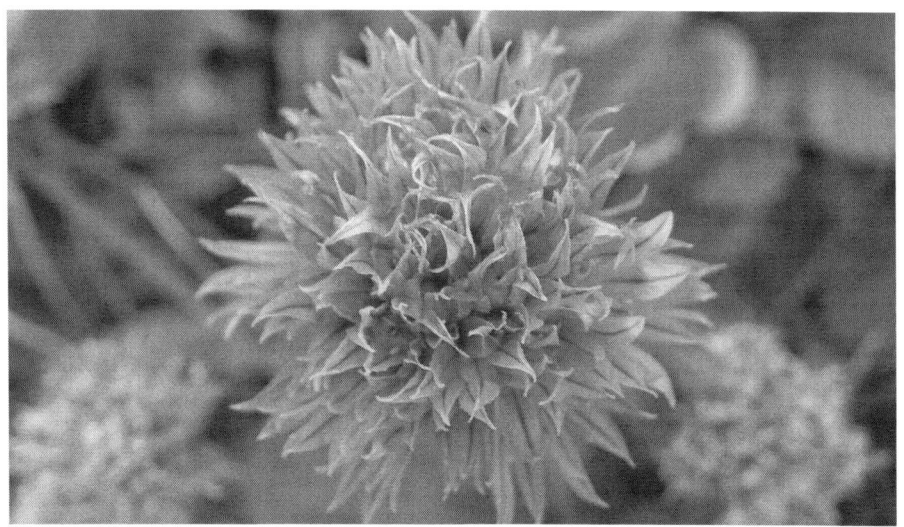
Chive flower

Onions have been used to relieve gas, eliminate worms, reduce edema or water retention, loosen sticky mucous associated with coughs and colds, control asthma, fight infections.

Externally, onions have been used for their antiseptic action in fighting fungal infections, warts, and earaches. For otitis, apply a roasted onion to the ear; while spastic neck tension responds better to a raw onion poultice. Corns and bunions find relief with a poultice of onions and vinegar, applied and changed three times daily.

Tincture of the red onion is a warming expectorant for chronic bronchitis or asthma, or a cold that is not feverish.

It's use for asthma was confirmed when scientists reported identifying a chemical in onions with moderate ability to prevent the chemical and biological steps that lead to inflammatory reactions. *Science News* June 16 1990; Dorsch et al, *European Journal of Pharmacology* 1985 107.

In one human trial, two 100 ml doses of onion alcohol extract suppressed both immediate and delayed asthmatic reaction in a female patient aggravated by dust mites. Dorsch, Wagner and Bayer, 1989.

The flavonoids quercetin and kaemperfol act as anti-inflammatory agents by inhibiting the activity of protein kinase, phospholipase A2, cyclooxygenase, and lipoxygenase, and the release of histamines from leukocytes.

Cepaenes are inhibitors of platelet aggregation probably by inhibition of the enzyme system cyclo-oxygenase responsible for formation of prostaglandins and prostacyclins.

Work by Corea et al, *J Ag Food Chem* 2005 53 found furostanol saponins responsible for the antispasmodic activity of Red Onions.

Onions can be mashed and applied to wounds and cuts, as well as swellings and contusions. The thin membrane that separates onion layers works as an antiseptic butterfly bandage.

Onion in rye will often relieve the phantom pain associated with amputated limbs(see below). In one clinical trial of 12 adults, topical application of a 45% ethanol extract inhibited allergic skin reactions.

Keloid tissue and recent scar tissue responds well to onion juice. In one study, a 0.5% water extract inhibited the growth of human fibroblasts and keloid fibroblasts.

Recent work by Hosnuter et al, *J Wound Care* 2007 16:6 found onion extracts helpful on hypertrophic and keloid scar tissue.

Fresh onion plant juice can be purchased commercially or made for oneself for increasing digestive juices, preventing fermentation and inhibiting the growth of harmful coliflora in the intestines.

In Russia, an alcohol extract of onion, called Allilchep is available in pharmacies, for treating flu, respiratory disease, nervous disorders, cancer, diabetes as well as skin and reproductive complaints. A saturated tincture of onion, made with good Holland gin, containing juniper berries, has been used traditionally for gravel and dropsy symptoms.

Onion juice is used as a diuretic and expectorant; to relieve cramps, strengthen the heart, and expel worms.

Onion juice was found, in a study by Serrame et al, to inhibit the development of liver tumours, but not skin tumours. *Philippine J of Science* 1995 124:3.

Kim et al, *Journal of the Pharmaceutical Society of Korea* 1994 38:5, looked at combining green onion (*A. cepa*) extract, with chitin derived from shellfish. The mixture was found to inhibit sarcoma 180 tumor growth by 52% in a dose dependent manner.

Work by Whanger et al, *J of Agric and Food Chem* 2000 48:11 looked at Ramps (*A. tricoccum*) grown in hydroponic and peat moss rich in sodium selenate. The bulbs concentrated organic selenium compounds up to 784 mg/kg; and when fed to chemical induced mammary tumoured mice, reduced them by 43% with no side effects. The organic selenium was found up to 28% more bio-available for regeneration of glutathione peroxidase activity than inorganic selenite.

Onions are active against viruses, as well as all the major bacteria including those responsible for peridonitis and dental caries. Even when highly diluted, onion is active against *Staphylococcus aureus*, *Brucella abortus*, *E. coli*, *Pseudomonas pyocyaneus*, *Salmonella typhi*, *S. typhimurium*, *Bacillus subtilis* and *B. communis*, as well as the fungi, *Candida albicans*.

Onion bulbs show activity against drug resistant strains of *Mycobacterium tuberculosis*. Gupta et al, *Ind J Med Res* 2010 131.

Onions are supportive of the immune system in a variety of ways; a powerful anti-oxidant that contains many anti-cancer agents. A 1989 study by You et al, reported in the *Journal of the National Cancer Institute*, found that eating onion significantly reduced the risk of stomach cancer. This was based on interviews with more than 560 patients with stomach cancer and over 1100 controls. Another study, by Dorant et al, in 1996 *Gastroenterology*, involved 120,852 subjects between 55 and 69 years of age.

This large scale Netherlands Cohort study showed a strong inverse association between the consumption of onions and reduced risk of stomach carcinoma.

Various studies indicate that those eating onions have decreased rates of various cancers such as: Colon-56%, breast 25%, prostate 71%, ovarian 73%, esophageal 82%, oral 84%, kidney 38%, endometrial 60%, pancreatic 54% and stomach.

A case control study in France on the protective nature of onion on breast cancer showed a positive correlation. Challier et al, *Eur J Epidemiol* 1998 14.

Onionin A, derived from onion suppressed tumor cell proliferation by inhibiting polarization of M2 alternatively activated macrophages. Mona El-Aasr et al, *J Nat Prod* 73:7.

Onions have significant hypoglycemic activity, comparable to the prescription drugs tolbutamide and phenformin. Bever et al, *Quarterly Journal of Crude Drug Res* 1979 17.

The active agent is believed to be allyl propyl disulphide, although quercitin may play a role. Clinical evidence suggests it lowers glucose levels by competing with insulin (which is itself a disulphide) for degradation sites, thereby increasing the half-life of insulin. Other mechanisms, such as increased liver metabolism of glucose or increased insulin secretion are less likely. Onion juice administered orally to diabetic patients reduced blood glucose levels. Water extracts had no such activity. James Duke suggests onions can reduce insulin resistance by up to 18%.

Recent work found methanol extracts of the outer scales of onion, which are high in phenolics, reduce diabetic neuropathy. Bhanot et al, *Pharmacog Res* 2010 2:6.

Quercitin has a number of key medicinal benefits, including tumour inhibition, reducing hypertension, relieving asthma, and reducing the inflammation of various bowel diseases.

Thiosulfates possess anti-tumour effect through induction of apoptosis or programmed cell death.

Sulphur is part of the composition of amino acids taurine, methionine, cysteine and cystine, a constituent of thiamine or B1, the growth factor biotin, the antioxidant glutathione and coenzyme A.

Red Onion skins are rich in quercitin, which helps promote the secretion of insulin, but are not as tasty, and quite dry. The skins also contain daidzein which activates estrogen receptors in young female mice. Airefaie ZA et al, *Can J Physio Pharm* 2011 89:11 829-35.

The peel possesses strong phosphodiesterase 5A inhibiting activity, important for treating erectile dysfunction. Lines et al, *Phytomed* 2006 13:4.

More recent work by Kumud et al, found an S-methyl cysteine sulphoxide (a sulphur containing amino acid) showed both anti-diabetic and anti-hyperlipemic activity. The effects were comparable to those of insulin and glibenclamide. *Ind J of Biochemistry and Biophysics* 1995 32:1.

A meta-analysis of various studies on onion and lowering blood sugar confirmed the obvious. Kook S et al, *J Med Food* 2009 12(3):552-60.

Allithiamines (B1) or benfotiamine is found in onions, garlic, shallots and leeks. This is a fat-soluble form of thiamine, which provides higher levels to the blood stream and tissues. Thiamine is not that well absorbed by the body, even though it is water soluble.

Benfotiamine enhances the activity of the enzyme transketolase, involved in glucose metabolism.

It prevents glucose from being metabolized in a manner that can cause cell damage, and can correct it by normalizing cell division rates and decreasing apoptosis or programmed cell death.

It may help diabetic neuropathy, as shown by several studies involving the supplement benfotiamine. Ironically, the diabetes drug metformin decreases B1 activity in body. Dilantin and some chemo drugs do the same.

Fructans play a key role in intestinal health, including the growth of healthy bacteria, and suppression of unhealthy fungi, yeasts and bacteria; laxative action, protection of hepatic function, lowering of blood serum cholesterol levels, hypertension and anti-cancer activity.

Onions help to improve kidney function, and lower both blood pressure and harmful cholesterol levels in the body. One study in India gave 10 men aged 35-50 years old, a daily supplement of 3.5 ounces of butter. As expected, cholesterol levels rose, while naturally occurring clot-busting activity dropped.

Then, over the next week, researchers added the juice of 2 ounces of onion to their diet, completely preventing the fat induced rise in cholesterol and increasing the activity of blood thinning by 16%.

Raw onions contain substances that reduce blood clots. Adenosine functions as an anticoagulant as effectively as aspirin. Both dimethyl and diphenyl thiosulphinates inhibit thrombocyte B2 biosynthesis in platelet rich human plasma and in pulmonary fibroblasts.

Boiled onions have little anti-thrombotic activity. Alliin is a potent platelet activating inhibitor and anti-thrombotic agent.

Methanol extracts of the outer scales and bulb markedly reduce cerebral infarction size and the attenuated impairment of short-term memory and motor coordination. Shri et al, *Fitoterapia* 2008 79:2.

Thiosulphinates inhibit anti-IgE induced release of histamine from peripheral granulocytes, and leukotriene biosynthesis.

In other words, they act as potent inhibitors in the prostaglandin cascade.

The anti-platelet activity of onions appears to be highest in the least pungent cultivars, such as Exhibition and 8155B. Adenosine is not destroyed by cooking, and is also present in scallions and shallots.

Research in the *European Journal of Nutrition* found in a study of 1400 people, that those who ate one or more servings of onions a week have a 22% less chance of having a heart attack.

The umbels of onions are an even more potent source of anti-platelet activity. Studies conducted by Goldman, *Hort Science* 1996 31:5 indicated the umbels were 336% higher in activity than the bulbs.

They help to remove heavy metals from the body, as well as parasites. They also increase appetite, and body heat.

Edgar Cayce believed that drinking onion juice builds blood, cures bronchitis, cancer and tuberculosis.

Many practitioners suggest that onion juice rubbed onto balding heads will result in new hair growth. This sounds unusual until you consider that cysteine, a sulphur amino acid is rich in onions and also a building block of hair.

Extracts of onion can be used to decrease scar formation, and is particularly useful in patients undergoing plastic surgery. *J Cosmetic Dermatology*.

Applied externally, onion juice cleans and heals infected wounds in a very short time.

Ambroise Pare's Onion Treatment for Burns was developed in the 16th century by a young surgeon looking for an alternative to the ointments of the day. Raw onions are simply mashed with a little salt and applied to affected area, helping heal burns without blistering.

Draelos et al, *J Cosmet Dermatol* 2008 7:2 on 60 patients with recent skin wounds showed improved scar softness, reduction of redness and texture from application of onion gel.

Raw onions enhance spermatogensis and help produce healthy semen, confirming the centuries long tradition of eating raw onions as an aphrodisiac. Onion consumption lowered risk of BPH by 59% in a study of 1800 men.

Onions may possess anti-depressant activity via the HPAA, or adaptogen mechanisms of the endocrine system. Sakakibana et al, *Biosci Biotech Biochem* 2008 72:1.

Research suggests onions may play a role in counteracting bone loss in menopausal women, based on rat studies by Huang et al, *Bone* 2008 42:6. Animals with ovaries removed and fed onion powder as part of diet, had significant benefit in serum calcium levels, similar to alendronate.

A gamma glutamyl peptide in onion has been found to significantly inhibit bone resorption of osteoclasts. Wetli et al, *J Ag Food Chem* 2005 53:9. This suggests use in preventing or treating osteoporosis.

A study in the journal *Menopause* found a 5% increase in bone density in women who ate one or more onions a day compared to those who ate once a month or less.

The green leaves contain flavonoids that are potent anti-oxidants with wide application for nutraceutical work.

These flavonoids affect immune function, capillary and brain blood flow, hepatic function, enzyme activity, platelet aggregation; as well as metabolic involvement with histamine, cholesterol, phospholipid and collagen synthesis.

Onions also induce phase II detoxification enzymes, helping neutralize and discharge harmful by-products from the body.

The young green onions are also warm and useful for treating colds, and symptoms such as nasal congestion, runny nose and headache.

The leaves of green onion are also used to treat colds, usually in the form of decoction.

This drink is used in China for treating stroke, painful sores and carbuncles, the latter as a hot mash applied directly on the affected area.

The slimy, inside of green onion leaf can be placed directly on bleeding wounds. Some practitioners heat the leaves first and replace them when cool, or the bleeding stops.

Modern medical and pharmaceutical journals have reported the use of green onions for treating colds, mastitis, indigestion in children, and pinworms; usually as part of herbal combinations.

The roots, resemble little beards, and are the only part of green onion not considered to be warming in nature. The roots are used to treat headache due to common cold, or injury due to frostbite, as well as sores in the throat. In the case of frostbite, the powdered, dried root is sprinkled on or the fresh root is decocted as a wash.

Green onion seeds invigorate the kidneys and improve vision. They are often used to treat impotence due to kidney deficiency, dizziness, seminal emission, and white vaginal discharges. Three to nine grams of the seed powder is taken with water.

Green onion juice, from the bulb or whole plant, is used to disperse blood stagnation, such as clotting, or black and blue marks on the skin, detoxify, and expel parasites.

And, of course, don't forget to stir fry the bulbs and apply them to the navel of men who suffer sudden exhaustion due to excessive sexual activity, which results in cold perspiration and feebleness. Several green onion bulbs are also mashed and cooked in wine and given to help restore Yang Chi.

The Welsh, or Japanese Bunching Onion *(A. fistulosum)* is well known in prairie gardens. The hollow leaves and stems are used early in spring as a chive substitute. Later, numerous green, flowering heads with black seeds form. The bulb is also used, and highly prized as scallion, a cross of onion and garlic flavors.

The seeds are used in Traditional Chinese Medicine, and known as **TSUNG TZU, CONG SHI** or **CHUNG TZU**.

They possess a pungent flavour with warm properties useful for supplementing the middle CHI, tonifying yang, clearing vision and supplementing deficiency of sperm.

The bulb is called **CONG BAI**, or **CHUNG PAI** in Mandarin, **CHAN BAAK**, in Cantonese, and **SOHAKU** in Japanese Kampo. It is considered a diaphoretic, nasal decongestant, expectorant, and analgesic with anti-bacterial (*Shigella dysenteriae*) and anti-fungal (inhibits white ringworm) properties. *In vitro*, the bulb extract inhibits *Trichomonas vaginalis*.

It is used at the onset of acute respiratory infections and bronchitis as a decoction or tincture, to induce sweating, and unblock the nose.

It is applied as a poultice to help drain abscesses, boils and open sores.

The roots of green onions are used for headaches and sore throat.

Fan et al, *Journal of the Chinese Agricultural Chemical Society* 1998 36:1 found ethanol extracts of the green leaves and white sheaths of Welsh onion showed anti-microbial activity.

Terao et al, *Biofactors* 2005 23:1 found Welsh Onion highly active as a novel anti-oxidant through glutathione peroxidase mimicry.

Water-soluble fractions showed no activity, whereas the oil soluble fractions showed inhibitory activity against *Bacillus cereus, E. coli, Lactobacillus plantarum, Pseudomonas aeruginosa* and *Proteus vulgaris*; as well as the fungi *Aspergillus niger* and *Saccharomyces cerevisiae*.

The roots or bulb contain steroidal saponins that may explain the Traditional Chinese use for preventing miscarriage.

The seeds contain anti-ischemic steroidal saponins fistulosaponins A-F.

Allium vegetables, especially garlic, are related to decreased rates of prostate cancer. Zhou et al, *Asian Pac J Cancer Prev* 2013 14:7 4131-4.

Garlic has been found protective of cardiovascular health in a number of studies, including reduction of hypertension and cholesterol. Generation of hydrogen sulfide and nitric oxide is one molecular mechanism, but regulating ion channels, modulating Akt signaling pathways, histone deacetylase inhibition and cytochrome P450 inhibition have been found potentially responsible as well. Khatua TN et al, *Can J Physiol Pharmacol* 2013 91:6.

A twelve week randomized, single-blind, placebo-controlled study of 70 type 2 diabetic patients with newly diagnosed dyslipidemia was conducted.

Garlic group significantly reduce serum total cholesterol and LDL and moderately raised HDL compared to placebo. Ashraf et al, *J Ayub Med Coll Abbottabad* 2005 17:3.

Aged garlic extract reduced blood pressure by nearly 12 mm Hg in twelve weeks compared to placebo. Ried et al, *Eur J Clin Nutr* 2013 67:1.

An earlier study by Ried et al on aged garlic also found it superior to placebo in lowering systolic blood pressure in a DB, PC trial of 50 patients. *Maturitas* 2010 67:2.

Sulfenic acid may be the active compound that makes garlic the most potent member of family. *Angewadte Chemie* 2009 January.

A meta-analysis of garlic trials showed positive effect on serum lipid levels. Ried K et al, *Nutr Rev* 2013 71:5 282-299.

Garlic is one of the most powerful herbs to induce cancer cell death via apoptosis. Chu YL et al, *J Tradit Complement Med* 2013 3:3 159-62.

The Garlic or Chinese chive *(A. tuberosum)* grows well in protected areas. The seeds are used in TCM in a similar manner to those of Welsh onion, with a few exceptions; and known in China as **JIU CAI ZI**. In Japan, the Chive is called **NIRA**.

The seeds are used for urinary incontinence exaggerated by damp and cold. There will be weakness of the knees and lower back, impotence, and loose stools associated with cold stomach.

The seeds are decocted and act as an aphrodisiac, and toner to the entire uro-genital system. Use same recipes as for Welsh onion seed.

Work by Guohua et al, *J Ethnopharm* 2009 122:3 on male rats seems to confirm the sexual potency of the seeds. At least in rats!

For men having strong erections with stinging pains in the penis, take 10 grams of ground seed powder with warm water three times daily.

For impotence and sexual weakness, simmer 15 grams of seeds in pint of water until reduce to one cup. Drink three times daily. Or take 20 chive seeds with salt water first thing in morning.

Chinese Chives are a rich source of both sulfur bearing compounds and steroidal saponins. In recent years, steroidal glycosides have attracted growing attention for their anti-diabetic, anti-tumour, anti-tussive, and platelet aggregation inhibitor activity.

The fresh leaves have been used for improving blood circulation, liver tonic, and anti-inflammatory.

For bruises, the leaves are applied externally, and a tea prepared for internal use. For nettle rash combine chives with a little salt, crush and apply to affected areas.

Thiosulfinates have been found to possess activity against cancer cell via apoptosis and anti-tumor pathways. Work by Kim et al, *Bioorg Med Chem Lett* 2008 18:11 found these compounds inhibit cell proliferation and induce apoptosis in PC-3 prostate cancer cell lines.

The seeds contain spirostane and furostane glycosides that possess properties such as froth formation, hemolytic activity, fish toxicity, and a complex formation with cholesterin.

At least twelve novel spirostanol saponins, tuberosides, have been isolated from the seeds.

A mannose binding protein or lectin isolated from Chinese chive has recently been found nearly identical to lectins from Snowdrop (*Galanthus nivalis*), and Daffodil (*Narcissus tazetta*). Work by Ooi et al, *J Agric Food Chem* 2002 50 suggests it may possess the same ability to agglutinate red blood cells.

Chives (*A. schoenoprasum*) themselves are warm in energy and act on the stomach caused by a cold nature. The Chinese use chives for enteritis, and weak stomach function.

The fresh juice can be drunk to relieve nosebleeds, taken cold for sunstroke.

The leaves can be crushed and applied to wounds, bruises, swellings and pain. In fact, chives are considered an important medicine for external injuries and pain with blood coagulation.

For this purpose boil small cut chives in water with wine and drink as a soup. It is a favourite of Chinese prison guards, who after beating confessions out of prisoners, give them chives with a meal to prevent internal hemorrhage and coagulations. How thoughtful!

One compound from the leaves, N-p-coumaroyl tyramine, is known to contain anti-platelet aggregation and cytotoxic effects.

Shallots (*A. ascalonicum*) have been shown in laboratory studies to exhibit significant anti-leukemic activity. Caldes and Prescott, *Planta Medica* 1973 23.

They are very high in phenolic content and the highest anti-oxidant activity. Yang et al, *J Ag Food Chem* 2004 52 of ten onions and shallots.

Western Yellow Onion was richest in flavonoids, with all plants exhibiting anti-proliferative activity against $HepG_2$ and Caco-2 cells.

Adeniyi et al, *Phytother Res* 18:5 found alcohol extracts of the leaf show activity against *Helicobacter pylori*, implicated in gastric ulcers.

Shallots appear to reduce toxicity to the kidneys associated with cyclosporine. Wongmekiat et al, *Food Chem Tox* 2008 46:5.

Shallots appear to increase glucose tolerance and reduce blood triglyceride levels. Jalal et al, *J Chin Biochem Nutr* 2008 41:3.

An epidemiological study in Shanghai found a significant reduction in risk of prostate cancer in those eating shallots on a daily basis.

Leeks (*A. porrum*) exhibit anti-mutagenic activity. Work by Carotenuto et al, in the *Journal of Natural Products* 1997 60:10 found porrigenins A and B (sapogenins) to have novel cytotoxic and anti-proliferative activity against 4 cancer cell lines.

Traditionally, in China, the leek was used medicinally for warming the central organs, opening up stoppages, cleansing the intestine and killing parasites.

It was used in treating tuberculosis related coughs, roundworm abdominal pain, as well as external ringworm, boils and other skin abscesses.

Leeks may be useful in dysphagia, which means difficulty or pain when swallowing, reduced appetite and diarrhea. Dysphagia is a common symptom in the elderly and requires special dietary approaches in extended care and long term care facilities.

In Kidney yang vacuity, with loss of libido, premature ejaculation, and lumbar pain, the vegetable may be added to diet. Do not use in cases of heat or general yin vacuity.

One to three leeks were simply chewed and swallowed. Leeks macerated in vinegar are applied to corns and calluses for 24 hours, and repeated if necessary.

Roasted Leeks is a traditional African Cape remedy for dropsy.

It has been shown to be strongly antibiotic against *Staphylococcus aureus*. An isolated compound, odorin, has been found, when heated to 60° Celsius for five minutes to inhibit *S. aureus* and *E. coli.*

HOMEOPATHY

Red Onion (Cepa) is indicated in acute sore throat, colds with runny nose, laryngitis with violent pain on coughing, and acute cystitis with a sensation of weakness in the bladder and urethra.

It is for the thread-like pain on facial neuralgia, flatulent colic, and neuralgia.

The symptoms are worse in the evening and in a warm room. Better in a cold room and open air. This is a specific remedy for the phlegmatic type, who suffer from colds in damp, cold weather.

It may help with the phantom pain associated with amputation, or where there has been injury to nerves.

DOSE-Third potency. The mother tincture is prepared from the fresh red onion.

Garlic reduces arterial hypertension in 30 to 45 minutes after 20-40 drop doses of the tincture. It is adapted to fleshy subjects with dyspepsia and catarrhal affection, especially meat eaters. Sensations of hair or tickling in mouth. Everything in stomach seems to drag downward. Swelling in breast after weaning. Obstinate coughs. Pains in hip and iliac muscles.

DOSE- Third to sixth potency. Proving by Petroz & Teste in France in 1852. Boericke, Hering and Mangialavori used clinical observations. More thorough materia medica in Plants, by Vermeulen and Johnson, volume one, pages 80-88.

MATERIA POETICA
Oh, my Darling, don't you cry
A flow of tears from your eye
A runny nose of acrid fire
Can burn the upper lip entire
The room is warm
Which makes things worse
And in the evening it's a curse
It all began inside your nose
On the left these ails arose
Spread to the ears, a headache rough
The larynx hurts with every cough
Or in a babe you just might be
A colic that grips painfully
Allium Cepa, here you are
Eating onions in the raw.
SYLVIA CHATROUX MD

ONION OIL

Research by Nepkar et al, in the Indian Journal of Experimental Biology 1981 found onion oil stops tumour growth in rats. Onion oil, freshly pressed, contains thiocyanic acid and allyl thiocyanate. Abu et al, *J Egypt Soc Paristol* 2005 35:2 found onion oil reduced the number of *Trichinella spiralis* worms in lab rats, particularly post infection.

The seed oil of *A. tuberosum* contains 57-71% linoleic acid, making it of important nutritional value.

ESSENTIAL OIL

Upon steam distillation, the bulbs of *A. cepa* yield up to 0.04% of a volatile oil with a specific gravity of 0.9960. The iodine value is 59.9 to 66.2.

Onion oil is brownish yellow, to pale yellow with a very strong odour that seizes the larynx. The flavour of onion oil is warm, aromatic, spicy, biting and pungent.

The composition is of various sulfur containing compounds, but without any terpenes or ally sulfides that are present in garlic.

In medical aromatherapy, the oil is considered diuretic, anti-inflammatory, anti-infectious including *Staphylococcus* species, expectorant, thyroid stimulating, hypoglycemic, anti-sclerotic, and anti-thrombotic.

It is used for patients with fatigue, edema, oliguria, diarrhea, obesity, impotence, prostate hypertrophy, genitourinary infections, respiratory infections, diabetes, arteriosclerosis, rheumatism and intestinal parasites.

The volatile oil has been found to kill *Staphylococcus aureus* and various protozoa at dilutions of 1:100,000.

The oil is active against *Aspergillus niger, Cladosporium werneckii, Candida albicans, C. lipolytica, Fusarium oxysporium, Saccharomyces cerevisiae,* and *Geotrichum candidum.*

It is used in the food industry for meats, sausages, soups, and sauces.

Very tiny amounts can improve rose, hyacinth, or violet perfume compositions.

An oleoresin is prepared from onion, which is sweeter than the essential oil, and a darker orangey brown. It is used widely in seasoning, pickles and sauces, as it is richer and fuller in flavour than the oil.

Chives essential oil contains 8-65% di-n-propyl disulphide and 20-23% methyl-n-propyl disulphide.

Chinese chives essential oil is very similar to Chives above, but with 16-27% dimethyl trisulphide.

The low content of diallyl monosulfide makes this oil of use in the treatment of the fresh water fish disease, *Flavobacterium columnare*. This is presently treated with oxy-tetracycline, and consumers are wary of antibiotic laden fish. Rattanachaikunspoon et al, *Fisheries Sci* 75:6.

Shallot essential oil shows significant effect against *Salmonella typhimurium, Listeria monocytogenes, Staphylococcus aureus* including methicillin resistant strains, as well as *Klebsiella pneumoniae, Pseudomonas aeruginosa* and *Acinetobacter baumannii.*

Scallion oil is similar in activity.

Welsh Onion (*A. fistulosum*) essential oil contains 28 compounds; the major ones being dipropyl disulfide (30.6%), 2-tridecanone, 7-53% methyl propyl trisulfide (12%) and dipropyl disulfide (12.3%).

Elephant Garlic essential oil contains 28-29% S-2-propenyl methane-sulfino-thioate; and 9-11% (Z, Z)-d, l, 2, 3,-dimethyl-1,4-butanedithial S, S'-dioxide, when analyzed by low temperature HPLC. By gas chromatography, the oil is 55% diallyl disulfide, and 31% allyl methyl disulfide.

Work by Rattanacallcunsopon et al, *Biosci Biotech Biochem* 2009 73:7 found the oil active against *Vibrio cholera*, a nasty food borne pathogen.

Leek essential oil is produced by steam distillation in Holland, and is used mainly by the flavour industry.

HYDROSOLS

Brunschwig, in Book of Distillation, wrote that onion water is good for growing hair on a bald head, and internally for thread worms.

Leek water is for cold blood, barren women, bleeding nose, and women's vagina be sore and broke after childbirth.

FLOWER ESSENCES

Hooker's Onion (*A. cernuum*) flower essence is primarily a remedy for Spirit. It has a direct impact on all seven major chakras, gently unfolding the full potential of each energy centre to work in harmony together. It creates a vital and harmonious link between heaven and earth. Hooker's Onion acts as a catalyst for creative expression and lightens the heart. It helps to dissolve writer's block.

This remedy also has the potential to release birth traumas. It dissolves the fear for both mother and child as physical separation occurs and helps to maintain the real connection at the level of Spirit. If is effective for post-partum depression. It resolves the emotional attachment- the "my child" syndrome- that inhibits a full and rewarding relationship between parents and children. **PACIFIC**

Allium wants to awaken in each of us the ability to be able to give of our substance to those who need it. It wants to eliminate needless suffering, to break down the Berlin Walls in all of us. The essence of Allium fully awakens our compassion, for as long as we are irritated by others and their differences, it shows us that our compassion has not blossomed far enough. **JADE MTN**

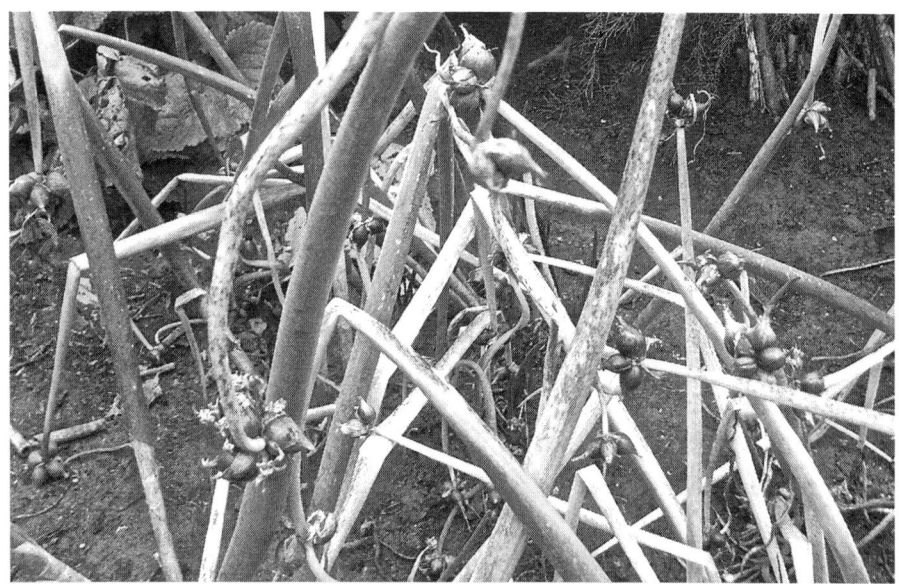

Egyptian Onion

Onion flower essence may help those who feel rejected, confused or disinterested in life. They may be needy, mistrusting, or lack sense of belonging. Lack of understanding self, or sudden crying and sadness from deep within. **LIVING FLOWER**

Onion flower essence assists all aspects of the grieving process, helping a person, first to access the emotion which is present, then to express it deeply and completely, and then to move the grief-emotion present out of the system. **DALTON**

Nodding Onion flower essence helps elevate one's sense of humor. **ROCKY MTN**

Textile Onion flower essence helps one deal with people who are coarse on the inside/outside but appear the opposite. **ROCKY MTN**

Chive flower essence helps to create new goals or targets after reaching one's objectives. It is for those individuals you have no sense of satisfaction after solving problems. **MIRIANA**

Onion flower essence strips away barriers that may exist between a therapist and client. It aids the counselor in gradually removing barriers the mind has built around itself for protection.

For a few individuals, onion will ease PMS.

This essence has many effects with plants. The most important of these is that the plant is able to assimilate the human's idea of correct growing more easily, and the correct ways to utilize minerals to understand and work with humanity, machinery, and other things that people may apply to plants.

The devic order associated with most plants will be slightly assisted by this flower essence. **GURUDAS**

Garlic flower essence is for those souls who have become too diffuse in their astrality and subject to influence by psychic forces and entities. It addresses nervous fear and protects from mediumism, and low-grade immune dysfunction. **FLOWER ESSENCE SOCIETY**

SPIRITUAL PROPERTIES

Years ago when I asked for a dream with this essence, I was visited by the Hooker's Onion Deva. She was clothed in shimmering pink and silver and moved like a light beam in the forest. She led me to a hallway where there were many doors. Each door was labeled with the particular creative venture to which it would lead. She said: " You are only limited by your thoughts of limitation. Leave these dense thoughts at the door and enter with expectation and joy."

SABINA PETTITT

Spiritually, there is a parallel to garlic in that there is assistance in the birthing process. Leek, in appearing as a cluster, can bring energy from the Earth more strongly into action, almost as if a birth is taking place. The energy is symbolized in the signature of the plant.

What occurs in spiritualizing the birthing process is an easing of the fears of expectant parents, a greater sense of calmness, and the sense that the life that has been before the birth will be continued into the birth.

After the birth, there is a tendency in some women to have what is termed 'postpartum depression' or difficulty after the birth relating to the loss of the connection, bonding, and deep sense of oneness with the child. Leek eases this, by enabling the mother to better see the continuum and understand that the child's life was very strong on a consciousness level, even before conception.   **GURUDAS**

The value of the onion lies in its content of sulphurous mustard oils which are present in the whole plant but especially in the bulb. These volatile essential oils are known to those who chop onions. These substances are of a sulphurous nature and therefore, belong to the realm of the flower. They are transformed substances belonging to the flower but submerged and hidden in the physiological interior of the plant.

This metamorphosis cannot but have a profound effect on the actual flower...It has small insignificant greenish-white flowers compressed into a spherical inflorescence.

The onion...provides itself with the necessary flowers with the minimal expenditure. Many small flowers...is a sign of the predominance of cosmic over earthly formative forces. It is completely self contained, a mirror of the cosmos on earth. **GROHMANN**

The starburst globe of the Allium flower is like an exquisite constellation of interconnected stars. Its spirit calls you to look at your awareness of how you fit into the bigger picture and feel part of a more open global consciousness... **ECLARE**

A common enough sin for the Alliaceae is sexual passion, with stink, sin and sex all linked together. There is both the arousing and the dampening of sexual interest.

It is an aphrodisiac, bewitching one into lascivious thoughts and actions as well as affecting fertility and pregnancy. To many it is a forbidden fruit, avoided to achieve sexual abstinence, purity and spiritual grace...Friend or foe? Sin or grace? That is the quandary for Alliaceae. **VERMEULEN**

PERSONALITY TRAITS

If all men will eat onions at all times, they will come into a universal sympathy. Look at Italy. I hope I am not mistaken as to the cause of her unity...All the social atmosphere of that delicious land is laden with it. In churches, all are alike; there is one faith, one smell.

C.D. WARNER

In Roman mythology, the onion was a symbol of human head sacrificed to Jupiter.

The legendary King Numa had been admitted in "celestial wedlock" to the love of the Goddess Diana (Egeria).

Because of this, Numa acquired blessedness and godlike wisdom; and therefore permitted to create rites approved by the gods.

This is a version of the universal archaic belief that no king can rule unless married to the Goddess of the land.

King Numa argued with Jupiter in an attempt to stop human sacrifice and heads. So eloquent were his pleas that he managed to persuade the God to accept onion heads and the blood of fish as a substitute.

WALKER

DOCTRINE OF SIGNATURES

The main signature is the odour and vapor that causes the eyes and nose to water, and help release sadness. The layers of onion can be peeled away to reveal another level of depth and realization.

The bulb and its growth are symbolic of the Light already within that spreads to all the outer layers as it grows in earth's darkness. The flower head represents the Light needed to shine forth on the outside as well as the inside.

The colour of the flowers, whitish pink with green stripe, corresponds to the seventh and fourth chakra. The white flower (seventh) balances physical power with spiritual guidance and wisdom.

The heart chakra (fourth) is the center where the union of what is above (spirit, light, wisdom and communication), meets what is below (matter, survival, procreation, knowledge, and personality).

The umbel represents group membership with its segments of six, needing each individual segment in order to form a group. In relation to the seventh chakra, we learn how we are an integrative system of energy within ourselves, and how each individual's energy system contributes to the larger system of energy.   **PALLASDOWNEY**

Onions look like body cells. They help clear waste from the body cells, and produce tears that wash the epithelial layers of the eyes.

MYTHS AND LEGENDS

A novice Buddhist monk once asked Lama Kalu Rimpoche whether eating garlic would prevent his attaining enlightenment. The Rimpoche replied with a parable. Many eons ago…a demon drank a magic elixir to increase his powers. He flew high among the clouds and changed the color of the sea. But the gods eventually shot him down. The demon's blood fell upon the earth, and from it sprouted garlic. This he said, was the birth of the Five Angry Vegetables doctrine, which prohibits Buddhist monks from eating not only garlic, but also onions, chives, spring onions and any member of the Allium family. **ALLEN**

An Onion pack sat on a bruised and sprained knee,
Then jumped on an earache and shouted "Whoopee!"
Comes a man using Onion for clogged chest and stuffed nose;
Put a slice on a bug bite and the pain quickly goes!

LALITHA THOMAS

ONION LAWS

Citizens of Grant's Pass, Oregon may throw onions at pushy salesman passed on a special town ordinance.

In Spades, Indiana, onions cannot be bought after 6 pm. without a doctor's prescription.

No female wearing a "hat that would scare a timid person" is permitted to be seen consuming onions in Blue Hill, Nebraska.

RECIPES

COUGH SYRUP- Thinly slice a medium sized onion and lay flat in a shallow dish. Cover with unpasteurized honey and leave overnight. In morning, a clear liquid will have pooled in the middle. Take one tsp. as needed. Repeat.

WELSH ONION SEED- 9-15 grams. Do not use when there is spontaneous sweating.

A. fistulosum bulb- **DECOCTION-**2-5 fresh bulbs for five minutes with lid on, drink hot.

Tincture- 2-4 ml.

ASIAN LEEK SEED DECOCTION- three to ten grams boiled for 10 minutes.

Tincture- 1-3 ml.

BULB DECOCTION- 2-5 fresh bulbs in a 5 minutes decoction . Drink hot.

BULB TINCTURE- 2-4ml. Onion tincture is made from 100 grams of onion in 300 grams of 70% ethanol and macerated for ten days.

FRESH GARLIC TINCTURE- Crush fresh, organic peeled cloves. Let sit ten minutes. Cover with 60% alcohol in a ratio of 1:4. Take 20-40 drops as needed in water.

Microwave extraction of anti-oxidant flavonoids can be achieved with microwave technology. Zill-E-Huma et al, J Chromatography A 2009 1216:45.

ONION IN RYE- Fill a bottle with onions sliced in rings, and pour a 40 proof rye whiskey over it and let stand in the sun or a warm place for ten days.

Then strain and rebottle. The liquid is rubbed on the amputated stump as needed. Combine this with a club moss pillow for maximum relief of phantom pain.

ONION HAIR LOTION- As onions contain significant amounts of sulphur, they help treat dandruff, disinfect, kill bacteria, and restore dry scalp and atrophied hair bulbs. The sugars in onions are used in fermentation to produce the hair lotion.

CAUTION- raw onions reduce iodine uptake by the thyroid (goitergenic). Onions may irritate baby's breastfeeding and are neuro-depressive and may exaggerate depression. Maybe.

Onions and garlic can increase clotting time, so caution is advised, especially in patients taking anti-coagulants.

NORTHERN PRICKLY ASH
TOOTHACHE TREE
(***Zanthoxylum americanum*** Mill.)
(***Xanthoxylum americanum***)
(***X. fraxineum*** Willd.)
PARTS USED- inner bark, berry

Xanthoxylum is derived from the Greek **XANTHOS**, yellow and **XYLON** in reference to the yellow colour of wood (xylem). Prickly refers to the sharp, scattered prickles on the branches. Zanthoxylum is preferred genus name.

The fresh leaves have a distinct lemon, orange scent, as do the small pale yellow flowers and black fleshy fruits and seeds.

Prickly Ash is fully hardy to the Canadian Prairies, with one cultivar by Skinner at Morden Research Station planted in 1964, recording a hardiness rating of 9.5. It is very frost resistant for a member of the citrus family.

Matthew Wood says, "prickly ash is as powerful a remedy as it looks and feels. The young branches have sharp thorns that rip the clothing and the skin. Any remedy that can inflict pain should be able to cure it."

Prickly Ash bark was infused by the Chippewa to treat colds, coughs and lung congestion. The root was decocted and used as a wash to strengthen legs and feet of weak children, or for paralysis of extremities. The fresh or dried bark was steeped in hot bear fat for several hours, strained and then used as a muscle rub.

The Fox tribe used both bark and berries for cough syrups, to treat tuberculosis, and to stop hemorrhage.

The Iroquois smoked the dried bark for toothache or neuralgia, decocted the bark for cramps, and infused it for anuria associated with gonorrhea. The Ojibwa used both berry and bark to treat tonsillitis and sore throat. A decoction of root and bark, along with wild ginger root, was used for colds and coughs.

In J. Carver's *Travels through the Interior Parts of North America*, a Winnebago chief is said to have cured a white trader of gonorrhea with a bark decoction.

The Pawnee found the fruit a good diuretic for their horses.

Jethro Kloss mentioned, "the berries are stimulant, antispasmodic, carminative acting mostly on the mucous membrane tissue removing obstructions in every part of the body." Both Felter and Lloyd considered the berries more carminative and anti-spasmodic, probably due to aromatic content.

I have found the twigs make excellent chewing sticks, a good wilderness toothbrush alternative.

In fall, the caterpillar of the Giant Swallowtail Butterfly (*Paplio cresphontes*), looking like a piece of bird poop, is found on the tree. If disturbed, the caterpillar shoots out a pair of red glandular "horns" which give out an odour like putrid citrus peels.

Originally from the south, where it lives on citrus groves, the butterfly has slowly moved north with this shrub.

MEDICINAL

CONSTITUENTS- bark- isoquinoline type alkaloids such as chelerythrine, nitidine, skimmianine, tambetarine, lauriflorine, candicine, magniflorine and tembetarine; malic acid, glucosides, essential oil, resins, fatty acids, berberine, methyl cinnamide, pyranocoumarins such as xanthyletin, xanthoxylin, xanthoxyletin, alloxantho-xyletin, and 8-(3,3-dimethylallyl) alloxanthoxyletin, dipelatine; lignans including asarinin and sesamin, tannins, resins, and an acrid volatile oil.
leaves- two furoquinolone alkaloids, gamma fagarine and skimmianine.

Dr. John King and other Eclectic physicians popularized Prickly Ash bark to treat cholera and typhus epidemics in the late 19th century.

Eclectic symptoms include skin that is dry but with spontaneous sweating. The patient may be thin, emaciated and tired, and yet sleeps poorly.

The herb was listed in the *US Pharmacopoeia* from 1820 to 1926, and in the *National Formulary (NF)* from 1926 to 1947. It is listed as GRAS in the US. The berries were official in NF from 1916-47.

The pungent bark is a terrific diffusive stimulant for peripheral circulation, aiding cold, deficient conditions of the extremities like cold hands and feet, including Raynaud's syndrome. Combine with scullcap for latter condition.

Work by Jia et al, *Phytomedicine* 2000 7:46 in two double-blind, placebo-controlled clinical trials, demonstrated improved venous circulation in patients with varicose veins.

It combines well with lesser periwinkle (*Vinca minor*), hawthorn or ginger root for peripheral circulatory insufficiency to extremities, including brain.

It increases both pulse and cardiac output slightly.

Cold, deficient conditions of the lungs especially clearing of damp conditions such as sinusitis, bronchitis and even tuberculosis, are helped.

This may be due to berberine content attributed to bark decoctions. For lungs and digestion, it combines well with angelica root.

In small doses, the herb helps relieve cold deficiencies of the intestine including diarrhea, digestive stagnation, and even gastric ulcers. It combines well with small amounts of goldenseal and cayenne to stimulate digestion, taken as a tincture in water before meals. It helps to increase GI secretions without irritating the stomach.

Hemorrhoids and varicose vein problems are reduced with continued use. It helps capillary engorgement in infected tissue, especially in the legs. Gangrene skin ulcers in diabetics, for example, may benefit from the herb as part of formula.

The herb will increase saliva production, and alleviate dry tongue associated with liver disorders. Cayenne is hot and drying, while prickly ash is even hotter but is moister in action.

It has proven invaluable in certain conditions associated with paralysis of the mouth and tongue. It both stimulates the nervous system, and helps to balance or equalize nerve pain or irritation.

One-sided paralysis, such as Bell's palsy responds to this herb, combining well with green, unripe cow parsnip seed.

Whenever nerves have been over-stimulated, or where nerve pain, tingling or numbness are present, remember prickly ash.

Neuritis, for example, or cases of paralysis associated with the after effects of stroke, or viral infections may be helped.

For toothache, one may chew the fresh bark, or apply the bark tincture to affected area. The herb will tone and reduce inflammation of gum diseases.

The herb stimulates kidney function; promoting elimination of uric and other acids associated with rheumatism, arthritis and gout.

For prostatitis associated with cold and damp conditions, combine the bark with thuja.

Poor skin tone, such as dryness and period rashes, are likewise relieved due to mild diaphoretic activity.

Prickly Ash combines well with crampbark, or thuja in treatment of delayed or absent menstruation, associated with illness, fear, or exposure to cold.

The herb may be useful for uterine cramping, neuralgia and dysmenorrhea with neuralgia as found in ovaritis and ovarian cysts.

For muscle cramping, fibromyalgia or chronic fatigue syndrome, combine with poplar bark or yarrow, the latter combination also useful for post-surgical recovery. It will increase peripheral circulation to the musculo-skeletal system.

It helps relieve persistent yeast infections, by neutralizing toxins, and disinfecting the terrain, as well as stimulating circulation to the pelvic region.

Chemical constituents that give the bark its heat, also kill food-borne bacteria and parasites. It is especially effective against roundworms.

Prickly ash in sesame oil stops pain from roundworms within a half hour, but is less effective in long-standing cases.

An enema of powdered bark helps eliminate pinworms in children.

The powdered bark is sprinkled on indolent skin ulcers, and scabies, a parasitic skin condition.

Prickly Ash may also be thought of as a Chi tonic, with direct nerve stimulation on the pituitary and hypothalamus. In turn, the immune system is balanced and optimized, and the nervous system brought back to balance. In this regard it is similar to schisandra berry and astragalus root as yang, or sympathetic deficiency tonic.

TCM use includes yang, chi or blood deficiency, with blood stasis from cold.

Generally speaking, prickly ash activity is directed towards the posterior lobe, while Walnut influences the anterior pituitary.

Larger doses have more effect in treatment of nerve and tonic conditions.

Chewing the bark, or placing a small amount of the powdered bark on the tongue helps alleviate insufficient salivary gland production. Consider using the herb for dry mouth caused by radiation.

Prickly Ash is one ingredient in famous Hoxsey Formula for cancer. Recent work appears to indicate cytotoxic activity from various coumarins and lignans in the bark.

The alkaloid chelerythrine possesses both anodyne and anti-inflammatory properties, while nitidine has been shown to possess hypotensive activity in mice. Lenfield et al, *Planta Medica* 1981 43.

Chelerythrine is active against threadworms, gram-positive bacteria and *Candida albicans*, with activity just 1/10th of lincomycin.

Nitidine inhibits synthesis of the RNS-dependant DNS polymerase (reverse transcriptase inhibition) responsible for reproduction of cancer viruses. Sethi et al, *J Nat Products* 1979 42.

Dipelatine is cytotoxic, with IC50 of 0.68 ppm against HL60 human leukemia cell lines. Ju et al, *Phytother Res* 2001 15:5.

Chelerythrine is found in greater celandine, bloodroot and other members of the Poppy family. It is a vasopression receptor ligand that may explain its anti-diuretic hormone activity. Candicine causes nicotine-like effects in the autonomic nervous system, first stimulating and then blocking ganglionic synapses.

Sesamin, also found in sesame seeds, reduces blood pressure in a DB PC crossover clinical trial of 25 patients for four weeks. Miyawaki et al, *J Nutr Sci Vitamin* (Tokyo) 2009 55:1.

Dr. Abayomi Sofowora, professor of Pharmacognosy at the University of Ife, Nigeria, suggests the herb may be of help in treating pain associated with sickle cell anemia.

This condition occurs mainly in persons of African descent with symptoms including anemia, leg ulcers, and sudden excruciating attacks of pain, associated with abnormal red blood cells. He found water extracts of powdered root, "will revert sickle-cell anemia... studies show that the extract of the root is not toxic orally."

It may combine well with Di Huang *(Rehmannia glutinosa)* prepared root.

Zinc supplementation helps affected children grow taller with stronger knees and arms. Zemel et al, *Am J Clin Nutr* 2002 75:2.

Prickly Ash bark provides temporary relief for abdominal pain associated with gall bladder and intestinal spasms. Apply as a plaster as needed.

Work by Ju et al, *Phytother Res* 2001 15:5 found various cytotoxic coumarins and lignans could be isolated from the plant. Dipetaline, a pyro-coumarin, was the most active against human leukemia cells, with an IC50 of 0.68 ppm. This was followed by alloxanthoxyletin, sesamin, asarinin, xanthoxyletin, & xanthylletin.

Katina et al, *J Nat Prod* 2013 76(11) identified cannabinoid receptor ligands in genus species, suggesting potential for type 1 diabetes.

The leaves are effective in treating this problem, which underwent clinical trials in Ibadan. Magnoflorine is associated with neuromuscular blocking activity, and laurifoline has been shown to lower blood pressure.

Nitidine possesses anti-tumour activity, and reverse transcriptase of RNA onogenic viruses.

The berries are active circulatory stimulants, and certainly more warming, aromatic, and pungent, making them a better choice for flatulence and intestinal spasms, as well as catarrhal lung conditions.

The fruit and leaves contain high levels of furanocoumarins, with anti-fungal activity found against 8 of 11 pathogens tested. Bafi-Yeboa et al, *Phytomed* 2005 12:5.

The follicular capsule, but not the seed, shows activity against *Staphylococcus aureus* and *Candida albicans*. The anti-oxidant level is significant 47,367 TE/100 grams. Burchardt et al, *J Med Plants Res* 2008 2:4.

HOMEOPATHY

Prickly Ash *(Xanthoxylum)* is helpful in mental depression, or when the patient is nervous or frightened. The head feels full, with pain and pressure over the forehead, nose and eyes.

Ringing in the ears, with a sick headache associated with dizziness and flatulence is also an indicator.

The lower jaw may exhibit neuralgia, with pharyngitis and dry mouth.

Griping abdominal pains with diarrhea may be present. In the female, menstruation is both painful and early with ovarian neuralgia especially on the left side extending down thigh.

Vaginal itching at menses, especially in the thin, neurasthenic patient, is an indication.

Sighing and constant desire to take a deep breath, with dry cough, day and night, is another.

The left side may exhibit numbness or paralysis with pain in nape of neck extending down back. Sciatica is worse in warm weather, with shooting electric-like nerve pains all over limbs.

Sleep may be un-refreshing with insomnia present in some neurasthenics. Dreams of flying are often present. Dreams of children, drowning, fear of being cheated.

DOSE- First to sixth potency. The mother tincture is made from the fresh inner bark before berries. First proving by Cullis with six provers and tincture in 1862. Proving by Southwick with three provers and tincture in 1884. Proving by Joshi with 17 provers at 30c in 1999. Clinical observations by Boger, Hering, Mangialavori.

BARK OIL

Steep one part of powdered bark in four parts of warm canola or olive oil for one week. Apply as massage oil to affected rheumatic pains, muscle pain and cold hands and feet twice daily as needed.

FLOWER ESSENCE

Prickly Ash essence strengthens light of the aura. It strengthens the immune system and gives protection from unwanted influences of the environment. This essence helps expand capacity for perspective, judgment and fairness.   **CLEAR PATH**

SPIRITUAL PROPERTIES

When there are too many spirits trying to communicate to you, burn Prickly Ash and the spirits will know to wait their turn to speak… When married couples were having difficulty, Prickly Ash was burned to help keep the peace and solve issues. It was also burned when clear decisions needed to be made.   **AVERSANO**

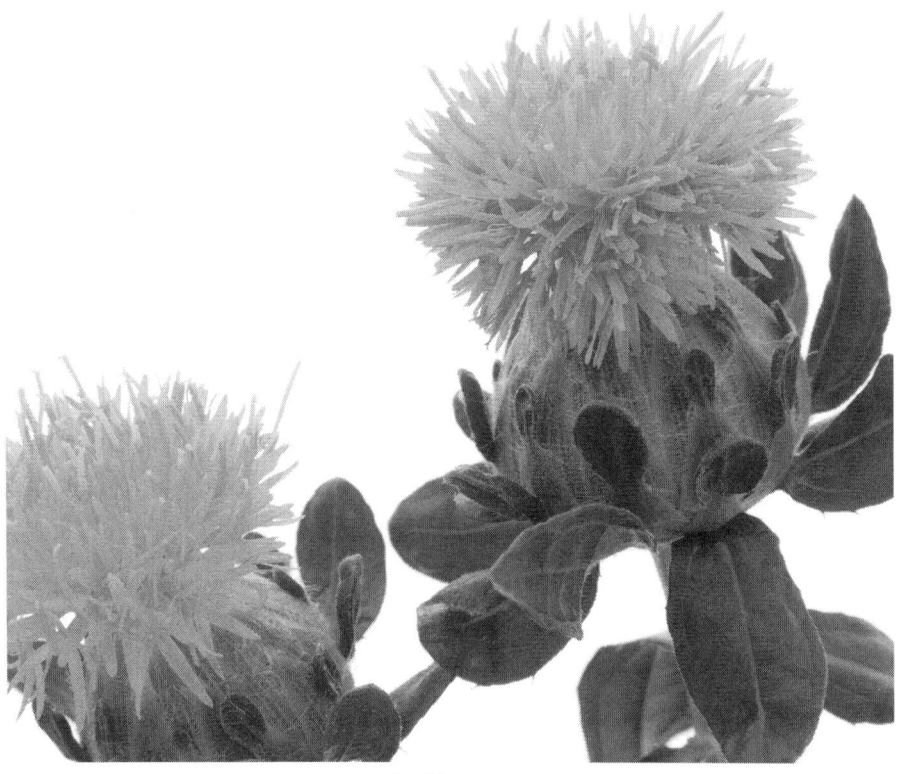

Safflowers

PERSONALITY TRAITS

The [Prickly Ash] patient is pale and lethargic; has sensations of cold in the hands and feet with occasional numbness or tingling; feels cold at the body surface; has recurring aches in the muscles aggravated by cold; has poor appetite; and sensations of cold in the epigastrium and abdomen that are aggravated by cold food and drinks.   **ROSS**

RECIPES

DECOCTION- 1-3 grams of bark in decoction, three times daily. The berry is decocted at 0.5-1.0 grams per dose.

TINCTURE- the dried bark tincture is taken 2-5 ml three times daily. It is prepared at 1:5 and 45% alcohol. The fresh bark is prepared 1:5 at 75% alcohol, both after flowering.

The berry is taken at 1-3 ml three times daily and prepared as the bark. Prepare at 1:1 in 45% alcohol.

CAUTION- Do not use during pregnancy, or combine with anti-coagulants. It may stimulate immune processes within the mother than may be detrimental to developing fetus. Potentiation of anti-coagulants is highly speculative, as the pyranocoumarins xanthyletin and xanthoxyletin do not possess anti-coagulant or anti-platelet effects.

People with acid indigestion, and hyperacidity of stomach should avoid the herb.

The herb is contraindicated in yin deficiency with heat, or true heat.

SAFFLOWER
(*Carthamus tinctorius*)
PARTS USED- seeds, leaves, root, flowers

You give your cheeks a rosy stain,
With washes dye your hair;
But paint and washes both are vain,
To give a youthful air.   **WM COWPER**

Carthamus is derived from Arabic **QUARTOM**, or Hebrew **QARTHAMI**, both meaning "to paint or the painted one". Tinctorius means, "of the dyer's".

Safflower descended from Middle English **SAFFLEUR**, and in turn the Old Italian **SAFFLORE**, due to its use as a poor substitute for saffron.

Safflower is an annual herb, extensively cultivated throughout the world. It is native to the East Indies, but traveled around the world. It was introduced into North America by Mormons in 1870s.

The Hopi then used it to colour their wafer bread -piki- a bright yellow. Amaranthus flowers were used for a red colour. See recipe below.

It has been grown commercially, and successfully in southern Alberta as an oil seed, as good seed set and high oil content is dependent on a dry atmosphere.

Safflower production in western Canada is confined to southern Saskatchewan and Alberta. Recent acreage is between 2000-5000 acres, but in the early 1990s it was up to 16000 acres. In the early 1980s, the crop was popular in Manitoba. The crop produces large seed harvest in climates with low humidity from time of flower formation to maturity.

A good crop should yield 1500 pounds of seed per acre, and about one-quarter higher with irrigation. Most is dedicated to the birdseed industry, as high oleic oil lines are not officially registered, or mature too late for our climate. One promising new addition is Lesaf 496, with about 40% oil yield.

The leaves and young shoots can be eaten as a potherb, something described by Dioscorides in ancient Greece. The women of that era used the flowers as a cosmetic stain. Pliny says it was imported into Rome from Egypt in his time, the flower for dye, and the oil of the seeds used as cathartic.

The seeds can be fried and made into chutney, or used like rennet to make cheese.

In Traditional Chinese Medicine, it was first described about 300 AD, but was introduced before 115 BC. They used the flower heads to dye silk.

In Tibet, the flowers are used to cure all types of liver disease, and close ruptures of blood vessels. The unsaturated fatty acids help reduce cholesterol levels and increase platelet linoleic acid levels associated with change in thromboxane B_2 levels.

It was well known to the Egyptians, who made garlands for mummies, and decorated religious feasts. Brilliant red linens were produced, found in graves dating back to 1st century BC.

Red colored tapes bound legal documents, hence, the original, annoying red tape.

Avicenna, the noted Arabian physician of the 10th century AD, used the seed, in those days called **KURTUM**.

In Mexico, it is called False Saffron, the dried petals ground as a substitute for expensive saffron stamens. The petals are infused and drunk hot to reduce fevers, or soaked in cold water to bring to surface, rash of measles and other eruptive childhood conditions.

The Malayans prescribe it for those suffering demonic possession. In India and Iran, the flowers have been used traditionally to treat digestive, kidney and pancreatic problems.

In the 19th century, in North America, safflower was used to encourage perspiration, to bring on menses and to promote the clearing of measles and other childhood diseases. The seed juice was added to chicken stock to relieve constipation and respiratory problems. It has been used to treat ear and menstrual problems, soothe bruises, wounds and painful or paralyzed joints.

Safflower can be a high value rotation crop, every 2-4 years, for farmers using no till or conservation tillage.

Donald Tanaka, in Mandan, North Dakota, says that safflower may be a good alternative to wheat because its deep roots take up water and nutrients that are out of reach of other crops. "Safflower is best suited to dry climates, such as those... in the western Great Plains", says Tanaka.

Research shows safflower roots descend to about seven feet, and may reach nutrients and fertilizers leached below the root zone of other crops.

Research shows up to 50% less nitrate in soil in years when safflower was planted in rotation with wheat.

Foliar application of zinc and manganese improve safflower seed yield and quality under drought conditions. Movahhedy-Dehnavy et al, *Ind Crops & Prod* 30:1.

Safflower encourages carbon sequestration, meaning it removes carbon dioxide from the atmosphere. Energy credits are given to companies removing CO2 they help create.

Safflower meal, after oil pressing, is commonly used for animal feed, but is too bitter and cathartic for humans.

An interesting study from China looked at ovarian disturbance in dairy cows. A control group of 47 cows was measured against 46 cows with ovarian cysts, quiescent ovaries and persistent corpus luteum, treating with a herbal mixture of angelica root, red sage root, motherwort and safflower. Blood samples before and after, indicated improvement in all cows, with most coming into estrus and pregnancy. *Chin J Vet Sci Tech* 1995 25:9.

Two phenolic glucosides, 2-hydroxyarctin, and matairesinol mono-glucoside are believed responsible.

Treatment of safflower meal with beta-glucosidase for two days, results in almost complete elimination of their bitterness and cathartic activity.

Carthamin, or carthemone, is a yellow to red preparation extracted from the flowers. Fresh yellow petals contain precarthamin which oxidizes to red colorant.

When dyeing silk, wool, and cotton, you can turn the light orange red into a deeper red by the addition of a small amount of diluted ammonia.

The powdered dried flowers are mixed with talcum or cornstarch powder to make rouge. The reddish colour is used in food, liqueurs, and dye silk.

In Japan, the flowers are chemically treated to remove the yellow pigment, and the red color is important pink dye for silk, and make-up. Hence, the name **KUCHIBENI** meaning, lipstick.

Diseased or fungal attacked safflower produces dehydro-safyrol, a phyto-alexin.

MEDICINAL

CONSTITUENTS- flowers contain a complex mixture of red and yellow pigments, including 20-30% safflower yellow (safflor yellows A&B), glycosides of quinone and chalcone including tinctormine; flavonoid glycosides including carthamin, carthamidin, isocarthamidin, neo-carthamin; quinochalone glycosides, erythro-alkane-6,8-diole, safflomin A&C, polysaccharides like xylose, fructose, galactose, glucose, arabinose, rhamnose and uronic acid residues; lignans such as tetracheloside, matairesinoside, and 2-hydroxyarctiin, fatty acids, dipalmitin.
Seed cake- 4,4"-bis (N-p-coumaroyl) serotonin, 4-{N-(p-coumaroyl) serotonin-4"-y}-N-feruloylserotonin, and 4,4"-bis (N-feruloyl) serotonin.
leaf- various flavonoids, including luteolin, quercitin, acacetin, and apigenin and their glucopyranosides.

The flowers diuretic and laxative in nature.

A hot tea is used for children with fevers, but with eruptive childhood illnesses, like chickenpox and measles, use a warm infusion to more quickly get by the infection stage, and resolve more quickly. Safflower tea will induce perspiration to detoxify the body of uric acid and alleviate colds and flu.

Hot infusions are used in muscular rheumatism and jaundice, both internally and externally; while warm infusions help bring on menstruation suppressed by cold.

Safflor yellow has immuno-suppressive and strong anti-coagulant activity, while the polysaccharides have immuno-potentiating effect. Tetsuya et al, *Cytotechnol* 1997 25.

Work by Caldes et al, *J Gen Applied Microbiology* 1981 27 found polysaccharides induce anti-body formation, and cross reacts with antisera, specific for *Streptococcus pneumoniae* type III and VIII.

Safflower extracts are cardiac and uterine stimulating, vaso-dilating, hypolipemic, hypotensive and interferon-inducing.

Water extracts of flowers potentiate cellular immunity, particularly Th1, by increased activation of macrophages. Choi et al, *Immunopharm Immunotox* 2007 29:2.

Safflower tea removes hard phlegm from the lungs, usually combined with other expectorants as hot infusion.

When the dried flowers are stored for a while they oxidize to create natural sugar-like compounds. These induce the adrenals to produce more adrenaline, and the pancreas to produce more insulin.

The flowers are a source of essential fatty acids, making them useful for those suffering gall bladder and biliary colic problems. They aid digestion of fats, helping to eliminate cholesterol from the system.

Safflower is used to treat constipation and fevers. In Japanese Kampo medicine, the flower is known as **MOGAMI-KOUKA** or simply **KOKA**, meaning Red Flower. In Korea, the plant is referred to as **HONGHWA**.

In Traditional Chinese Medicine, the flowers are known as **HONG HUA** or Red flower. In Tibet, a rare and special variety called **TSANG HONG HUA**, is considered to be of the highest quality.

Carthamus flower is considered a vasodilator that causes blood vessels to expand. Safflower was therefore used traditionally to open the blood vessels of the scalp for treating hair loss.

A mouse study appears to support the use of flower extracts as a hair-promoting agent. Junlatat J et al, *Phytother Res* 2013 Dec 11.

Massaging the scalp with safflower powder, or added to shampoos would help achieve the desired effect. For hair loss associated with nervous tension, James Duke suggests dried flowers in vegetable oil (safflower?) applied as a hair paste that is rinsed out after a half hour.

The tincture is used on sprains and wounds, to decrease inflammation, and for bruises and trauma in a manner similar to yarrow or arnica.

The flowers are good for abdominal pain in women due to blood coagulation, dysmenorrhea and menopause. They combine well with red peony root for these purposes as well as amenorrhea, and chronic menorrhagia associated with congested uterine conditions.

Recent work by Zhao et al, *Zhongguo Zhong Yao Za Zhi* 2007 32:5 found flowers have both estrogenic and anti-estrogenic influence, depending upon the internal levels already present. The study found Dodder seed possesses similar activity.

Ethanol extracts of flowers inhibit 5 alpha reductase, similar to prostate drug finesteride. It showed potent hair growth promotion, which would be expected. Kumar et al, *J Ethnopharm* 139:3 765-771.

Safflower is anti-inflammatory, analgesic, and inhibits carcinogenesis on the skin.

Safflor yellow A has demonstrated pain-killing action of a longer duration than morphine in mice studies. When combined with barbitol, it increases inhibition of the central nervous system.

The flowers show over 30% inhibition of acetyl-cholinesterase activity, a possible link to the reduction or treatment of Alzheimer's disease. Ingkaninan et al, *J Ethnopharm* 2003 89:2-3.

Some naturopathic practitioners have noted positive effects on hysteria and mental-related seizure activity with warm safflower tea taken three times daily, empty stomach.

Zhao et al, *J Ethnopharm* 2009 124:1 found ethanol extract of flowers possess novel monoamine inhibition that may, through regulation, improve neuro-psychology. The extract also regulated dopamine and serotonin levels.

The flowers are helpful in relieving insomnia. Chen et al, *J Clin Pharm Ther* 2009 34:5.

The flowers contain a novel serotonin transport inhibitor, suggesting use in depression. Zhao et al, *Eur Neuro-psychopharmacol* 2009 19:10.

Safflower herb can help expand coronary arteries and prevent angina pectoris, activate the blood and bring down blood pressure. In small doses it stimulates the heart, and inhibits it when dosage increases. Water extracts cause coronary dilation, increase tolerance to oxygen starvation, and prolong survival time in animal studies. It is combined with Red Peony root for chest pain due to obstructed Qi in chest.

In one study on patients with coronary heart disease, 41% showed ECG improvement in only one month, and after four months, 90% of the patients were able to stop using nitroglycerin.

The quinochalone glycosides (tinctormine) have a potent Ca 2+ antagonistic effect, and exert anti-hypertensive effect by reducing plasma renin activity and angiotensin II levels.

Siow et al, U of Hong Kong, found activation of Stress Activated Protein (SAP), a major complication in ischemic heart disease, inhibited by 95%. Un-treated ischaemic/reperfused hearts showed 57% elevation in activity of SAP kinase.

In other studies, the herb prolonged blood coagulation time and inhibited platelet aggregation. It lowers cholesterol and triglyceride levels.

A trial of 316 Thai patients with dyslipidemia, compared safflower petal tea at six grams per day, with gemfibrozil at 600 milligrams per day. The drug provided greater total cholesterol and triglyceride reduction, while the safflower tea induced greater HDL-C levels. Kamkaen et al, *Trad Med & Nutraceuticals* 2005 6.

He et al, *Phytother Res* 2008 June 20 found hydroxysafflor A improves cardiac insufficiency in diabetic conditions.

The flowers scavenge free radicals and mediate PI3K signaling pathways associated with cardiac risk. Han et al, *Phytomed 2009* April 23.

Clearly this is a valuable cardiovascular herb. In China, 50% injection solutions are used for cerebral thrombosis, diluted with 10% glucose solution for intravenous infusion.

Safflower is mentioned for hypoglycemic patients who are prone to painful muscles due to lactic acid buildup. In Matthew Wood's latest great book, The Earthwise Herbal, he mentions a patient who pointed out this specific symptom to him many years ago.

It is used to treat various types of cancer. Yasukawa et al, found safflower tincture stopped formation of skin tumours induced by chemicals. *Oncology* 1996 53:2.

This may be due, in part, to the modulating effect on B lymphocytes by safflower petals; and/or the stimulation of Tumour Necrosis Factor, a chemical produced by macrophages and activated T cells that kills cancer cells by attacking their blood vessels.

Shi et al, *Zhongguo Zhong Yao Za Zhi* 2010 35:2 found safflower polysaccharides inhibit T739 lung cancer cell lines.

The flowers appear to increase efficacy of chemotherapy drugs in multi-drug resistant cancers. Increased synergism from 2.8 to 4 fold suggests adjunct usage in stubborn malignancies. Wu JY et al, *Afr J Trad Complement Altern Med* 2013 10:4 36-40.

Safflower breaks down fibrin, the protein that cancer masses use to grown their own blood vessels, and thus prevent their spread.

Safflower extracts may be of great benefit in the treatment of chronic pain conditions, including back pain, neck pain associated with cervical spondylosis, carpal tunnel syndrome, wrist tendosynovitis, costo-chondritis and rheumatoid arthritis.

All of these conditions are governed by the Wood element, or liver health. Safflower helps to cleanse the blood, increase portal circulation and improve circulation in the pelvic region.

Work by Takii et al, *Int Immunopharmacology* 2003 3 found inhibition of pro-inflammatory cytokine production. Hanania et al, *Integrative*

Medicine 2005 4:3 looked at the patented safflower extract Zolacet and its treatment for back and neck pain, carpal tunnel and tendonitis. Sixty-six subjects with mean age of 64 years applied the concentrated safflower extract on affected areas, 3-4 times daily for four weeks.

Overall, 86% reported moderate or greater relief, with 80% suffering back pain reporting benefit.

Safynol, found in safflower infected by fungi, and occurring naturally in various *Centaurea* species, inhibits COX and 5-LOX, perhaps explaining in part, the anti-inflammatory properties.

Carpal tunnel patients reported 100% improvement. Matthew Wood reports on a patient with severe Raynaud's disease that responded well to the herb, suggesting an alternative or possible synergy with prickly ash.

Zhao et al, reported safflower markedly inhibits lens aldose reductase, and may be beneficial in prevention or treatment of diabetic retinopathy.

Hong Hua, 2 ml injection ampoules, are used for intra-muscular injections in the treatment of neuralgic dermatitis or pain of hematoma swelling.

Blaszczyk et al, *Phytotherapy Research* May 2000 found safflower possessed the highest activity against *Aspergillus fumigatus* of 56 Chinese herbs tested.

Methanol extracts of leaf and flower exhibit activity against *S. aureus, Bacillus subtilis, B. cereus, E. coli,* and *Candida albicans.* Akroum et al, *Eur J Sci Res* 2009 31:2.

The petals show cytotoxicity against gamma herpes virus infection. Lee H et al, *J Microbiol* 2013 51(4): 490-8.

Safflower petals are a potential adjuvant for the treatment of multi-drug resistant cancers.

Work by Wu JY et al, *Afr J Tradit Complement Altern Med* 2013 10(4): 36-40 found the herb increased chemo-sensitivity from 2.8 to 4 fold and general synergism in cytotoxic effect.

A serotonin derivative, N-p-coumaroyl, isolated from safflower oil cake, has been shown to stimulate growth-promoting activity for fibroblasts.

Takii et al, *Journal of Biochemistry* (Tokyo) in May 1999, found normal human fibroblasts were stimulated, but it did not affect normal or tumour cells. This serotonin derivative is present in the oil. This suggests safflower derivatives may play a role in connective tissue synthesis and regeneration.

Safflower seeds are used in TCM to promote blood circulation and detoxify, and for measles or chicken pox that fail to erupt.

Hot water seed extracts appear to be anti-adipogenic, suggestive of use in weight loss.

Recent *in vivo* work suggests safflower seeds protect from bone loss caused by estrogen deficiency, with substantial effect on the uterus. The seeds have been used clinically in Korea to promote bone formation and prevent osteoporosis. Kim et al, *Calcif Tissue Int* 2002 71:1.

Yuk et al, *Am J Chinese Medicine* 2002 30:1, found the seed inhibited bone resorption, and may be useful in elevated bone loss. Work by Jang et al, *Nat Prod Res* 2007 21:9 found seed extracts produce significant osteoblast formation.

Safflower extracts protect against stress-induced damage to osteoblasts. Choi et al, *Phytother Res* 2009 Dec 3. Toxicity is low; LD50 of carthamin greater than 8 grams/kg.

Methanol seed extracts induce apoptosis in glucose-deprived HT29 colon carcinoma cells lines. Son, Eun-Soon et al, *J Med Plants Research* 2011 5:19.

A Calgary company, SemBiosys Genetics, studied safflower with its potential for medicinal and other applications.

They grafted recombinant protein to oilseed protein, and later extracted it with the oil after harvest. The process was believed to lower the cost of producing, collecting and purifying peptides and proteins, for vaccines, pharmaceutical, industrial enzymes, cosmetics and nutritional products.

They showed the ability to produce insulin in commercial quantities using GMO safflower in fields in Washington State, Chile and Arizona. Phase 2 clinical trials began in early 2008, but alas, never made it to market.

Another protein, Apo A1, from safflower has shown in clinical trials to clean plaque from heavily blocked coronary arteries. Unfortunately, this will probably not reach market.

Their patented Stratosome™ Biologics System attaches genetic protein to oleosin, the protein coating of the oilseed. There are several advantages to this system including stabilization of intracellular accumulation of foreign protein.

Growing transgenic safflower in southern Alberta is feasible, as there are no native relatives that could help spread the genes through wild populations.

Low tendency to weediness, and seed dormancy, combined with high self-pollination make this a good choice for bio-pharming.

A water emulsion of the non-transgenic safflower oil bodies forms a milky cream called Dermasphere™. This product has potential for the personal skin care industry, as evidenced by a 2004 license agreement with Lonza, Inc.

Botaneco offers several safflower oleosome products to the cosmetic market. The latest, SF2, has ecocert status and can be used from pH 3.5-9 for hand sanitizers, etc.

Kanehira et al, *Planta Medica* 2003 69:5 found kinobeon A from safflower cell culture, a potent natural tyrosinase inhibitor. The study indicated more potent inhibition for both mushroom and human tyrosinase than kojic acid, arbutin or L-ascorbic acid. This may lead to an avenue of application in cosmetic formulations.

The leaves contain a variety of flavonoids that exhibit anti-oxidant activity. Lee et al, *Arch Pharm Res* 2002 25:3.

One GMO crop by Enlay and Associates inserted growth hormones from carp into safflower. This experiment was approved by the USDA and grown on eleven acres in North Dakota and Nevada, during the summer of 2003.

SEED OIL

Safflower seed oil consists of approximately 75% linoleic acid, 13% oleic acid, 6% palmitic acid, and 3% stearic acid.

Various genotypes have large variation in oil composition, with some containing over 80% oleic acid, and others with 83% linoleic. This makes plant breeding with safflower most interesting! Specific gravity is 0.927, saponification is 192 and iodine value is 145.

Safflower oil contains long chain triglycerides, which exerts some effect on the reticulodendothelial (immune) system.

It can effectively decrease the severity of clinical auto-immune encephalomyelitis by enhancing T cell proliferation, and has been used clinically in the treatment of chronic nephritis and lupus.

Linoleic acid is converted into immuno-suppressants, prostaglandin E2 and 1-2 within the prostaglandin pathway.

An experiment in 1982, by Bell et al, at Iowa University involved safflower oil emulsion infused intravenously to low-birth weight babies. The increase in energy intake allowed more energy for growth.

The oil has been compounded with glycerin, and rose oil as an external massage lotion.

Topical administration is, however, a poor substitute for ingestion. The plant is used traditionally in India, known as **KOOSUMBHA**. The oil is used as the base of a number of Ayurvedic medicinal body oils.

Safflower oil, with some wheat germ oil, is a good combination for sunburned skin, helping both heal and reduce the pain and damage caused.

Safflower oil contains Vitamin F, an essential fatty acid needed for both skin regeneration and reducing allergy symptoms from corn, wheat, dust, feather or wool allergy, according to Dr. Lepore.

In one study, switching from other oils to safflower for 8 weeks, reduced total serum cholesterol levels by 9-15% and LDL cholesterol by 12-20%.

The seed oil can become rancid very quickly if not refrigerated, and is not suitable for deep-frying, as flavour is not stable at high temperatures.

The oil cake contains seven anti-oxidative serotonin derivatives. Zhang et al, Nagoya City University, Japan 1997.

Linoleic acid decreases neurotoxicity caused by lithium carbonate. Lieb, *Prostaglandin and Medicine* 1980 4.

Safflower oil is a good substrate for the production of CLA, or conjugated linoleic acid, used in weight loss and cosmetic applications.

An isomerized safflower oil product, Safflorin™ has been shown, in clinical studies to benefit the human immune system.

The enrichment of the trans 10 cis 12 isomer to the cis 9 in CLA (conjugated linolenic acid) gives a unique proprietary product.

One double-blind study found Safflorin, taken for twelve weeks, increased levels of IgA and IgM compared to placebo group of healthy people. The first group maintained higher antibody levels for 12 weeks after supplementation, suggesting long-term benefit.

In another study, 71 healthy volunteers were repeatedly exposed to a vaccine containing part of the hepatitis B virus. After 85 days, the active component of Safflorin boosted induction of virus specific antibody levels in a dose dependent manner. *Eur J Clin Nutr* 2003 57. Other studies indicate benefit against the rhinovirus, and other flu conditions.

Safflorin™ was effective in reducing symptoms of rhinovirus infection, sore throats and cough, in a double-blind placebo-controlled study of 50 volunteers. *17th Int Conf on Antiviral Research* May 2004 Tucson, Arizona.

CLA was used as treatment for Crohn's disease in an open-label study. It may also be useful in irritable bowel syndrome and colitis, due to the fact that healthy flora in colon produce CLA locally and suppress inflammation. For more info go to www.vt.edu.

Recent work by Arcadia Biosciences has achieved a GLA content of 65% in safflower seed oil. This is a significant breakthrough that is sure to affect other sources of gamma linolenic acid such as borage, evening primrose and black currant seed.

FLOWER OIL

The petals of safflowers contain 4.0-5.8% lipids consisting of C32 and C29 iso-paraffins (2-methyltriacontane and 2-methyl-octacosane), free fatty acids, mainly consisting of palmitic acid, and alpha linolenic acid; but also containing 2-3% gamma linolenic acid, GLA.

The petals contain 33 esters of phytol, esterified with three groups of fatty acids- paraffinic, isoparaffinic and monoenoic of the C9-C26 series.

Also present are small amounts of beta sitosterol and beta-D-glycopyranoside.

The petals and seeds both contain waxy matter. In India, the oil is boiled in earthenware vessels for 12 hours, and then placed in flat dishes partly filled with cold water. This solidifies into a thick jelly-like mass called **ROGHAN**. It is used in the manufacture of African wax linoleum, as well as for drawing artistic designs on woven cloth. Finely pointed staves are dipped in the Roghan, drawing it out into very fine threads which are deposited on the cloth as indelible patterns.

ESSENTIAL OILS

Safflower produces an absolute that is used in the perfume and fragrance industry. It is a deep orange-red colour as would be expected.

RECIPES

TINCTURE- 2-4 ml as needed, Tincture is made at 1:5 from dry petals in 45% alcohol. The flower heads are picked in late summer when yellow blooms begin to change to red.

INFUSION- 4-8 ounces at a time, made by infusing 6-8 grams of flowers in 250 ml of boiling water.

DECOCTION- 3-9 grams, 12-15 grams is a large dose. For blood tonic only 1-1.5 grams in decoction.

SAFFLOWER CHEESE- To 100 ml of whole milk, add 10 grams of defatted meal from safflower seeds. This is incubated at 50° C for ten minutes. Then it is drained in a cheese cloth and salted.

PIKI (PAPER BREAD)- Crush corn kernels between stones, and toast in pottery to prevent burning and then toast twice again. Mix with cold water and then boil. When cool, the batter is cooked on hot stones, using crushed squash or sunflower seeds as an oil. This bread cooks immediately. Safflower petals are added during boiling for yellow colour.

DYE- A yellow dye is made by soaking the flowers in vinegar overnight, and using alum as a mordant.

To get red, the flowers from the yellow dye bath are rinsed and soaked again for a few hours in ammonia or washing soda. Then vinegar is used to neutralize the dye bath and turn it brilliant red.

EXTRACTION- A simple, fast, sensitive and accurate reverse phase HPLC method for safflower flavonoids is described in *Acta Pharmaceutica Sinica* 1997 32:2.

Those interested in growing safflower may contact the Alberta Safflower Growers Association Box 822 Lethbridge, Alberta T1J 3Z8.

CAUTION- Do not use during pregnancy or with ulcerative, menorrhagic or hemorrhagic conditions. In small doses, the flowers cause rhythmic contractions of the uterus, and when the dose is increased the tone of contraction also increases until convulsions. Traditionally, the flower tea was given to new mothers about two weeks postpartum to ensure the uterus was cleansed. Some pharmacists suggest avoiding the herb during vaccinations.

SPRING ADONIS
FALSE HELLEBORE
(*Adonis vernalis* L.)
SIBERIAN ADONIS
(*A. sibir* Attan.)
(*A. siberica* Patrin ex Ledeb)
AMUR ADONIS
(*A. amurensis* Regel & Radde)
PARTS USED- whole plant w/o root

Adonis is from the Phoenician **ADON** meaning, ruler or lord. It is a common Proto-Semitic title of respect. Adonia was an annual feast in Greece, where women wept over his death for eight days and

268

then rejoiced at his resurrection. Adonis was the handsome lover of Aphrodite. Adonai is a name of the Lord in the Old Testament, worshipped in a former sanctuary of Adonis in Bethlehem.

The god's thorny crown of myrrh was assimilated into Christian legend, and Adonis' mother was the virgin Myrrha, or Myrrh of the Sea. The name was re-applied, by early Christians to Mary, mother of Jesus.

Vernalis is from the Latin meaning "of the springtime". Amur is derived from the river separating Russia and China.

Spring Adonis is one of our earliest perennials to bloom. Its buttercup-like yellow blooms are matched to delicate, fern-like foliage. It opens to the sun, but when it clouds over the petals fold up.

By mid-summer, the blooms and leaves practically disappear until the following spring. It originated in the steppes of Russia, and around the Black Sea. It is rare and legally protected in Europe; the root often used in place of Black Hellebore; thus called False Hellebore.

According to Grieve, the plant contains a glycoside Adonidin, with action almost identical to digitalis, but much stronger and no accumulative toxicity.

It appears to be ten times stronger than digitoxin, and has been prescribed in past instead of digitalis, or where there is kidney disease, or digitalis does not work well.

Today, because of its powerful and somewhat poisonous nature, it is best used as a homeopathic preparation.

Siberian Adonis is a hardier perennial that adapted very well to the prairie climate. It is hardy to zone 2, while its cousin requires zone three.

So too, does Amur Adonis, native to Manchuria, Korea and Japan. In the latter country, the plant is known as **FUKUJUSO**, meaning wealth and happiness.

One Ainu legend, from northern Japan tells of a Goddess turned into a plant when she refused to marry the god of her father's choice; very similar to the Greek legend of Adonis.

There are several related annual species including Summer Pheasant's Eye (*A. aestivalis*), Autumn Pheasant's Eye (*A. autumnalis*) and Annual (*A. annua*). They all contain adonidin, but have not been studied as well. In fact, all three may be variants of one species, rather than separate species. Summer Pheasant's Eye has been implicated in poisoning of three horses from hay containing plant. All died. Woods et al, *Vet Pathol* 2004 41:3.

An insecticide called Hellebore is made from the roots and sold as a dry powder. Only potent when fresh, it is rather pricey, but can be used on ripening fruit and vegetables.

It is a slow stomach poison for insects and especially useful against currant worms, and chewing insects like beetles, caterpillars, grubs, cutworms, and grasshoppers. It is usually mixed with flour or hydrated lime and used as a dust, or mixed with water as a spray.

MEDICINAL

CONSTITUENTS- *A. vernalis* leaf- cardiac glycosides of cardenolid type (0.2-0.5%) related to digitalin: adonidoside, adonivernoside, adonivernith, cymarin, ribitol, 16-hydroxy-strophanthidin, and adonitoxin; as well as 2,6-dimethoxybenzoquinone.
Various water-soluble polysaccharides include D-glucose, D-galactose, L-arabinose, D-xylose, L-ribose, and L-rhamnose.
Seeds have greater amount of glycosides.
root- vernadin, a coumarin derivative.
A. aleppica- various cardenolide oligoglycosides including alepposides, and adoligoses, consisting of rare didesoxy sugar. Spring Adonis is toxic, so be extremely careful.
A. amurensis- cymarin (which hydrolyzes into cymarose and cymarigenin), adonin, adonitoxin.

Adonis vernalis is used in several commercial German preparations for heart complaints and low blood pressure. Bechterew's Mixture, a Russian formulation for heart conditions of nervous origin, contains the herb.

The herb is used for cardiac insufficiency, irregular or rapid heartbeat, mitral stenosis and edema related to heart failure.

Perhaps best stated, it is a cardiac sedative. The action of the herb does not last long, has an absorption rate of 15-37%; and is primarily excreted via the kidneys.

Dr. Weiss rated Adonis more of a cardiac sedative than Lily of the valley, which is high praise indeed. He recommended it be used in functional heart disorders, with nervous tachycardia, extra systoles and in post-infectious cardiac debility.

Dr. Bastyr suggested Adonis for cardiac incompetence, shallow electro-cardiogram, poor amulation, dyspnea, and fluid retention with albuminuria present.

The herb is used in cases of asthma where there is cardiac weakness and in other neuro-circulatory asthenia.

Animal tests have shown that *Adonis sibir,* whose glucoside composition is similar to *A. vernalis*, exerts cardiotonic, diuretic and sedative action.

Studies conducted in Russia by Maksiutova et al, *Farmakol Toksikol* 1978 41:2 223-6 found activity of *A. sibir* meets requirements of *State Pharmacopoeia X* for *A. vernalis*.

In fact, by comparison, the Siberian species displays more pronounced sedative properties, is less cumulative, is absorbed at a slower rate, and produces a greater slowing down of the cardiac rhythm.

Unlike Digitalis, the effect on the heart is slightly sedative, and used where the patient's heart is beating too fast or irregularly. It stimulates the vagus nerve and increases the contractibility and work output of the heart, but is more toning than stimulating in quality.

In certain cases, it can be used in treating constitutional low blood pressure, but not conditions of a toxic or infectious origin. These patients are usually asthenic with myocardial weakness, and in need of motor stimulation and at the same time sedation of the autonomic nervous system. The diastolic is shortened, with venous fullness and stasis, and a feeble, irregular, intermittent pulse.

For functional heart problems, it combines well with lily of the valley, or hawthorn, depending upon the whole picture person. It combines well with motherwort in cases of high heartbeat, and with astragalus root in cases of myocardial inflammation associated with cox-sackie viral infections.

False hellebore is strongly diuretic and can be useful in pulmonary edema, and other poor circulatory function.

Note that the composition of chemicals is complex. The chief active constituent is cymarin, which can be hydrolyzed to K-strophantidin and D-cymarose. It occurs alongside adonitoxin, which yields L-rhamnose and adonitoxigenin.

Cymarin has a direct action on the heart, causes contractions and acts through control of the vagus nerves. It dilates coronary blood vessels to increase blood flow.

Cardenolides are interesting steroidal compounds. They are chiefly recognized as cardiac glycosides used to treat congestive heart failure. At low levels they show cytotoxic activity against human cancer cell lines.

The 2,6-dimethoxybenzoquinone, that is present in aerial parts of *A. vernalis*, and wheat, has been found cytotoxic, *in vitro*, against P388 lymphatic leukemic cells.

Adonivernith is present in Green Foxtail (*Setaria italica*) as well.

Amur Adonis (*A. amurensis*) is used in Traditional Chinese Medicine and known as **PIN LIANG HUA,** or **FU SHE TSAO**.

A local medical clinic in northeastern China has found the plant has therapeutic effect on rheumatic heart diseases, particularly those resistant to digitalis.

The plant extracts are quick acting and have low toxicity. They act through control of the vagus nerve, in some unspecified manner. In one study, water extracts, tincture and powder were prepared as heart stimulants, strengthening the contraction of the heart muscles and possibly dilating the coronary artery.

In 32 cases of varying forms of cardiovascular problems in patients ranging from 16-51 years of age, 34% showed positive effects in three days, 56% in one week and 9% showed no effect after the week. In 29 cases, edema was a concern, and in 14 this was reduced or disappeared. The plant is effective as a diuretic and tranquilizing agent.

Those interested in the pharmacognosy and clinical use can look up an article by Fu Xiang et al, *Journal of Plant Resources and Environment* 1995 4:3.

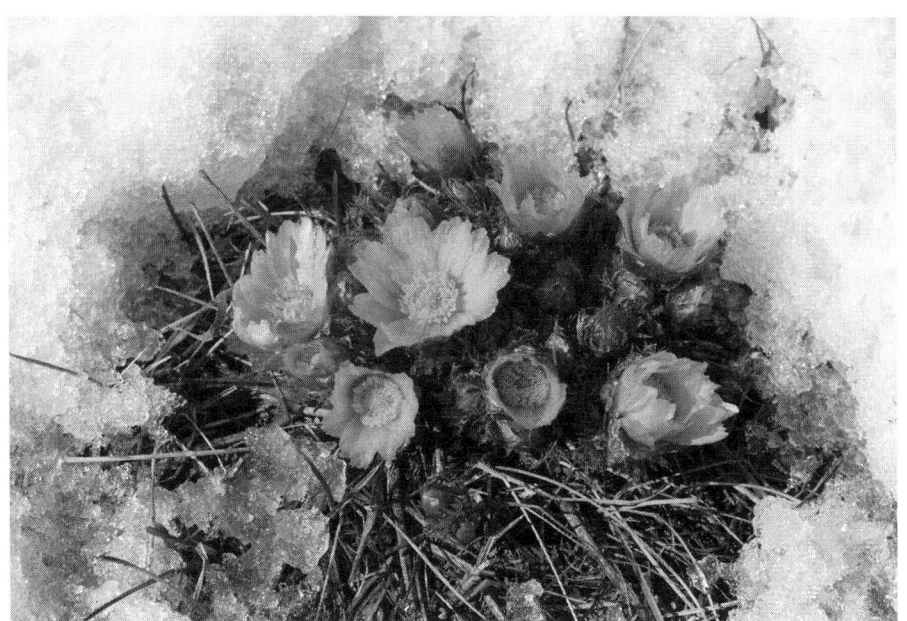
Adonis vernalis

The roots contain pregnane tetraglycosides that show activity against HSC-2 human oral squamous cancer cell lines. Kuroda et al, *Steroids* 2010 75:1 83-94.

The leaves of *A. mongolica* contain olitoriside and gluco-olitoriside.

HOMEOPATHY

Adonis vernalis has action similar to digitalis, without the cumulative effects. It is useful in arrhythmia, endocarditis, and even rheumatism with cardiac involvement.

In the heart, sensations of pressure, palpitations, pain, anxiety and gulping for breath are all noted. There may be a pressure towards the sternum, pulse can be changeable, or irregular. Pains in the left arm with crawling sensation should be noted.

It should be considered in conditions of fatty degeneration of the heart, cardiac dropsy, and Bright's disease.

There may be irritability, difficulty in falling asleep, or restlessness with terrifying dreams.

In the evening, coughing and violent left sided headaches, may accompany cold hands and feet, with heat in the head and perspiration.

Spinal irritation is present with pain in the nape of the neck, back and sacrum; and stiffness along whole length of spine. The left arm and shoulder have pain, and the left elbow has pain producing loss of sensation in the hands.

There may be sensation of nausea and periodic shooting pains in the upper abdomen. The urine is increased, with stabbing pain, strong urging, and in women a feeling of heaviness in lower abdomen.

The auditory muscle is energized. Exothalmic goiter may be involved.

It may be tried in Parkinson's disease, if some of the above symptoms also fit.

DOSE-5-10 drops of the mother tincture.

The mother tincture is prepared from the fresh flowering plant, without the roots. Use the 30X potency for dyspnea.

Adonidin is a cardiac tonic and diuretic. It helps to increase arterial pressure, and prolongs the diastolic, thus favoring an emptying of engorged veins. It is an excellent substitute for Digitalis, and is not cumulative in action.

DOSE- One-quarter grain; or two to five grains of 1x dilution.

MYTHS AND LEGENDS

Adonis is a handsome youth in Greek myths who spent half the year above ground, and then plunged into the underworld during winter.

Adonis was borrowed by the Greeks via Asian and Middle Eastern fertility myths.

Akkadian Adon Tammuz was the lord of agriculture. He represented a spirit of vegetation that is born and dies, and is born again the next spring.

Adonis personifies the cycle of the year, and the changing seasons.

The Rite of Adonis involved the carrying of effigies of dead youth by mourning women.

The Gardens of Adonis were ancient Greek vases and crocks filled with plants and placed by doorways, or rooftops.

Adonis was personalized by the Greeks. Instead of vegetation gods appearing and disappearing, the Greeks came to see Adonis as a handsome youth loved equally by two powerful Goddesses. Aphrodite, the goddess of earthly love enjoyed Adonis for the spring and fall.

Persephone, love goddess of the underworld, claimed him for fall and winter.

Ares, the Greek God of War, was jealous of Aphrodite's love of the young Adonis. He disguised himself as a wild boar and gored Adonis to death. As he is dying, blood soaked nearby flowers and stained the blossoms of *A. annua* red.

Of course, our Adonis is yellow, but who am I to ruin such a good story with logic.

ASTROLOGY

The pheasant's eye is the only buttercup species that forms a genuine calyx, from which a radiant corolla emerges. Unlike the buttercup, it has real petals, which is the annual species that flower in summer— *Adonis flammeus* and *Adonis aestrivalis*—form a five-parted corolla and thus manifest Venus in their perfect form.   **KRANICH**

RECIPES

FLUID EXTRACT- 1-2 drops as needed.

TINCTURE- 3-6 drops as needed. The tincture is made from the fresh aerial plant in full flower at 1:4 and 60% alcohol. Combine in equal parts with Lily of the valley and valerian root for functional heart disorders.

Felter suggested ten drops in four ounces of water, and take one teaspoon every two hours. British law restricts plant use to 100 milligrams at one time, and 300 milligrams as maximum daily.

INFUSION- Seven grams of herb to one pint of boiling water. Steep. Strain. Give one tablespoon every three hours.

CAPSULES- 60-300 mg twice daily. Maximum dose is one gram single dose and no more than 3 grams daily. Oral overdose can cause vomiting, nausea and palpitations.

INSECTICIDE- One ounce to two gallons of water as a spray for insects.

CAUTION- Small doses can cause cardiac paralysis. If poisoned use activated charcoal, a cathartic; and follow with atropine to restore arterial activity and raise heart rate at dosage of 0.6 mg IV for adults, 0.05 mg/kg/dose IV for children. Hyperkalemia should be monitored and treated with Kayerlate (R), or glucose and insulin.

Individuals taking Digoxin should avoid Adonis. It may interact with Lasix and other diuretics, laxatives, quinidine, and prednisone.

YARROW
(***Achillea millefolium*** L.)
(*A. millefolium ssp. millefolium*)
(*A. millefolium ssp. lanulosa* Nutt.)
(*A. millefolium ssp. borealis* Bong.)
SIBERIAN YARROW
MANY-FLOWERED YARROW
(*A. sibirica* Ledeb.)
(*A. multiflora*)
(*A. borealis* Bong.)
PINK YARROW
(*A. millefolium var occidentalis*)
(*A. millefolium var. rubra*)
(*A. millefolium f. rosea*)
GOLDEN YARROW
YELLOW YARROW
(*A. clytedata* Sibth & Sm.)
PARTS USED- leaves, flowers, root, stalks
Yarrow away, yarrow away, bear a little blow?
If my lover loves me, my nose will bleed now.   **OLD SAYING**

Thou pretty herb of Venus' tree,
They true name is Yarrow,
Now who my bosom friend must be,
Pray tell thou me to-morrow.   **ENGLISH POEM**

"I ate of Qeisun (Yarrow) when they left us, I found it sweet, but the parting bitterness not to be borne".
    PALESTINIAN FUNERAL SONG

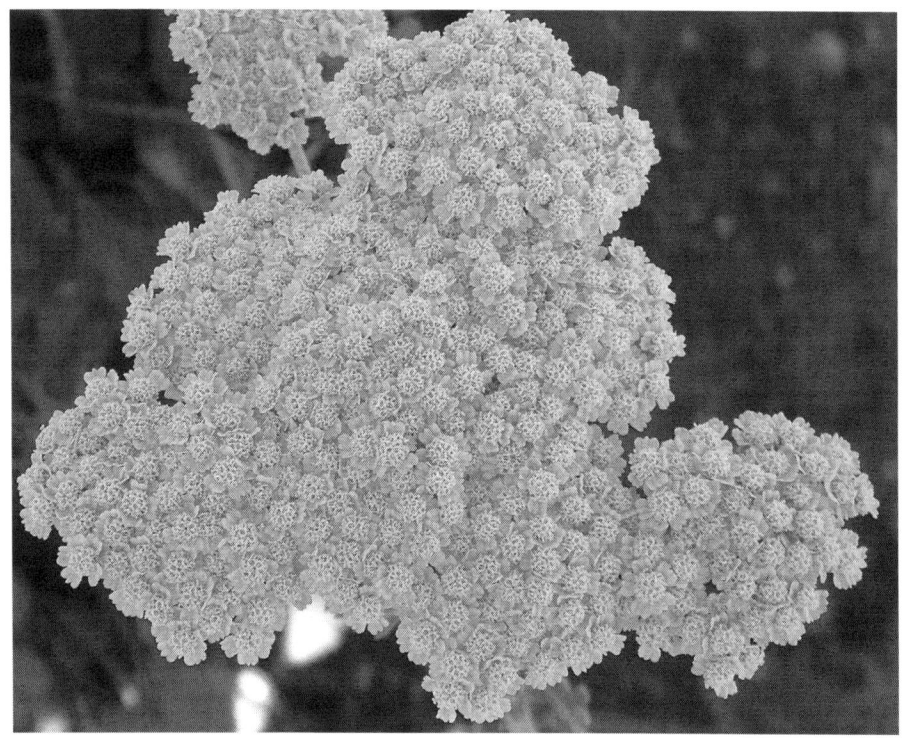

Golden Yarrow

Achillea is named in honour of Achilles, who used yarrow to heal his soldier's wounds. Or it may be named after Achilles, a Greek doctor who recorded the medicinal uses of the plant. Achilles was dipped into the river Styx, by his mother/goddess Thetis, to coat and protect his body with a magic shield. Paris learned of this during the Trojan War, and shot an arrow into his heel, the only vulnerable part of his body. Don't you just hate that!

Millefolium (myllophullon) is from the Latin, meaning thousand-leaved, and refers to the lacy leaf structure.

Yarrow is believed derived from the Dutch **YEWR**, the German **GARWE,** or Anglo-Saxon *GEARWE*, "to repair", or prepare. It may derive from **HIERA**, meaning Holy Herb.

The Druids used yarrow stems to divine seasonal weather. One ancient Gaelic name is **ATHAIR THALMHAINN** meaning earth/ground father.

Kathleen Wilkinson, in her excellent Wildflowers of Alberta, suggests yarrow is derived from the name of a Scottish parish. We can surmise this was much later.

In medieval manuscripts it shows under the name **SUPERCILIUM VERNERIS**, the eyebrow of Venus, suggestive of benefit to women's health, and affairs of the heart. It is dedicated to the spilling of blood in honor of Mars, god of war, but also predicts the favors of Venus, goddess of love.

Yarrow is a common native/introduced circumpolar perennial.

Like the leaf reference, yarrow has a thousand uses.

Fifty stalks, stripped of leaves and dried, have been used for thousands of years for casting the I Ching, or Chinese Book of Changes.

Originally, the stalks would be passed through incensed smoke, and the participant would face south, and repeat the question many times before casting.

Dioscorides suggested yarrow be made into a suppository with wool and inserted vaginally to slow down excessive menstrual bleeding. If you look carefully, you will see the stalks streaked with red, looking like venous or arterial blood.

In 16th century Germany, the seeds were added to wine barrels as a preservative. It is well known that yarrow excretes into the soil a toxin that restricts it's own growth. In 1891, Frank Bolles wrote "The Yarrow: As disagreeable among flowers as a cynic is among men".

A field of yarrow in flower on a hot day is very strong scented, making one feel somewhat delirious. In England, the name yarrow was given to men who were too talkative or boastful.

This same property is used in compost to increase the breakdown of plant material. Throw a handful of yarrow into your compost every week. Sometimes, yarrow is planted among other plants to increase their resistance to disease; or made into an insecticide spray.

The leaves are spicy, and have been substituted for nutmeg, cinnamon and pepper. The sharp flavour was also used in many countries in beer, and often preferred over hops. Field Hop was another name.

Yarrow seed was traditionally added to wine for flavour and preservation.

A flower extract is used today in one brand of soft drink.

The fresh leaves are used in a German dish called **GRÜNDONNERSTAG SUPPE**.

It is one of the nine green herbs eaten in spring as a folk food.

Linnaeus called the plant **GALENTARA**, causing madness, "stirring up the blood, and makes one lose balance".

In anthroposophic terms, the content of sulphur was fortuitous. "The spirit moistens its finger with sulfur in order to work in the physical world".

On the Isle of Skye, the herb was boiled together with quartz in milk for consumption.

Yarrow, however, grows where the earth's energy is moving downward, a natural grounding spot, for meditation and stone circles. The herb has been found in 60,000 year old gravesites in northern Mesopotamia, in digs directed by Ralph Solecki.

The Swiss flavour vinegar with the flowers for added zest; and in bitters and vermouth.

Common yarrow (*A. millefolium*) is introduced or circumpolar, while Many Flowered Yarrow is native. They may be used interchangeably.

Russell Willier of Sucker Creek, a native Cree medicine man, calls yarrow, Morning Flower. He uses the flower for bee sting, to soothe the area and draw out the venom.

Traditionally, the Cree call yarrow, **WAPANEW-USKWA**, or "bee plant". The entire plant was used in cold water for burns, and earache. Hot infusions were given to promote menstruation, relieve stomach pain, and control tuberculosis fevers. Around Lesser Slave Lake, the leaves are infused for treating late onset diabetes.

The Wood Cree call it **KA-WAPISTIKWANIKAPAT**. They used the dried flowers to disguise the scent of traps used for lynx. Yarrow flower tea, or better yet, the fresh root was rubbed into the gums to relieve teething pain. Cree from different locations have a various names for yarrow.

WAPANOWASK, meaning "white flower"; **ASTAWESKOTAWAN**, meaning "to put out a campfire", or burning pain; **MISKIGONIMASKI**, meaning Heart Medicine; **MISTIGONIMAS-KIGAH**, Head Medicine, and **OSGUNIM-ASGIGAH**, for Bone Medicine; are all variations. Another Cree name is **AMOWASK**.

Bone Medicine refers to the use in arthritic baths or applied as poultice on affected areas. The Métis refer to the plant as **LARBADEN** or **KÂ-WÂPISCIKWÂNIYÂSIKI**.

Distinction between *A. millefolium* and *A. sibirica* is seldom noted, with similar uses for both. The Chipewyan of northern Alberta used yarrow, or **T'ANCHAY DELGAI**, "holy flower", in bundles on hot rocks for inhalation to treat lung conditions.

In Alaska, the Dena'ina used Northern Yarrow (*A. borealis*) for sore eyes and skin. It was given to new mothers for internal cleansing, and for kidney and bedwetting problems. The flowers were gently steamed and the rich vapors inhaled for stuffed sinuses. The Chugach of the Kenai Peninsula used a tea internally for measles and other eruptive diseases.

The Wet'suwet'en decocted **BI'IL YESONE** as a skin wash to treat itching.

The Blood chewed the flowers for swollen glands, and decocted a stronger tea from the stems only was used for liver sickness, sore throats, and reducing the pain of childbirth. They referred to the plant as "Having a Pine Stem".

The neighboring Blackfoot drank a whole plant tea as a laxative; while the leaves and flowers only were used for tuberculosis, headaches and digestive troubles. For headache, the fresh plant may be poulticed and applied to the neck and temples.

Many tribes chewed the root for toothache, or dried the flowers for smoking mixtures. The dried flowers are also added to lynx bait. The Flathead of Montana rubbed the flower underarms as a natural deodorant.

The Thompson of British Columbia call it "little soak root" or "little chipmunk tail", and used the plant for many of the same ailments as above. The Makah used yarrow for childbirth, the Nuxalk for bronchitis, and the Saanich to stop bleeding.

Further east, the Iroquois combined it with Dock (*Rumex* species) as a cold decoction for treating diarrhea, and with Meadowsweet species for nausea. The Chippewa call it Squirrel Tail, or **ADJID AMO-WAMO**. An Ojibwa name is **WA'BIG WUN**.

The Crow call it Chipmunk Tail or **CHIBAAPOOSHCHISHGOTA**, due to resemblance of first year leaves with drooping top.

The Forest Potawatomi name is **NOKWE'SIKÛN** or perfume reviver. The herb was placed on coals to revive patients and keep evil spirits away.

The Prairie Potawatomi name is **KÎSHKATOA'SOANÛK** meaning flying squirrel tail.

One Onondaga name means "looking like frosty or cold weather", in reference to the flower appearance.

The Spanish name in the American Southwest also alludes to the fine, soft leaves, **PLUMAJILLO**, meaning little feather.

Another Spanish name **YERBA MUELA** means "molar tooth herb", suggesting its use for toothache.

The Navaho drank an aphrodisiac tea or chewed the raw yarrow stem several hours before sex.

The Ute tribe name means wound plant, similar to the Woundwort from medieval Europe. Likewise, the Lakota call it **TAOPI PEJUTA** meaning, "wound medicine".

The Osage name is **WETSA8IND-SEEGON**.

Early Ukrainian settlers used infusions as a wash for vaginal yeast infections.

Maurice Mésséque, the famous French herbalist, called yarrow, "the iodine of the meadows and fields", and "as a specific for wounds, its praise is justified, it is not exaggeration to say it is a panacea for sores, ulcers, bruises, and minor hemorrhages such as nosebleeds. Less well-known as an antiseptic, it stops infection as well."

In Brazil, yarrow is used for toothaches, hemorrhoids and rheumatism. Italians use the fresh juice for varicose veins, and applied to sore nipples. In the Orkney Islands of northern Scotland, the tea is often given to those suffering melancholy, and in Germany, the beer for its mood elevating properties.

Dr. Ellingwood, one of the great Eclectic Physicians, wrote that Dr. Cole noted when there is raised temperature, Achillea has a diaphoretic effect, but when normal temperature, it has a diuretic activity. Ellingwood also noted in intermittent or bilious fevers, yarrow causes profuse sweating that actually stains bed sheets.

The herb was widely used in Europe and North America, and later in China. The aerial parts are known as **YANG SHI CAO**, and used to clear exterior wind, tonify deficiency and clear Heart phlegm associated with high blood pressure and cholesterol.

The acrid and cooling nature of yarrow helps resolve wind papules, and clears and dispels heat from the upper burner. The bitter, acrid property helps drain liver fire and relieve depression. It also relaxes sinews and muscle that are painful due to heat and obstruction, such as rheumatic arthritis.

The strong bitter and cooling nature, taken in cold water, or as a cold infusion is best for promoting urination.

Traditional Chinese Medicine uses Siberian Yarrow (*A. sibirica*) for stomach ulcers, amenorrhea, abdominal cramps, abscesses, bleeding and to reduce inflammation.

It goes by many names such as Sky Flying Centipede, or **FEI-T'IEN WU-SUNG**; Centipede Grass, **WU-SUNG TS'AO**; or Unkempt Hair, **LUAN-T'OUFA**.

Facial steams made from the fresh or dried flower heads are good for oily skin. The infused tea is a stimulating hair tonic that can be poured on and rubbed in well as a final rinse.

Hildegard, the 14th century Abbess, recommended that all patients undergoing cancer operations do so under the protection of yarrow. For three days before, and eight days after take yarrow powder, and "metastases almost never develops, and the wound heals smoothly and quickly without infection".

Other herbalists disagree, claiming yarrow encourages circulation in smaller veins and capillaries, and may help feed tumours and cancers already present. The latter is highly unlikely.

Hildegard also recommended two parts yarrow and one part fennel in a summer insomnia poultice placed on the temple and head.

Maria Treben wrote "yarrow works on the bone marrow and thus stimulates blood renewal is not well known."

Root and flower extracts are highly prized in cosmetics for anti-inflammatory and anti-wrinkle action. It is even said to prevent baldness if washed with plant decoctions.

Seventeen plant patents are filed for yarrow, ranging from cosmetics, shampoos and mouth care products; to anti-tumour agents.

A recently excavated grave near Shanidar in modern Iran, held the pollen grains of eight medicinal plants- yarrow among them- to accompany the dead on their journey.

Yarrow contains some highly unsaturated amides with insecticidal properties. The compound, pellitorine (N-(2-methylpropl) -(e, E)-2,4-decadienamide) from the leaves has been found at five parts per million to kill 98% of mosquito larvae. *J of Chem Ecol* 1980 6.

Work by Tunón et al, *Economic Botany* 1994 48:2 found ethanol extracts of the plant a good mosquito repellant. Further fractionation identified several compounds with activity similar in activity levels to toxic Deet.

Work in Hungary shows that chamazulene has excellent phyto-toxic activity against weeds such as lamb's quarters, thistles, sow thistle and chickweed.

Yarrow leaf steeped in warm water for several days, make an excellent protective spray against damping off by mildew, and copper rich water for fertilizing.

The Alberta Research Council recommends yarrow as a native reclamation plant.

The plant produces small seed (5.5-6.0 million per kilogram) that is often part of seed mixtures. Early experiments conducted by Frank Burcik in Leadville, Colorado indicate that yarrow may also be an excellent plant for phyto-extraction of heavy metals. Recent work suggests it hyper-accumulates cadmium.

Given the value of the essential oil (see below), it could probably be grown as a single crop on some waste and restoration sites; for both soil stability and essential oil production. Yarrow is said to increase the essential oil content of other plants grown among them.

Yarrow grows easily from seed, and competes well with weeds, after first year. If planted in rows two to three feet apart, you can pull small machinery through. Do not expect much of a harvest the first year, but after that you have a hardy perennial crop. The seeds should be stratified for a month before sowing, and even then a rate of 70% is high. Germination occurs in one to two weeks, thin to one foot apart.

Yarrow is extremely variable in chemical composition. Consistency of chamazulene content in essential oil is needed to compete in the aromatherapy world. Yarrow is influenced by warm and sunshine, with greater intensity of taste associated with higher levels of sunshine. Northern Alberta, for example, with 16-20 hour days in June and July, is a great environment to grow high quality herbs.

Rudolf Steiner used yarrow in his compost preparation that he referred to as geographic medicine, or forces for balancing earthly and cosmic energy. Steiner, of anthroposophic fame, called yarrow a "true marvel in the plant world", due to its ability to balance sulphur and salts. See recipe below.

The various colored hybrids in gardens contain no medicinal value.

When ill, sheep seek out yarrow as medicine. Work by Grela et al, *Zootechnica* 2000 18 looked at a mixture of yarrow, nettle, garlic, juniper berry, plantain, and couch grass root as a feed supplement to growing pigs. The herb mixture not only matched the growth rate of commercial probiotics, but increased polyenoic fatty acids content in back fat and decreased the LDL serum levels of the finishing pigs.

Polish studies on chickens fed yarrow, nettle, and St. John's Wort water extracts showed yarrow increased body fat, nettle produced the leanest bird, and the latter herb produced the best quality meat.

In another study involving young chickens, it was found that yarrow and other herbs increased hemoglobin and leukocyte counts.

And in cows aged 3-12 years with various degrees of endometrititis, an herbal uterine infusion with yarrow and other herbs resulted in higher and quicker pregnancy rates than those treated with penicillin, nystatin, DES, vitamin A and E.

Bears seek out yarrow for maintaining good health.

Yarrow and sage make a good electrolyte tea for people or horses suffering heat stroke. It is served at room temperature and taken slowly in small sips.

Yarrow is also useful to racehorses suffering from hemorrhagic pulmonary edema, from overly strenuous workouts.

Yarrow can also be smudged and inhaled for those suffering lung problems involving bleeding. If the smoke is irritating, simply steam with the herb and boiling water under towel.

The powdered flowers kill tick larvae in less than an hour. The fresh herb juice can be applied to livestock coats as protection from flies, and other insects.

Yarrow water extract is a significant anthelmintic for parasite infections in ruminants. Tariq et al, *J Helminthol* 2008 82:3.

Sneezewort (*A. ptarmica*) has a leaf pattern that conforms exactly to the Fibonacci sequence. This 13th century mathematician found the numerical sequence generated by the so-called "golden ratio" or Phi from the twenty-first letter of the alphabet.

The golden ratio (numerically approximately 1.618034...) is the foundation of organic harmony, beauty and balance found in nature.

Cosmos, sunflowers, and daisies follow the geometric pattern known as the golden ratio spiral, as do cacti and butterfly wings. Even the overtones generated by the full spectrum harmonic sounds of ocean waves and wind exhibit the same golden ratio.

The sequence of numbers is the sum of the two preceding (1,1,2,3,5,8,13, 21,34, etc), and governs much of early Greek art and architecture. The so-called Fibonacci numbers ratio to each other all come very close to the golden ratio or mean.

Fibonacci is a contraction of **FILIUS**, meaning "son of", and **BONACCIO**, his family name. Another name was Leonardo Pisano, as he lived in Pisa, famous for a leaning tower, or Leonardo Bigollo, which means either a traveler or good-for-nothing.

Fibonacci, as he came to be known, introduced the Hindu Arabic numbering system to Europe, and published the *Book of Calculating* in 1202 AD. He proposed a problem for his readers to practice. "A pair of rabbits are put in a field, and if rabbits take a month to become mature and then produce a new pair every month after that, how many pairs will there be in twelve month's time?" The answer, assuming none die, is a series of numbers that is the sum of the previous two.

A 19th century French mathematician Edouard Lucas saw the importance of his work and named them Fibonacci numbers.

If you divide each number by the one preceding it, the answer is always the same- 1.618, the golden number or golden mean. It is interesting that in a floral spiral, each neighbor is positioned approximately 0.618 of a turn from the preceding one, so if you go from the centre to the outside there are 1.618 florets per complete turn of the spiral.

This spiral is found throughout nature, including pine cones, sunflowers, and the Tai Chi symbol of TCM.

MEDICINAL

CONSTITUENTS-149 constituents such as the alkaloid achillein, numerous sesquiterpene lactones including, achillicin (0.05%) millifin, estafiatin, leucomisin, axillarin, artecanin, and balchanolide; thujone; apigenin; luteolin, aconitic/ salicylic/ acetic/, achimillic and iso-valerianic acids, asparagin, inulin, stachydrin, (-)-betonicine, cale divian (bitter), beta-sitosterol, tannins (3-4%), campesterol, stigmasterol, alpha-amyrin, alkamides, prunasin (leaves) pontica-epoxide, rutin, rupicolin, 11,13-dehydrodeacetyl-matricin, essential oils and various alkaloids. In bloom, yarrow contains 15.2% protein (10.7% digestible), with good levels of iron (100 ppm) and manganese (71 ppm).
A. sibirica- d-camphor, desacetyl-matricarin, chamazulene.
A. filipendulina- flowers- esculetin and dihydrocoumarin.

Hot yarrow tea induces perspiration, and combines well with elderflower and wild bergamot or wild mint for breaking fevers in both young and old. The tea helps resolve childhood ailments like the mumps, measles and chickenpox, by encouraging faster eruption, and thereby relieving the itch.

A hot bath, followed with a cup or two of hot infused yarrow leaves and flowers, will induce sweating and break the first signs of colds and flu.

Even inhaling the vapors will clear stuffed sinus. In Norway, a body liniment with yarrow as a main ingredient is used for these purposes.

For hot, inflamed lungs with excessive mucus, combine with Scullcap and pleurisy root. Work by Raju et al, *Arch Appl Sci Res* 2009 1:2 suggests yarrow is useful for asthmatic conditions.

The fresh leaves can be chewed for inflamed gums, toothache, even rolled up and inserted into the nostrils to stop nosebleeds.

Chewed leaves relieve spider bites, bee and wasp stings,

The root is also analgesic, and chewed on for tooth pain. Jeremy Ross mentions chewing the fresh leaves to reduce effects of altitude, sunstroke and dehydration, as well as help concentration and memory.

A cooled infusion applied externally will relieve severe sunburn and dry, scaled and irritated eczema.

The leaves can be dried and powdered as an excellent styptic with mildly antiseptic, analgesic, astringent and hemostatic activity. It can be sprinkled on open wounds, especially the shallow scrapes, burns and popped blisters.

The powder has enough anti-infective action to use as a binding agent with the yellow serum leaking from shallow wounds. This helps form a dark, hard scab that protects from infections and contact destruction.

The alkamines, also found in Echinacea, may help to reduce inflammation. Muller-Jakic et al, *Planta Medica* 1994:60.

This includes reduction of vascular inflammation, noted in work by Dall'Acqua et al, *J Ethnopharm* 2011 18:12 1031-6.

Matrin, for example, is a proprionic acid analogue that yields chamazulene carboxylic acid. This compound is a COX 2 inhibitor with activity similar to ibuprofen.

Yarrow is a universal regulator of the female reproductive system. For amenorrhea, irregular menstruation, or to calm the hot flushing of peri-menopause, yarrow and it's mildly progesterone influence has few equals. Take cold to prevent aggravating night sweats or hot flushes. Yarrow was at one time considered to cause temporary sterility, and in mice studies yarrow extracts show anti-spermatogenic action.

Inflammation of the ovaries, prolapsed uterus, fibroids and numerous spasmodic pelvic conditions respond to yarrow sitz baths, combined with internal use. It also helps decrease the length of heavy menstrual bleeding, shortening it by two to four days. It combines with Shepherd's Purse for excessive menstruation, or blood in the urine or stool. More specifically however, yarrow is for hemorrhage with bright, red blood; whereas dark, coagulated blood is best served with shepherd's purse. Therefore, consider the type of flow during period. Uva ursi may be added for severe pain associated with strangury.

Yarrow is a useful pelvic decongestant for use in cervicitis, uterine fibroids and endometriosis. This fits in with the theory that yarrow's main action is on connective tissue of the venous system. Combine yarrow and hawthorn for those individuals suffering blue veins on the hands and feet, especially in the elderly.

Matthew Wood has found that yarrow counters the hot flashes associated with the use of the cancer drug Tamoxifen.

Work by Innocenti et al, *J Phytomed* 14:2-3 found apigenin and luteolin activate alpha and beta estrogen receptor sites.

Yarrow has been used traditionally for stimulating uterine contractions associated with abortifacient activity. One strange rat study fed 56 times the daily human dose to pregnant animals and found it reduced fetal weight and increased placental weight. The authors concluded that the dose used was not materno-toxic, with no increase in pre- or post-implantation losses suggesting yarrow was neither abortifacient nor contraceptive. IN RATS! Boswell-Ruys et al, *Birth Defects Res B Dev Reprod Toxicol* 2003 68:5.

It has an interesting blend of bitter and sweet, making it useful for numerous digestive conditions, including anorexia nervosa. It both aids digestion, and stimulates appetite. This may be due to the flavonoids that help the body produce prostaglandins that control smooth muscle contractions, and thereby provide relief, and cure from gastrointestinal distress, such as Crohn's disease, diverticulitis and ulcerative colitis.

Recent work suggests water extracts of yarrow reduce the capacity of dendritic cells to induce Th17 response, suggesting a damping down of immune pro-inflammatory response and possible use of the herb in rheumatoid arthritis, multiple sclerosis, asthma and irritable bowel diseases. Jonsdottir et al, *J Ethnopharm* 136:1. See Astragalus in Immune book regarding balance of Th1 and Th2, and role of Th17 in both.

In France, it is used for gallstones; while Russian herbalist have used it mainly for gastric ulcers, inflammation, colds and coughs. Apigenin, for example, is anti-spasmodic.

The German name **BAUCHWEHKRAUT** means "belly ache weed".

Work by Benedek et al, *J Phytomed* 13:9-10 found a 20% alcohol extract stimulates bile flow, thus suggesting choloretic effect. This is more due to the content of di-caffeoy-quinic acid. Further work by the author suggests inhibition of elastase for skin health.

Warm decoctions in the morning on an empty stomach are for digestive toning and appetite, and cold infusions for those convalescing from night sweats, fevers and nervous exhaustion. The herb is cold and dry, but its actions are modified by temperature of preparation. Cold and dry are symptoms of the melancholic temperament, which yarrow can help to balance.

And although mainly a liver herb, it is useful in both acute and chronic rheumatic and neuralgic complaints, due in part to salicylic acid and other compounds.

According to Sama et al, in 1976, yarrow constitutes one of the components in a LIV 52, used in the therapy of acute viral hepatitis.

Yarrow is used extensively in Ayurvedic medicine, and known as **GANDANA**. Yarrow has been used in Europe in the treatment of chronic hepatitis. Harnyk, *Lik Sprava* 1999:7-8.

Yarrow tincture can be diluted with water for external treatment of varicose veins and bleeding hemorrhoids by encouraging better circulation to the smaller veins. The liniment also relives inflammation of joints, ligaments, shin splints and bone spurs.

Achillein is a nerve relaxant with an affinity to the heart, and in combination yarrow is useful for treating high blood pressure. It combines well with nettle and sweet clover for preventing cerebral and coronary thrombosis, due in part to blood thinning coumarins and salicylic acid.

Work by Yaeesh et al, *Phyto Res* 20:6 found yarrow is liver protecting due to its calcium channel blocking activity in a manner similar to verapamil.

Achillein increase the ability of the blood to clot 60% more efficiently than calcium chloride, a salt often used in allopathic medicine.

Achillein has been found to have protective properties in cases of coronary thrombosis. Work by Miller et al, *J Am Chem Soc* 1954 76 found achillein to decrease clotting times in rabbit studies, with hemostatic action persisting for 45 minutes with no toxic effect.

At the turn of the 20th century, achillein was isolated and used as a quinine substitute for malarial fevers.

Trigonelline, present as well in fenugreek seeds, helps balance blood sugar, while stachydrine and betonicine contribute hypotensive properties. Both are present in Betony species, with stachydrine specifically lowering systolic levels, and betonicine also reducing inflammation.

Armentin decreases angiotensin II and the herb as a whole reduces vascular inflammation. P. de Souza et al, *Phytomed* 18:10 819-25 and Stefano Dall'Acqua et al, *Phytomed* 18:12 1031-6.

Yarrow tea can be very helpful for those suffering hypoglycemia and the dropping of blood sugar that causes restless sleep and insomnia. A cup of tea before bedtime will help maintain blood sugar levels during the night.

Chamazulene inhibits the formation of leukotrienes that trigger inflammation.

Axillarin, found in Chamomile and some Artemisia species, possesses anti-viral activity.

It can be combined with couch grass, and goldenrod for persistent bladder infections or acute inflammation and bleeding from the kidneys; but is better to drink as a cool tea for these conditions.

Drinking several litres of cold yarrow infusions daily for up to a week will often help to dissolve and eliminate ovarian cysts.

Like many herbs, the temperature at which yarrow preparations are taken influence the activity and organ systems affected. When taken cold, the lymphatic system is more stimulated, while at body temperature the digestive and kidney influence is more noted. For flu and fever, accompanied by chills, the hot tea is more recommended.

The herb that yarrow is combined with also influences activity. For increased diaphoretic effect or circulatory stimulation use with Prickly Ash; for hemostasis, or anemia with Shepherd's Purse or Cranesbill; while for severe fever take cold in combination with Pleurisy Root.

It combines well with Elder flowers, peppermint and Boneset for fevers, and combines with Hawthorn, and Linden Blossoms, for treating hypertension. Wormwood and Yarrow are a good combination for digestive toning, while yarrow and sage are good for headache and muscle ache associated with flu. Yarrow combines well with gold thread or Oregon grape root for congestive prostatitis.

Yarrow most specifically lowers elevated diastolic blood pressure, while dandelion leaf is more useful for elevated systolic, especially in the elderly.

Externally, yarrow combines well with fireweed and Toadflax for hemorrhoid salves and boluses; and internally for varicose veins. When there is acute inflammation of the veins, use a tincture of yarrow, arnica and St. John's Wort as a topical compress.

Plaque formation and gingivitis are helped with yarrow mouth rinses. Van der Weijden et al, *J Clin Peridontol* 1998 25:5.

Recent studies have demonstrated the antibiotic properties of yarrow. Some practitioners feel that the root is superior for blood cleansing purposes; and skin conditions like acne.

Yarrow up-regulates melanocortin receptor-2, and u-opioid receptor-1, in human skin.

In vivo, a two-month treatment of 2% extract significantly improved the appearance of wrinkles and pores compared with placebo. Results were directionally better than glycolic acid. Pain S et al, *Int J Cosmet Sci* 2011 33:6.

Yarrow has been investigated in Lithuania for its possible anti-tumour activity. Studies by Tozyo et al identified three new anti-tumour sesquiterpenoids (achimillic acids) in yarrow active against mouse P-338 leukemia cells in vivo. *Chem Pharm Bulletin* 1994 42:5.

Work in Hungary by Csupor Loffler et al, *Phytother Res* 2008 23:5 identified the compound centaureidin as extremely potent against HeLa and MCF-7 cancer cell lines. The IC_{50} of the former is 0.0819 uM, and latter just 0.1250. Other compounds such as casticin and paulitin were still cytotoxic but less potent.

As a general tonic, the fresh plant juice, or frozen ice cubes of the freshly squeezed plant, can't be beat.

Recent studies in India have shown achillin fed to rabbits, almost immediately lowers their body temperature, and the alkaloids have been shown to decrease blood-clotting time.

In a double blind, randomized, crossover study of 35 patients with osteo-arthrosis, a mixture of feverfew, aspen poplar, and yarrow (2:2:1) provided the same subjective pain relief as 400 mg of ibuprofen when taken three times daily. Ryttig et al, *Ugeskrift for Laeger* 1991:153.

The anti-inflammatory activity may be due, in part, to the presence of rupicolin and 11, 13-dehydro-deacetyl-matricin. Zitterl-Eglseer et al, *Plant Medica* 1991:57.

Yarrow flowers contain 7 fractions with anti-inflammatory activity similar to indomethacin. Choudhary et al, *Nat Pro Res* 2007 21:11.

Aerial parts inhibit xanthine oxidase, suggesting use internally and cool footbaths for gout. Owen et al, *J Ethnopharm* 1999 64 149-60.

Ethanol/water extracts may be gastro-protective, due to anti-oxidant activity. Potrich et al, *J Ethnopharm* 2010 Apr 24.

Recent research suggests the anti-inflammatory properties may be due, in part, to anti-protease activity.

Dr. Gary Null mentions in his interesting book, Secrets of the Sacred White Buffalo, that yarrow tea, sweetened with honey, is beneficial for glaucoma.

Axillarin, found in both yarrow and some artemisia species has been found to reduce lens aldose reductase associated with diabetes and cataract formation. Yarrow also contains compounds that strengthen the ciliary muscles, helping improve focus and clarity of vision.

Aerial parts extracted with ethanol, methanol, as well as the essential oil, show activity against *Candida albicans*. Candan et al, *J Ethnopharm* 2003 87; Kumar et al, *J Ethnopharm* 2006 107.

You will occasionally encounter a patch of naturally occurring pink yarrow (see flower essences below). Ryan Drum, noted herbalist, believes the pink variety contains alkaloids that improve trans-cranial circulation. Susanne Fischer-Rizzi prefers the pink flowering plants for treating gynecological diseases.

Pink Yarrow was known to the Lakota, as Wound Medicine, or **TAOPI PEZUTA**.

Yarrow tinctures have an influence on mood similar to diazepam, but not mediated by $GABA_A$/BD2 neuro-transmission. Baretta et al, *J Ethnopharm* 2011 December 6.

Recent work found yarrow to inhibit acetylcholinesterase activity, suggestive of use in brain dysfunction. Mekinic IG et al, *Nat Prod Commun* 2013 8:4 471-4.

Work by Stognii et al, *Rastitel'nye-Resursy*, 2000 36:1, found high levels of low molecular weight antioxidants and/or SOD in the seeds of yarrow grown in low precipitation and high air temperatures.

The seeds of White Sweet Clover exhibit a similar pattern.

Yarrow grown at higher elevations does not appear to contain alpha and beta thujone.

A great review of yarrow is Applequist & Moerman, *Econ Botany* 2011 209-225.

HOMEOPATHY

Millefolium (Yarrow) is an invaluable remedy for various hemorrhages, where the blood is bright red, and accompanied by high temperatures. For nosebleeds, profuse menses, or bloody urine, yarrow is appropriate. There may be a cough with blood expectoration; or hemorrhoids that continue to bleed.

The head may feel full of blood, or there may be vertigo and dizziness when moving slowly. Sensations of forehead being contracted and drawing skin upward.

DOSE- Tincture to the third potency. The mother tincture is prepared from the fresh plant while in flower. Initial proving by Schreter and Nenning 1833; then Hering with four male provers as tincture and 1x in 1851; then Keil tincture 1854, then Mure, Hering, Mangialavori and Kent's Repetory.

ESSENTIAL OIL

CONSTITUENTS- *A. millefolium-* 42 constituents including various monoterpenes like limonene, germacrene, pinenes, camphene and sabinene (9-17%); sesquiterpenes like chamazulene, achilline and dihydroazulene; 1,8-cineole, bornyl acetate, achillicin, iso-artemisia ketones, p-cymene, eudesmol, (E)-nerolidol, and beta thujone. The variation is huge.
Monoterpenes make up 56-90+% of the aerial parts, in headspace studies; while the roots are 40-63% non-terpenes.
A. sibirica- beta pinene (16-32%), beta elemene (5-13%), 1,8-cineole (10-16%), germacrene A (5-13%), germacrene D (5-6%), chamazulene (7-9%), (E)-nerolidol (2.4-3.6%), carophyllene oxide (0.8-3.6%), as well as minor amounts of viridiflorol, gamma cadinene, beta bourbonene, limonene, sabinene, and terpineol.
A. lanulosa- chamazulene
A. ligustica- 96 constituents including santolina alcohol, borneol, sabinol, trans sabinyl acetate, alpha thujone, terpinen-4-ol.

The essential oil is steam distilled from the whole plant. The oil obtained from the flowers and leaves is a beautiful dark blue flower; from the stem greenish-white; and from the root- colour-less to slightly yellow. Yield averages 0.2% from the whole plant; and has a specific gravity of 0.926.

When cold, the oil has a buttery consistency, tasting similar to the plant.

Being related to chamomile, it contains chamazulene, one of the strongest anti-inflammatory plant products in the world. It is sedative, cooling, protective, and anti-allergenic for various skin disorders; unless you are one of the rare individuals allergic to the plant itself.

Although considered a minor essential oil, annual production is about 800 tonnes, with a value of $ 88 million.

Dr. Daniel Penoel feels that yarrow oil is both stimulating to the liver, is anti-catarrhal, and beneficial to the female reproductive system. It strengthens the nerves, and reduces painful neuralgia.

It is useful oil for cellulite, bleeding hemorrhoids and varicose vein therapies, combining well with an infused carrier oil like St. John's Wort, or Toadflax oil.

Use this type of mixture on sunburn, irritated skin, or as an aftershave and hair restorative. It combines well with birch leaf oil in shampoos for supporting new hair growth.

Work by Candan et al, *J Ethnopharm* 2003 87:2 found both anti-oxidant and anti-microbial activity, the latter including *Streptococcus pneumoniae, Clostridium perfringens, Candida albicans, C. krusei* and *Mycobacterium smegmatis.* Other studies indicate anti-microbial activity against *Bacillus subtilis, E. coli, Shigella sonnei* and *S. flexneri.* Sant'Anna et al, *Phytother Res* 2008 September 19, found yarrow extracts active against *Aspergillus nidulans.*

For bronchitis, and bronchial asthma, the oil can be diffused or applied as a chest rub, combining well with balsam poplar bud carrier oil. The oil exhibits both expectorating and anti-tussive properties.

During the menopausal transition, yarrow oil helps keep both physiologic and psychological balance. At this time in life, the emphasis is shifting from a caregiver and life creator, to more inward energies. Yarrow oil will help this transition.

Yarrow can be used for its soothing, warming and penetrating influence on muscles.

One study found the essential oil useful for wound healing associated with napalm burns. Popovici et al, *Rev Med* 1970 16:3-4.

Yarrow oil and rosewater combine for an excellent douche for vaginal irritations and infections. Rub into the affected areas for ovarian inflammation, or fibroids. For heavy and painful menstruation apply two drops yarrow and one drop of mint oil to the inner portion of a sanitary napkin.

Males can also benefit from the oil, as it helps reduce inflammation associated with benign prostatic hypertrophy.

The anti-inflammatory nature of oil is due to down-regulation of iNOS, COX-2, TNF-alpha, IL-6 and heme oxygenase expression. Chou ST et al, *Int J Mol Sci* 2013 14:7.

Psychologically, yarrow can be diffused throughout a room, or applied to a Kleenex and inhaled for clearing confusion, ambivalence and depression.

The oil also offers protection to those exposed to radiation; and aids those undergoing detoxification like drug and alcohol withdrawal.

The oil is less relaxing than chamomile, but has a more powerful effect upon the respiratory system.

Yarrow oil is added to cosmetics, to increase the whitening property of face creams. It is worth noting that many sub-types of *A. millefolium* contain little or no trace of azulene.

The essential oil suppresses melanin production by decreasing tyrosinase activity through regulation of the JNK and ERK signaling pathways. The potential to treat hyper-pigmentation is obvious. Peng HY et al, *PLoS One* 2014 9:4 April 17.

Proazulene levels tend to be related to the soil levels of phosphates, magnesium, and manganese.

It appears that the greater the intensity of the sun, the greater the essential oil content of the plants.

The time of year can greatly influence the scent and composition of yarrow essential oil. For example, the same fields harvested in July and September show very similar composition but different amounts. Cineole is nearly 14% in July, and only 7% in September. Beta caryophyllene is 39% in July and only 26% later. Beta bisabolene is 0.4% in July and not detectable later.

During flowering, monoterpenes like cineole dominant, while during the vegetative period, the oils are mainly sesquiterpenes, with germacrene D dominating. Oil content can vary as well, with full bloom averaging yields of 0.34%, and the vegetative stage only 0.13%.

Pink Yarrow has similar variability, with beta pinene decreasing and E nerolidol increasing with the intensity of color. In fact up to 32% nerolidol has been found in the flowers in work by Judzentiene et al, *Centr Eur J Bio* 2010 Feb 11.

Other species, such as *A. ligusta* have oil with a pale, sapphire quality, as well as *L. moschata* which is high in cineole and used to prepare the medicinal apertif, Iva liquor.

The cultivated *A. ligusta* is rich in linalool, viridifloral, beta pinene, 1,8-cineole and terpinen-4-ol. It shows inhibition of *Streptococcus mutans* and moderate activity against four cancer cell lines.

DOSE- Due to the presence of beta iso-thujone in the essential oil, it can be considered toxic at levels of 30mg/kg thujone. Do not use internally, and avoid during pregnancy, or with babies.

There appears to be a correlation between the presence of prochamazulene and the chromosome number of the plant.

Only tetraploid plants, such as *A. lanulosa* and *A. collina* contain procham-azulenes (up to 50%), while others are azulene free. Oswiecimska, *Planta Med* 1974 25.

Our true Yarrow (*A. millefolium*) is hexaploid and relatively azulene free.

Octaploid species contain monoterpenes mainly linolool, while hexaploid type contains 40-50% mono and sesquiterpenes, and no chamazulene. Kastner et al, *Sci Pharm* 1992 60:87.

Chemotyping is crucial for commercial yarrow plantations that are geared to production of quality essential oils.

Work in Norway by Rohloff et al, *J Ag Food Chem* 2000 48 looked at some of the challenges involved in production of the essential oil. They are many, but worthwhile.

FLOWER OIL

Combine one part of fresh flowers only with five parts of canola oil in a crock pot or double boiler and simmer at 115 F degrees for at least 24 hours.

This strained oil can be used for various aching muscles, or respiratory rubs, or combined with Toadflax, Fireweed and/or Agrimony plant oils for hemorrhoids and varicose veins externally.

HYDROSOL

Yarrow hydrosol is very medicinal smelling, not even that pleasant. It has a pH of 3.6-3.9, quite acidic, and is quite stable.

Like the herb, it is a good digestive tonic, if you can get past the odour.

Suzanne Catty says that animals like the smell, and the water can be used for healing skin and digestive problems.

It soothes the itching associated with eczema and psoriasis and helps promote new skin cell growth.

The distilled water can be used as a compress or in a sitz bath for hemorrhoids, cellulite or varicose veins. It also gives relief in PMS, due to mild anti-spasmodic activity.

Viaud wrote that yarrow hydrolat is useful for easing circulation problems in women.

Jeanne Rose recommends the hydrolat for acne and damaged skin.

"Distilled water of yarrow heals all internal injuries. It will dissolve clotted blood, stop excessive flower of the menses and white discharges, and kill tapeworms, provided half a gill is drunk every morning and evening. When the mouth is rinsed with yarrow water, it will heal scurvy of the gums and festers on the gums and in the throat. If a small piece of linen is moistened with yarrow water and laid warm over the privates, it will heal the injury".   **SAUER**

Yarrow water is distilled from the herb and stalk. It is useful for the heart and stomach, taken internally as well as rubbed on. It kills worms in the belly, and helps those who have lost too much blood and lack color. It is used to wash fresh wounds, and cleans and purifies the blood.   **BRUNSCHWIG**

FLOWER ESSENCES

Yarrow flower essence strengthens the light of the aura to protect against disharmony and negative environmental influence. It builds a strong psychic shield; helping protect those who take on the problems and illness of others.   **FLOWER ESSENCE SOCIETY**

Pink yarrow flower essence is for the psychic sponge that absorbs the emotional; and gives a greater sense of emotional clarity.
          FLOWER ESSENCE SOCIETY

Yarrow flower essence gives off a strong aura of protective energy. Its powerful vibration reflects that quality of our energies back to us, helping us connect more deeply with our own sources of light.
          ALASKA

Pink yarrow flower essence is for someone who identifies with the emotions of those around them to an uncomfortable extent, and lacks the boundaries to separate themselves from other's extremes.
          RUNNING FOX FARM

Golden Yarrow is for those who easily lose sense of self, or harden themselves to cope with vulnerability. The essence helps one stay open and balanced.   **FLOWER ESSENCE SOCIETY**

SPIRITUAL PROPERTIES

Yarrow offers protection from negative influences such as radioactive fallout, or psychic attack by enhancing and strengthening the aura. It stabilizes those working with the emotionally disturbed, so that they do not become too empathetic.

Yarrow balances the upper and lower poles of the body. Rudolph Steiner said that the upper pole relates to sensory and nervous activity and the lower pole to metabolism. **GURUDAS**

Yarrow is a plant that is much needed by mankind at the present time, due to its ability to release the dreaming consciousness from the lower astral regions.

Many souls are drawn to the lower astral in the dream state because of the coarse vibrations that surround them in the waking hours. The dream experience can be quite unsettling, even terrifying- particularly if the dream episodes are clearly recalled upon waking.

To use yarrow, simply cut the head off, and pour near boiling water on it to make tea. Let it cool, and then drink, just before retiring.

HILARION

Yarrow stalks for divination are best snapped off at the ground at the full moon just after most flowers are pollinated. These flower stalks are hung tied together in bundles of 11, 13, or 21, butts up, to dry, after cutting off the flower tops.

After drying, gently strip leaves from stalks; store stems as fine medicine. These active constituent loaded stalks will add clarity when used to consult the oracle (I Ching) due to palmar percutaneous perfusion of bioactive molecules. The almost two hour time period when the stalks are actually in the hands of the seeker permits both warming of the stalks and the mixing of palmar skin oils with the oil soluble resins and terpenes of the yarrow stalk surfaces. Fifty of the stalks are taken up and divided, and arranged according to an elaborate preparatory ritual.

The movement of even modestly psychoactive substances into the body through the palmar surfaces helps to calm the mind, improve peripheral circulation and enhance concentration. **RYAN DRUM**

The hardy yarrow loves dry heights. From the first its leaves are so fine and aromatic that flowers are expected, but leafing continues into high summer, culminating in the spicy umbel, which blooms well into fall. This slow development allows full absorption and maturing of the season's elements, blending earthly salt with silica and sulfur.

MURPHY

In calling on the spirit of the plant, an innocent and gentle female spirit comes floating towards me. She is very ethereal, wearing a covering of white satin pressed against her long golden hair. She carries with her a harp, very surreal and enchanting. Upon hearing the healing cries of the yarrow plant, she gracefully sets herself down upon the earth in the midst of a lush green garden. Surrounding her are beautiful plants of yarrow that immediately become hypnotized by her majestic presence.

AVENSARO

The essential oil has slightly spicy notes beneath a fresh, green, herby scent…The Chinese have also recognized its powerful spiritual qualities, which create balance between the yin and yang forces. Its sacred nature opens the recipient to intuitive perceptions. It brings about change through harmony, brings equilibrium to instability, and centers and stabilizes scattered energies. Its nature is to open the way to celestial flow, drawing in the energies of the sun, moon and stars.

CLARE GOODRICK-CLARKE

PERSONALITY TRAITS

I will pick the smooth Yarrow, that my figure may be more elegant, that my lips may be warmer, that my voice may be more cheerful; may my voice be like a sunbeam, may my lips be like the juice of the strawberries.

May I be an island in the sea, may I be a hill on the land, may I be a star when the moon wanes, may I be a staff to the weak one: I shall wound every man, no man shall wound me.

GAELIC FOLK CHARM

Whenever I come upon it in meadows or along roadsides, Yarrow always carries itself with a certain refinement. Its feathery leaves drape across the long stem like an elegant scarf swept to the side.

Yarrow holds its flower head high, always rigid and looking above the tall grass in search of people who will notice and admire it.

The other plants may think yarrow is putting on airs, but it stays resolute in its desire to be a little more educated than the other plants, and perhaps rise above its "weed" standing. Yes, if yarrow were a person, I have a feeling it would listen to Vivaldi, crave appetizers such as hearts of palm and asparagus tips, and read only the classics.

DEWEY

The warrior, no matter what his status in modern life, wants to be on the winning side. The warrior may experience resentment and anger from a wounding, whether this is the result of physical or metaphorical injury. He hates to be thought of as weak and finds it hard to heal with feelings of vulnerability. These reactions stimulate existential questioning: "Is life worth the struggle?"

Yarrow, while gently nurturing and providing protection, may bring dreams and visions, putting the individual in touch with an intuitive understanding of their illness or situation in life.

GOODRICK-CLARKE

Yarrow's keyword is determination. Yarrow encompasses two realms. It functions on the physical level as courage. When used in a tincture it manifests as the determination to push through to accomplishment.

When used as a flower essence it functions in the white realm and has to do with discernment of the truth. Yarrow functions in two dimensions; one horizontal and the other vertical. Invaluable for people who have difficulty making choices.   **EVELYN MULDERS**

The Romans believed that yarrow could be used to court the favor of Venus, the Roman goddess of love, who intervenes in affairs of the heart.

The characteristic love theme of yarrow is of the "my heart bleeds for you" variety; this type of passion is imbued with a subtle subtext of violence. A yarrow type typically sees courtship as a process of "winning her hand". In other words, love is not unlike war, because it involves tactical maneuvering and the feeling of I must have her, I cannot lose, or I will be mortally wounded. Think of yarrow for blood feuds over love. Romeo and Juliet is a play with yarrow undertones.

Yarrow oil is specific for the individual for who life is a form of combat. Love, family, career all engender battles. The yarrow type tends to be an intellectual idealist who opts for the road less traveled... The world is not kind to idealists who are willing to put it all on the line, and inevitably the yarrow type does have to fight a lot of battles and suffer many wounds.

The cumulative effect of these struggles and wounds wears the yarrow type down, and he can become debilitated and angry, bitter, melancholy and filled with self-doubt. The yarrow oil picture has the symptoms fear of heights and dreams of falling.

BRUCE BERKOWSKY

Yarrow is almost always indicated by an elongated, pointed, reddish tongue (the classic indication for heat), but with a blue undertone or middle, indicating venous stagnation. The tongue is usually dry in the center, indicating that heat is driving off fluids.   **WOOD**

Yarrow is a really nice herb at high doses for opening and relaxing the mind to make it easier to discern patterns in the world around you that were harder to see when your thoughts were whirling about.

SEAN DONAHUE

DOCTRINE OF SIGNATURES

The red colour runs in streaks up the stem. It looks like blood in veins or arteries...the whole plant is covered in fine white hairs. **BURGESS**

Yarrow is often called a warm, stimulating botanical. However, its indications actually contradict this designation. A medicinal that is bitter and acrid can be somewhat stimulating without being warming. Acridity, if sufficient in any plant, can be stimulating, as acridity has a dissipating and moving action. Even a bitter flavor can be stimulating without warming the system; in fact, it cools the system. Dissipating medicinals are Yang. However, upon closer examination, it is clear that the overall picture of yarrow is cooling due to its overwhelming bitterness and its ability to clear heat and even drain fire.

GARRAN

MYTHS AND LEGENDS

Achilles was the greatest hero of the Trojan War, and the son of Peleus and Thetis, who dipped him into the River Styx, rendering him invulnerable except in the spot where she held him, the heel.

He withdrew from the war when Agamemmnon commandeered his war prize, the young Briseis, but re-entered the conflict after Hector slew his friend Patroclus. Achilles killed Hector, and was slain by Paris, which fulfilled the prophecy that he would lead a short, heroic life. **HATHAWAY**

ASTROLOGY

"Being an herb of Dame Venus," as Culpepper quaintly puts it, the plant governs the reproductive cycle of women. Venus, the evening star and the only planet easily visible with the naked eye, is the light of this plant. It tunes the individual into balance. It also suggests that war is not always the best way to win what we want from life. Venus is love, and love can disarm the warrior.

Mars, the god of war, was the lover of Venus, goddess of love. In a beautiful painting by Sandro Botticelli called Venus and Mars (1485), a sleeping Mars is watched over by Venus, who is alert and composed. This throws light on how Venus might rule a knight's wound remedy. When the warrior is thrown back on his own resources, the light of Venus, goddess of love, is there to bring healing and peace.

GOODRICK-CLARKE

BOTANICA POETICA
If you go out to the Battlefield
As in the days of old
Put Yarrow in your knapsack
It's worth its weight in gold
Yarrow for your bleeding wound
A poultice for your knee
Or for a painless hemorrhage
You'll want to drink the tea
For diaphoresis it's the King

The stem, the leaf, the flower
Reduce your fever, sweat full fling
We're talking Yarrow power!
Achillea Millefolium
An astringent disinfectant
A urinary healer
Hemostatic and protectant
It's an aromatic bitter
If you lose your appetite
Have spasmodic ailments
Or your tummy is uptight
If it's good enough for Achilles
Of Greek Mythology
To stop his bleeding wounds
Why, it's good enough for me!
SYLVIA CHATROUX MD

Yarrow sings of fevers, of cold sores and of flus,

And to intestinal pain he certainly rues.

Songs of rashes and scratches, clean blood and short fasting,

For help with all these, Yarrow tea is quite lasting.

LALITHA THOMAS

RECIPES

INFUSION- Add one ounce of chopped leaves and flowers to one pint of boiling water, and steep twenty minutes. Drink hot for fevers, and cool for toning and digestive effect.

HOT WRAP- Place a hot, strained tea compress on stomach for 20-30 minutes to help stimulate digestion, relieve constipation, stimulate liver function, relieve depression.

TINCTURE- 2-4 ml up to three times daily. Make the tincture 1:5 at 45% alcohol from dried herb; or 1:2 at 70% with fresh plant. Latter is best. Use only flower and leaves, toss stems.

OINTMENT- Take ten ounces of fresh leaves and flowers. Crush, and add to fifty ounces of canola oil and heat very slowly for one hour.

Remove from heat and let sit overnight. In morning strain and add enough beeswax to desired texture. Clinical trials show topical ointments containing 2% extracts are not generally irritating or phototoxic.

BLACKHEADS- Soak four tablespoons of chopped yarrow in four ounces of cold milk and refrigerate overnight. Heat and strain. Bathe face in warm, enriched "milk".

FRESH JUICE- One tsp 3x daily. In some sensitive individuals, a mild skin rash may appear for a day or two.

HARVEST- The flowering tops are best gathered on cool, cloudy days, or before 9 AM on sunny days. Save the larger flower heads, which are probably polyploids with higher than average levels of psychotrophic molecules, and best used for yarrow tea. Dry them at 70-90° F for five to ten days, in shade.

NOTE- Commercial yarrow has higher content of fat and saturated fatty acids, proteins, ash, energy value, sugars and flavonoids. Wild yarrow has higher levels of carbohydrates, organic acids, unsaturated fatty acids, tocopherols and phenolic acids. The bioactivity of the alcohol, infused and decocted herb is reported by Dias et al *Food Chem* 2013 141:4. 4152-60.

BIODYNAMIC COMPOST- YARROW FLOWERS- PREPARATION 502

"Like sympathetic people in human society, who have a favourable influence by their mere presence and not be anything they have to say, so Yarrow in a district where it is plentiful works beneficially by its mere presence."

This preparation has a quickening effect on the soil, where the spiritual can penetrate into substance. The compost and the earth where it is applied are given new power. It permits the plants to attract trace elements in extremely dilute qualities for their best nutrition.

The flowers are packed into the bladder of a stag, hung in a sunny place for the summer, and buried in the ground overwinter. This preparation helps regulate the potassium and sulphur processes.

CAUTION- Should perhaps be avoided during first trimester of pregnancy due to uterine stimulation from essential oils, but this is questionable. Yarrow is probably safe throughout pregnancy. Contraindications are based on a single low quality rat study with no significance to humans. Wendy Applequist et al, *Economic Botany* 652 207-23.

The herb is probably safe for later pregnancy (if no heart problems) and during lactation, in small doses. Avoid combining with potassium supplements.

It may also interfere with anticoagulant medication (due to coumarin content); hemophiliacs and perhaps in certain cases of epilepsy. Brinker believes it may interact with antacids and gastric acid secretion inhibitors, particularly H2-receptor antagonists.

In TCM, the herb is not to be used by those with interior cold, and cautiously with Qi vacuity.

ABOUT THE AUTHOR

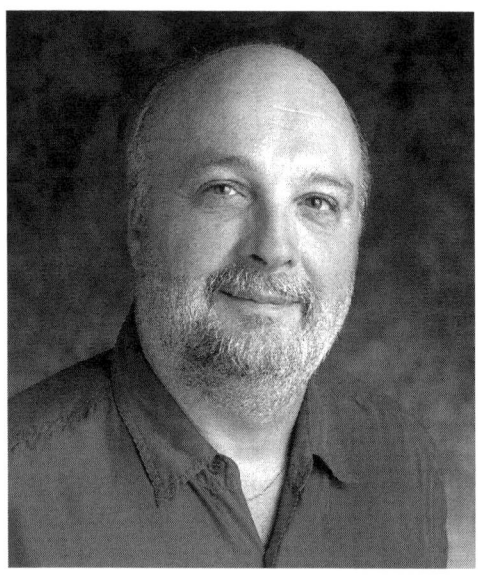

Robert Dale Rogers has been an herbalist for over forty years. He has a Bachelor of Science from the University of Alberta, where he is an assistant clinical professor in Family Medicine. He teaches plant medicine, including herbology and flower essences at Grant MacEwan University, as well as Earth Spirit Medicine at the Northern Star College of Mystical Studies in Edmonton, Alberta, Canada.

Robert is past chair of the Alberta Natural Health Agricultural Network and Community Health Council of Capital Health. He is a Fellow of the International College of Nutrition, chair of the medicinal mushroom committee of the North American Mycological Association and on the editorial board of the International Journal of Medicinal Mushrooms, and Discovery Phytomedicine.

Robert co-hosts The Alberta Herb Gathering held every second year (www.albertaherbgathering.com)

He lives on Millcreek Ravine in Edmonton with his beautiful and talented wife, Laurie Szott-Rogers and out of control cat Ceres.

You can email him at scents@telusplanet.net
or visit
www.selfhealdistributing.com

BIBLIOGRAPHY

Abbe, Elfriede, The Fern Herbal, Cornell University Press, Ithaca, 1981

Acorn, J. Bugs of Alberta, Lone Pine Publishing, Edmonton, AB, 2000.

Adams, J. Les Plantes Medicinales. Bulletin 23, Agriculture Canada. 1916

Adams, Jean. Insect Potpourri, Adventures in Entomology. Sandhill Crane Press, FL. 1992

Aggarwal, Bharat. Healing Spices. Sterling Pub. New York 2011.

Albert-Puleo, Michael. Economic Botany, 32, Jan-Mar, 1978.

Allaby, Michael. Temperate Forests. Facts on File. New York. 1999.

Allen, D & Hatfield, G. Medicinal Plants in Folk Tradition. Timber Press, Portland. 2004

Allen,E, Morrison,D, &Wallis,G. Common Tree Diseases of B.C. Canada Forest Service, '96

Allende, Isabel. Aphrodite- A Memoir of the Senses. Harper Flamingo. New York. 1998.

Alstat, Ed. Electic Dispensatory of Botanical Therapeutics. Ecl Med. Oregon. 1989.

Anderson, Anne, Some Native Herbal Remedies, Pub 8A, Devonian Botanical Gardens 1980
_____ Plants in Cree. Duval House Pub. Edmonton AB 2000.

Anderson, C.&Tischer,T. Poinsettias, the December Flower, Waters Edge Press, CA, 1997

Andoh, Anthony. The Science & Romance of Selected Herbs used in Medicine and Religious
      Ceremony. North Scale Institute. San Francisco. 1986.

Andre, Alestine & Fehr, Alan. Gwich'in Ethnobotany. Gwich'in Social and Cultural Institute,
      Box 46, Tsiigehtchie, NWT, X0E 0B0, fax 1867-953-3820.

Andrews, Tamra. Nectar and Ambrosia. ABC-CLIO Box 1911 Santa Barbara CA. 2000.

Andrews, Ted. Animal Speak- The Spiritual and Magical Powers, Llewellyn. Minn. 1996.
_____ Animal Wise, DragonHawk, Jackson, TN, 1999.

Antol, Marie. The Incredible Secrets of Mustard. Avery Pub. New York. 1999.

Aronson J K Ed. Meyler's Side Effects of Herbal Medicines. Elsevier Amsterdam. 2009.

Arrowsmith, Nancy. Essential Herbal Wisdom. Llewellyn Pub. Woodbury, Minn. 2009.

Arsdall, Anne Van. Medieval Herbal Remedies. Routledge, New York. 2002.

Arvigo & Balick, Rainforest Remedies, Lotus Press, Twin Lakes, WI. 1993

Arvigo & Epstein. Rainforest Home Remedies, Harper SanFrancisco, 2001.

Assiniwi, Bernard. La Medecine des Indiens d' Amerique, Guerin Literature, 1988

Atal C.K. & Kapur B. Cultivation and Utilization of Medicinal Plants, Jammu-Tawi, 1982

Attenborough, David. The Private Life of Plants. Princeton U Press. Princeton NJ 1995.

Ausubel, K. Seeds of Change The Living Treasure. HarperSanFrancisco, 1994.

Aversano, Laura. The Divine Nature of Plants. Swan•Raven & Co. Columbus, NC, 2002.

Ayensu, Edward,S. Medicinal Plants of the West Indies, Reference Publications, 1981

Baïracli Levy, Juliette Herbal Handbook for Farm and Stable, Faber&Faber, London, 1952

Baker, Phil. The Dedalus Book of Absinthe. Dedalus 2001.

Barl, Branka et al, Saskatchewan Herb Database, U. of Sask. Saskatoon, 1996.

Barlow, Max. From the Shepherd's Purse. 1990

Barnes J, Anderson L, &Phillipson J. Herbal Medicines, A guide for healthcare professionals.
      Pharmaceutical Press, London, 2002.

Barnett, Robert A. Tonics, Harper Collins, New York, N.Y. 1997

Bartram, Thomas. Bartram's Encyl. of Herbal Medicine, Robinson Pub. London, 1998.

Bascom, Angella. Incorporating Herbal Medicine into Clinical Practice. F. Davis Co. 2002

Beals, Katherine, M. Flower Lore and Legend, Henry Holt, 1917

Beers, Susan-Jane. Jamu The ancient Indonesian Art of Herbal Healing, Periplus, 2001.

Belcourt, Christi. Medicines to Help Us. Gabriel Dumont Instit. Saskatoon, SK 2007.

Béliveau, R & Gingras,D. Foods That Fight Cancer. McClelland & Stewart Toronto. 2006.

Belsinger S & Dille C. Cooking with Herbs. CBI- Van Nostrand Reinhold, N.Y. 1984.

Benjamin, D.R. Mushrooms: Poisons and Panaceas. WH Freeman, San Francisco, 1995.
Bennet, Doug & Tiner, Tim. Up North. Reed Books Canada. Markham, Ont. 1993.
_____ Up North Again. McClelland and Stewart. Toronto, 1997.
Bennet, J & Rowley S. Uqalurait An Oral History of Nunavut. McGill Queens, Mont. 2004
Benyus, Janine. Biomimicry Innovation Inspired by Nature. William Morrow. 1997.
Berenbaum,May R. Buzzwords, A Scientists Muses on Sex, Bugs and Rock N Roll, Joseph
        Henry Press, Washington, D.C. 2000.
_____ Bugs in the System. Helix Books, Addison-Wesley Pub. 1995.
Beresford-Kroeger, Diana. The Global Forest. Viking Penguin. 2010.
_____ Arboretum Borealis. U Michigan Press. 2010.
Berliocchi,Luigi. The Orchid in Lore and Legend. Timber Press, Portland Oregon, 2000.
Berlund B & Bolsby C. The Edible Wild Pagurian Press, Toronto, Ont. 1971.
Berkowsky, Bruce. Mount Julius Flower Remedies. Mt. Vernon Washington, 1986
Bermejo, J & Leon,J. Neglected Crops-1492 ... FAO Series 26, United Nations, Rome, 1994.
Bernhardt, P. The Rose's Kiss, A Natural History of Flowers . Island Press, Covelo CA 1999
Bianchi, Ivo. Geriatrics and Homotoxicology. Aurelia-Verlag GmbH, Baden Baden, 1994.
Bianchini, F. The Complete Book of Health Plants. Crescent Books, New York, 1975.
Biship, Carol. The Book of Home Remedies &Herbal Cures, Jonathan-James, Toronto, 1979.
Bisset, Norman G. Herbal Drugs and Phytopharmaceuticals. 2nd Ed. CRC Press, 2001.
Blackburn, Thomas. December's Child: A Book of Chumash Oral Narratives , U of California
        Press, Berkeley, 1975.
Blanchan, Neltje. Nature's Garden. Doubleday, Page&Co. New York, 1900.
Bland, John. Forests of Liliput. Prentice Hall, Englewood Cliffs, New Jersey, 1971.
Bliss, Anne. Rocky Mountain Dye Plants. Juniper House, Boulder, Colorado, 1976
Blouin, Glen. Weeds of the Woods. Goose Lane, Fredericton, New Brunswick 1992.
_____ An Eclectic Guide to Trees, east of the Rockies. Boston Mills, 2001.
Boas, F. Ethnology of the Kwakiutl. Bureau of Am. Ethnology, 35th annual report, 1921.
Boericke, Wm. Materia Medica with Repetory. B. Jain Publishers. 1976
Boik, John. Natural Compunds in Cancer Therapy. Oregon Med Press, Princeton,Minn 2001
Boland, Bridget. Gardener's Magic &Other Old Wives' Lore. The Bodley Head, London, 77.
Bolton, Brett L. The Secret Powers of Plants. Berkley Pub Co. New York. 1974.
Bolton, J.L. Alfalfa, Botany, Cultivation &Utilization. Interscience Pub, New York, 1962.
Bone, Kerry. A Clinical Guide to Blending Liquid Herbs. Churchill Livingstone. 2003
Borrel, Marie. Healing Plants. Cassell & Co. Wellington House, London. 2001.
Bouchardon, Patrice. The Healing Energies of Trees. Journey Editions, Boston, 1999.
Bossenmaier, Eugene. Mushrooms of the Boreal Forest. U. of Saskatchewan Press, 1997
Boulos, Loutfy. Medicinal Plants of North Africa, Reference Pub. Algonac, Mich. 1983
Bowles, E. Joy. The Chemistry of Aromatherapeutic Oils. Allen & Unwin, Crow's Nest,
        Australia, 2003.
Bowman, Daria. Hydrangeas. Friedman/Fairfax Pub. New York. 1999.
Bradley, Peter. British Herbal Compendium Vol 2 Brit Herb Med Assoc. Bournemouth 2006.
Brahmachari, Goutam Ed. Natural Products, Alpha Sci Int Ltd. Oxford UK 2009.
Brandeis, Gayle. Fruitflesh. Harper Collins, San Francisco. 2002.
Brennan, M. Complete Holistic Care & Healing for Horses. Trafalgar Sq. Pub. VT. 2001.
Bringhurst, Robert. A Story as Sharp as a Knife. Douglas&McIntyre Vancouver, 1999.
Brinker, Francis N.D. Herb Contraindications and Drug Interactions .Third Edition Eclectic
        Medical Publications, Sandy, Oregon, 2001
_____ The Toxicology of Botanical Medicines, revised 2nd. Eclectic Med, Oregon, 1996.
_____ Eclectic Dispensatory of Botanical Therapeutics, Vol 2, Ecl. Med . Oregon, 1995.
Brodo, Irwin & Sharnoff. Lichens of North America. Yale University Press, 2001.

Brown, Deni. Enclyclopedia of Herbs and Their Uses. Reader's Digest Press, Que. 1995.
Bruneton, J Pharmacognosy, Phtyochemistry, Medicinal Plants, Lavoisier Pub. Paris, 1995
_____ Toxic Plants Dangerous to Humans and Animals. Editions TEC&Doc, Paris, '99.
Brunschwig, Hieronymus. Book of Distillation. Johnson Reprint Co No. 79. New York, 1971.
Bubar, Carol et al. Weeds of the Prairies. Alberta Agriculture Pub. Edmonton, 2000.
Buchanan, Carol. Brothers Crow, Sister Corn. Ten Speed Press, Berkeley, 1997.
Buckle, Jane. Clinical Aromatherapy. 2nd ed. Churchill Livingstone, Toronto, 2003.
Buhner, Stephen H. Sacred and Herbal Healing Beers, Siris Books, Boulder, Co, 1998
_____ Sacred Plant Medicine. Robert Rinehart, Boulder, Co. 1996.
_____ Herbal Antibiotics. Storey Books, Vermont, 1999.
_____ The Lost Language of Plants. Chelsea Green Pub. White River, Vt. 2002
_____ Secret Teachings of Plants. Bear & Co. Rochester, Vt. 2004.
_____ The Natural Testosterone Plan. Healing Arts Press, Rochester VT. 2007
Burbridge, Joan. Wildflowers of the Southern Interior of B.C. U. of B.C. Press, 1989.
Burger, W. Flowers- How they changed the world. Prometheus Books. Amherst NY 2006.
Burgess, Isla. Weeds Heal. Viriditas Pub Group. Cambridge NZ 1998.
Burlando, Bruno et al, Herbal Principles in Cosmetics. CRC Press Boca Raton 2010.
Caius, Rev. Fr. Jean F., The Medicinal and Poisonous Plants of India, Scientific Pub, 1986.
Cameron, Elizabeth. A Floral ABC. John Wiley and Sons. Toronto. 1980.
Carpenter D. Snr Pub. Nursing Herbal Medicine Handbook, Springhouse Corp. 2001.
Carpinella, Maria et al. Novel Therapeutic Agents from Plants. Sci Pub. Enfield NJ 2009.
Carr, Emily. Wild Flowers. Royal BC Museum, Victoria, B.C, 2006
Carroll, Roisin. The Crane Bag Celtic Tree Ogam Oils , Feasibility Pub. Dublin
Carter, Bernard F. The Floral Birthday Book. Bloomsbury Books, London. 1990.
Casselman, Bill. Canadian Garden Words. Little, Brown & Co. Toronto, 1997.
Castleman, Michael. The Healing Herbs. Bantam Books. 1995.
Castro, Miranda. The Complete Homeopathy Handbook. MacMillan, 1990
Catty, Suzanne. Hydrosols the next Aromatherapy, Healing Arts Press, Vermont, 2001.
Cavers, Paul ed, The Biology of Canadian Weeds 62-83,Ag Institute of Canada, Ottawa, 1995
_____ 84-102 Ag Inst. of Canada, Ottawa, 2000.
_____ 103-129 Ag Inst. of Canada, Ottawa 2005
Ceres. Herbal Teas for Health and Healing. Healing Arts Press, Rochester, Vermont, 1984.
Chan, K, and Cheung L. Interactions between Chincese Herbal Medicinal Products and
    Orthodox Drugs. Harwood Academic Publishers, Canada, 2000.
Chandler, F. Herbs-Everyday Reference for Health Professionals, Can. Pharm Assoc. 2000
Chang & But. Pharmacology &Applications of Chinese Materia Medica, World Scientific, 86
Chang Chao-liang et al, Vegetables as Medicine, Pelanduk Pub, Malaysia, 1999.
Chappell, P. Emotional Healing with Homeopathy. North Atlantic Books. Berkeley, 2003.
Chase, Pamela & Pawlik, J. Newcastle Trees for Healing , Newcastle Pub. Van Nuys,1991
Chatroux, Sylvia. Botanica Poetica. Poetica Press 2004 1-877-POETICA.
_____ Materica Poetica. Poetica Press 1998.
Chen, John K & Chen, Tina T. Chinese Medical Herbology & Pharmacology. Art of Medicine
    Press, City of Industry, CA 2004.
Chevalllier, Andrew. The Encyclopedia of Medicinal Plants. Reader's Digest, 1996.
Chishti, Hakim. The Traditional Healer, Healing Arts Press, Vermont,1988.
Clark, Ella E. Indian Legends of Canada. McClelland & Stewart. Toronto, 1960.
Coats, Peter. Flowers in History. Weidenfeld and Nicolson, London. 1970.
Coffey, Timothy.The History and Folklore of North American Wildflowers, Houghton-Mifflin,
    1993.
Cohen, Kenneth. Honoring the Medicine. Random House, Toronto. 2003.

Conrad, Chris, Hemp for Health, Healing Arts Press, Rochester, Vermont, 1997.

Cook, Wm.H. The Physio-Medical Dispensatory. 1869. Reprinted by Eclectic Medical Publications, Portland, Oregon, 1985.

_____ A compendium of the new Materia medica together with additional descriptions of some old remedies. Wm. Cook Publisher, Chicago, 1896.

Cooper, J.C. Dictionary of Symbolic & Mythological Animals, Thorsons, London, 1992.

Cormack, R.G.H. Wild Flowers of Alberta. Hurtig Publishers, 1977

Coupland, Francois. The Encyclopedia of Edible Plants of N. America. Keats Pub. 1998.

Cousin, Pierre J. Eat Well, Be Well. Thorsons, London. 2001.

Cowan, Eliot. Plant Spirit Medicine. Swan Raven & Co. Box 726 Newberg, Oregon, 1995.

Cowan, Thomas. The Fourfold Path to Healing. New Trends Pub. Washington DC 2007.

Crane, Eva. Honey- A Comprhensive Survey , Heinemann Pub. London 1975.

Craydon D. & Bellows W. Floral Acupuncture. The Crossing Press Berkeley CA 2005.

Creekmore, H. Daffodils are Dangerous. Walker and Co. New York. 1966.

Crow, Tis Mal. Native Plants, Native Healing. Native Voices Book Pub. Box 99 Summertown, Tennessee, 2001 1-888-260-8458.

Crowell, Robert L. The Lore & Legends of Flowers. Thomas Crowell, New York, 1982.

Crowfoot & Baldensperger. From Cedar to Hyssop. Sheldon Press, London, 1932.

Cruden, Loren. Medicine Grove. Destiny Books. Inner Traditions Vermont. 1997.

Cummings, S. and Ullman, Dana. Everyone's Guide to Homeopathic Medicines, St. Martins

Cupp, Melanie. Toxicology and Clinical Pharmacology of Herbal Products. Humana P. 1999

Curtin, LSM. Healing Herbs of the Upper Rio Grande. SouthWest Museum, Los Angeles 1965

Cutler & Cutler Eds. Biologically Active Natural Products: Agrochemicals, CRC Press 1999.

Dai Yin-fang&Liu Cheng-jun. Fruit As Medicine. Rams Skull Press, Kuranda, Aust. 1987

Dalton, David. Stars of the Meadow. Lindisfarne Books. Great Barrington, Mass. 2006.

D'Amelio Sr. Frank. Botanicals A Phytocosmetic Desk Reference CRC Press, Boca Raton, 99

Darby,Wm et al. Food: The Gift of Osiris, Vol 1. Academic Press, San Francisco, 1977

Darwin, Tess. The Scots Herbal, the Plant Lore of Scotland. Birlinn Ltd, Edinburgh 2008

Davidow, Joie. Infusions of Healing, A Treasury of Mexican-American Herbal Remedies, Fireside Books, New York, 1999.

Davis,W. El Gringo, New Mexico and Her People. Harpers, New York, 1857.

Demargaux, N. Phytotherapy. Herbal Health Publishers Ltd. 1989

De Bairacli Levy, Juliette. Herbal Handbook for Farm and Stable, Faber and Faber 1952

Deer Lame, J & Erdoes, R. Lame Deer Seeker of Visions. Washington Sq Press, 1976.

Deer, Thea Summer. Wisdom of the Plant Devas. Bear&Company Vermont 2011.

De Smet et al. Adverse Effects of Herbal Drugs. Springer-Verlag, Berlin. 1997.

Der Marderosian, Ara & Liberti L. Natural Product Medicine, George Stickley Co, Philadel.

Diederichsen, Axel. Coriander. Int. Plant Genetic Resources Institute. Rome, Italy. 1996.

DeRios, Marlene D. Hallucinogens: Cross Cultural Perspectives. U. New Mexico Press, 1984

DeSmet, P. et al. Adverse Effects of Herbal Drugs. vol 2 Springer-Verlag

Devi, Lila. The Essential Flower Essence Handbook. Crystal Clarity Pub. Nevada City 2007.

Dewey, Laurel. Plant Power- revised. Safe Goods/New Century Pub, Markham Ont, 2001.

Dewick, Paul M. Medicinal Natural Products.3rd Ed John Wiley and Sons, West Sussex, 2009.

Dixon, Bernard.Power Unseen, How Microbes Rule the World. W.H. Freeman, Oxford, 1994

Dow, Elaine. Simples and Worts. Historical Presentations, Topsfield, MA. 1982.

Duke, James. Handbook of Medicinal Herbs. CRC Press, Boca Raton, Florida, 1985

_____ Handbook of Edible Weeds. CRC Press. 1992

_____ The Green Pharmacy, Rodale Press, Emmaus, Pennsylvania, 1997.

_____ The Green Pharmacy Herbal Handbook, Rodale Press, 2000.

_____ Anti-aging Prescriptions. Rodale Press. 2001.

Dumas, Anne. Book of Plants and Symbols. English Ed. Octopus Pub. London 2004.

Dymock,Wm. Pharmacographia Indica, Vol 2, Kegan Paul, Trench, Trubner and Co. 1891

Earle, Liz. Vital Oils, Ebury Press, London, 1991.

Eason, Cassandra. Fabulous Creatures, Mythical Monsters... Greenwood Press, CT. 2008.

Eastman, John. The Book of Swamp and Bog... Stackpole Books, Mechanicsburg, Penn, 1995

Ebadi, M. Pharmacodynamic Basis of Herbal Medicine, CRC Press, Boca Raton. 2002.

Eckey, E.W. Vegetable Fats and Oils, Rheingold Publishing Co, New York, 1954.

Eclare, Melanie. Flower Spirit Cards. Quadrille Publishing, London, England, 2004.

Edwards, Lawrence. The Vortex of Life. Floris Books. Edinburgh 2nd Ed. 2006.

Eisner T et al. Secret Weapons. Belknap Press, Harvard U Press. Cambridge & London 2005.

Ellingwood F. American Materia Medica, Eclectic Med. Pub. Portand, Oregon, reprint, 1983

Elliot, Douglas B. Roots . Chatham Press, Old Greenwich Conneticut.

Ellis, Hattie. Sweetness & Light. Hodder and Stoughton, London, 2004.

Erdoes & Ortiz. American Indian Myths and Legends, Pantethon Books, New York, 1984.

Erichsen-Brown,Charlotte. Use of Plants for the Past 500 Years, Breezy Creeks Press, 1979

_____ Medicinal and Other Uses of North American Plants, General Pub, 1979.

Erickson, David, Wai Kit Nip Food uses of whole oil and protein seeds, Amer. Oil Chemists Society, 1989.

Eskin, N. A. Michael, Tamir, S. Dictionary of Nutraceuticals and Functional Foods. CRC Press, 2006.

Etkin, Nina. Edible Medicines, An Ethnopharmacology of Food. U Arizona Press. 2006.

Evans, W.C. Trease and Evans' Pharmacognosy. WB Saunders Co. Toronto, 2000.

Fang Jing Pei, Dr. Natural Remedies from the Chinese Cupboard. Weatherhill, 1998.

Farmer-Knowles,Helen. The Healing Garden. Sterling Publishing, New York, 1998.

Fielder, Mildred. Plant Medicne and Folklore, Winchester Press, New York, 1975.

Felter, Harvery and Lloyd, John. King's American Dispensatory . 1898.

Reprinted by   Eclectic Medical Publications, Portland Oregon, 1983.

Ferguson, Gary. Spirits of the Wild. Clarkson Potter/Random New York, 1996.

Fernie, W.T. Dr. Old Fashioned Herbal Remedies. Coles Pub. Toronto, 1980. Reprint.

Fingerman M. et al editors. Bioremediation of Aquatic and Terresrial Ecosytems. Sci Pub. Enfield NH 2005.

Fischer-Rizzi, S. Complete Aromatherapy Handbook, Sterling Pub. New York. 1990.

_____ The Complete Incense Book, Sterling Pub. New York. 1998.

_____ Medicine of the Earth, Rudra Press, Portland, Oregon, 1996

Florey, H.W. et al. Antibiotics vol 1. Oxford University Press. London 1949.

Ford, Gillian. Plant Names Explained. Friends of the Devonian Botanic Garden, #16, 1984

Foster, Steven. Herbal Renaissance, Gibbs Smith Pub. Salt Lake City

_____ & Yue Chongxi. Herbal Emissaries, Healing Arts Press, Vermont, 1992

_____ & Johnson R. Desk Reference to Nature's Medicine. Nat Geographic. Washington, D.C.

Fox, H. M. Gardening with Herbs. Macmillan Pub. New York 1933.

Freeman, D. & Mongeau D. Nettles and More...Vol One. Self published 2nd printing 2009.

Freeman, Lyn. Mosby's Complementary & Alternative Medicine.3rd Ed. Mosby Elsevier 2009

Friedman, Sara Ann, Celebrating the Wild Mushroom, Dodd, Mead & Co. New York, 1986

Friend, Tim. The Third Domain: the Untold Story of Archaea. Joseph Henry Press. 2007.

Fugh-Berman, Adriane. The 5-minute Herb &Dietary Supplement Consult. Lippincott Williams &Wilkins, Philadelphia 2003.

Gaertner, Erika. Reap without Sowing. General Store Publishing, Burnstown, Ont. 1995

Galun, Margalith. Handbook of Lichenology, CRC Press, 1988

Garran, Thomas. Western herbs according to Traditional Chinese Medicine. Healing Arts Press. 2008.

Garrett, J.T. The Cherokee Herbal. Bear&Company, Rochester, Vermont. 2003.

Genders, Roy. Floral Scents of the World . St. Martin's Press, London, 1977

Geuter, Herbs in Nutrition. Bio-Dynamic Agricultural Assoc. London. 1978.

Gildemeister, E. The Volatile Oils. John Wiley and Sons, New York. 1916

Gifford, Jane. The Wisdom of Trees. Sterling Pub. New York 2000.

Gill S. & Sullivan I. Dictionary of Native American Mythology. Oxford U Press 1992.

Gilmore, M.R. Uses of Plants by Indians of the Missouri river region. 33rd Annual Report Bureau American Ethnology, 1911-12, Washington D.C. 1919.

Gladstar R & Hirsch P. Planting the Future. Healing Arts Press, Rochester, Vt. 2000.

Gladstar, Rosemary. Family Herbal. Storey Books, North Adams, Mass. 2001.

Glasby, J.S. Dictionary of Plants Containing Secondary Metabolites, Taylor & Francis, London 1991.

Godfrey, A & Saunders P. Principles and Practices of Naturopathic Botanical Medicine, Vol 1, CCNM Press Toronto ON 2010.

Goodrick-Clarke, Clare. Alchemical Medicine for the 21st Century. Healing Arts Press. 2010.

Gordon, David G. The Compleat Cockroach. Ten Speed Press, Berkeley, CA. 1996.

Gordon, Lesley. The Mystery and Magic of Trees & Flowers. Grange Books. London 1993.

Gottesfeld, Leslie M. Johnson. Plants, Land and People, A Study of Wet'suwet'en Ethnobotany.U of A, 1993.

Grae, Ida. Nature's Colors, Dyes From Plants. Macmillan Pub. New York, 1974.

Graham, Frances K. Plant lore of an Alaskan Island. Alaska Northwest Pub. 1985

Grange, Michael etal, Handbook of Plants with Pest Control Properties, J. Wiley& Son 1988

Gray, Bev. The Boreal Herbal. Wild Food & Medicine Plants of the North. Aroma Borealis Press 2011

Green, James. The Male Herbal . Crossing Press, Freedom, California, 1991.

_____ The Herbal Medicine-Maker's Handbook. Crossing Press, Freedom CA 2000

Green, Jonathan. Consuming Passions. Sphere Books, London, 1985.

Grey Wolf. Earth Signs, Raincoast Books, Vancouver, B.C. 1998.

Grieve, M. A Modern Herbal. Jonathan Cape. 1931

Griffiths, Deirdre. Elk Island National Park. U. of Alberta Press, 1979.

Grigson, Geoffrey. A Herbal of All Sorts. Phoenix House, London

Grimaud, Baptiste,Paul. TAROT DES FLEURS, France Cartes, France 1989

Grimshaw, John. The Gardener's Atlas. Firefly Books, Willowdale, Ont. 2002.

Grohmann,Gerbert. The Plant Vol 2, Bio-Dynamic Farming & Gardening Assoc. 1989.

Gruenwald et al, Ed. PDR for Herbal Medicines. 4th Ed. Thomson Pub. 2007.

Guillet, Alma. Make Friends of Trees and Shrubs. Doubleday & Co. New York, 1962.

Gumbel, Dietrich. Principles of Holistic Skin Therapy with Herb Essences. Haug Pub. Heidelberg 1986.

Gurudas. The Spiritual Properties of Herbs , Cassandra Press, 1988

_____ Flower Essences and Vibrational Healing, Cassandra Press, 1983

Hageneder, Fred. The Spirit of Trees. Continuum. NY and London. 2005.

Hale, Mason. The Biology of Lichens. Edward Arnold Pub. London, 1967.

Hall, Dorothy. Creating Your Herbal Profile , Keats, 1988

Hallworth, B & Chinnappa CC. Plants of the Kananaskis Country U of A Press 1997.

Hanchuk, Rena. The Word and Wax. Can Inst of Ukrainian Studies Press, Edmonton, 1999.

Hanson, J, & Morrison D. Of Kinkajous, Capybaras, Horned Beetles...Harper Collins, NY '91

Harbourne & Baxter. The Handbook of Natural Flavonoids Vol 1&2. John Wiley & Sons, 1999

_____ Phytochemical Dictionary. Taylor & Francis 1993.

Harrington, Geri. Growing Your Own Chinese Vegetables, MacMillan, N.Y. 1978.
Harrington, H.D. Edible Native Plants of the Rocky Mtns. U. of New Mexico Press, 1967.
Harris, Ben C. Eat the Weeds, Keats Pub. New Cannan, Conneticut 1973.
_____ Make Use of Your Garden Plants. General Pub. New York. 1978.
Harris, Marjorie. Botanica North America. Harper Collins, New York, 2003.
Harrison, Nora. Flower Remedy Rhymes , self published, England, 1990.
Hart, Jeff. Montana Native Plants and Early Peoples, Montana Historical Society Press. '92
_____ The Ethnobotany of the Northern Cheyenne Indians of Montana. Journal of
    Ethnopharmacology 1981 4.
Hartung, Tammi. Growing 101 Herbs That Heal. Storey Books, Pownal, Vt. 2000.
Hartwell, Jonathan, Plants Used Against Cancer. Quarterman Pub. 1982
Hartzell, Jr. H. The Yew Tree A Thousand Whispers. Hulogosi, Box 1188, Eugene, OR 1991.
Harvey, C & Cochrane A. The Healing Spirit of Plants. Godsfield Press, Sterling Pr N.Y. 1999
Harvey Clare. The New Encyclopedia of Flower Remedies. Watkins Pub. London 2007.
Hatfield, Gabrielle. Encyclopedia of Folk Medicine. ABC CLIO Santa Barbara. 2004.
Haughton, Claire. Green Immigrants. Harcourt Brace Jovanovich. New York and London.
Hawksworth, Frank & Wiens, D. Dwarf Mistletoes, Ag Handbook 709, USDA, Wash, DC, '96
Health Canada, Native Foods and Nutrition. Medical Services Branch, 1995.
Heatherington, M. and Steck,W. Natural Chemicals from Northern Prairie Plants, Ag West
    Biotech Publishers, Saskatoon, Canada. 1997.
Heilmeyer, Marina. The Language of Flowers-Symbols & Myths. Prestel Pub. Munich 2001.
Heinerman, John. Encyclopedia of Nuts, Berries and Seeds, Parker Publishing, 1995.
_____ Encyclopedia of Healing Herbs & Spices. Parker Pub. N.Y. 1996.
Heinrich, Bernd. Winter World The Ingenuity of animal survival. HarperCollins. NY 2003.
Heinrich, Clark. Magic Mushrooms in Religion and Alchemy. Park St. Press, VT. 2002.
Heiser, Charles B. Jr. Of Plants and People. U. of Oklahoma Press, 1985.
Hellson, John C, Ethnobotany of the Blackfoot Indians No. 19, National Museums of Canada,
    Ottawa 1974.
Henderson, Robert K. The Neighborhood Forager. Key Porter Books, Toronto, 2000.
Hendrickson, Robert. Encycl of Word and Phrase Origins. Facts on File Inc. NewYork, 1997.
Hendry, G. Natural Food Colorants , Blackie and Son, Glasgow Scotland, 1992.
Henry, J. David. Canada's Boreal Forest. Smithsonian Institute. 2002.
Hilarion. Wildflowers, Their Occult Gifts. Marcus Books, Queensville, Ont. 1982.
Hobbs, Christopher. Usnea : The Herbal Antibiotic. Botanica Press. 1986.
_____ Medicinal Mushrooms, Botanica Press, Santa Cruz, 1995.
Hoffman, David. The Holistic Herbal. Findhorn Press, 1983.
_____ Welsh Herbal Medicine. Abercastle Publications, Dyfed, 1978.
_____ Medical Herbalism. Healing Arts Press, Rochester, VT, 2003.
Hole, Lois. Favorite Trees and Shrubs. Lone Pine Pub. Edmonton Alta. 1997.
_____ Perennial Favorites. Lone Pine Pub. 1995.
Holm, LeRoy G. World Weeds, John Wiley and Sons, 1997.
Holmes, Peter. The Energetics of Western Herbs, Vol 1 and 2, Artemis Press, 1989.
_____ Jade Remedies, Vol 1 and 2, Snow Lotus Press, Boulder 1996.
Hopman, Ellen. A Druid's Herbal, Destiny Books, Rochester, Vermont. 1995.
Howarth, D& Kahlee Keane. Wild Medicines of the Prairies Self Published, 1995.
_____ Native Medecines Self Published , 1995
Hozeski, Bruce. Hildegard's Healing Plants. Beacon Press. Boston, Mass. 2001.
Hsu, Hong-Yen. Oriental Materia Medica, Keats Publishing,Connecticut, 1986.
Huang, Kee Chang. The Pharmacolocy of Chinese Herbs. 2nd Edition, CRC Press, 1999.
Hu-Nan. A Barefoot Doctor's Manual. Running Press, Philadelphia, 1977.

Hudson, James B. Antiviral Compounds from Plants, CRC Press, Florida, 1990
Hudson, Rick. A Field Guide to Gold, Gemstone and Mineral Sites. Orca Pub, Victoria, 1999
Hurley, Judith. The Good Herb Wm. Morrow and Co. New York, 1995.
Hutchens, Alma. Indian Herbology of North America. Merco. 1969
Ingram, Cass. Supermarket Remedies. Knowledge House, Buffalo Grove, Ill. 1998.
Inkpen W & Van Eyk, R. Guide to the Common Native Trees and Shrubs of Alberta,
    Government of Alberta, Environmental Protection, 1995.
James & Keeler, Poisonous Plants- 3rd Int. Symposium, Iowa State U. Press, 1992.
Jason, Dan & Nancy. Some Useful Wild Plants, Talon Books, Vancouver, 1972.
Jiao Shu-De. Ten Lectures on the Use of Medicinals. Paradigm Pub. Brookline, Mass. 2003.
Johnson, Kershaw, MacKinnon & Pojar Plants of the Western Boreal Forest and Aspen
Parkland, Lone Pine Press, Edmonton, Alberta 1995.
Johnson, L. Tending the Earth A Gardener's Manifesto. Penguin Books, Toronto, 2002.
Johnson, Leslie. Journal of Ethnobotany and Ethnomedicine. 2006 2:29.
_____ Health, Wholeness & the Land: Gitksan Traditional Plant Use and Healing. U of
    Alberta 1997.
Jones, Alison. Larousse Dictionary of World Folklore. Larousse, New York, 1995.
Jones, Pamela. Just Weed, History, Myths and Uses. Prentice Hall Press, Toronto, 1991.
Kamm, Minnie W. Old Time Herbs for Northern Gardens Little Brown & Co. 1938.
Kane, Charles W. Herbal Medicine of the American Southwest. Lincoln Town Press. 2007.
_____ Herbal Medicine: trends and traditions. Lincoln Town Press 2009.
Kapoor, L.D. CRC Handbook of Ayurvedic Medicinal Plants, CRC Press, Boca Raton, 1990.
Kari, Priscilla. Tanaina Plantlore. National Park Service, Alaska Region 1987.
Kaur, Sat Dharam. The Complete Natural Medicine Guide to Breast Cancer. Robert Rose Inc
    Toronto, 2003.
Kavash E, Barrie & Barr K, American Indian Healing Arts. Bantam Books, Toronto 1999.
_____ The Medicine Wheel Garden. Bantam Books, N.Y. 2002.
Kay, Margarita Artschwager. Healing with Plants in the American and Mexican West, The
    University of Arizona Press, Tucson. 1996
Kays, S & Nottingham S. Biology and Chemistry of Jerusalem Artichoke. CRC Press 2008.
Keane, Kahlee & Howarth,D. The Standing People. Saskatoon, Saskatchewan. 2003.
Kee Chang Huang, The Pharmacology of Chinese Herbs, 2nd Edition, CRC Press, 1999.
Kemp, Cynthia. Cactus and Company. Desert Alchemy, Tucson, Arizona, 1993.
Kenner D &Requena Y. Botanical Medicine: .Paradigm Pub. Brookline, Mass, 1996.
Kerik, Joan. Living with the Land:Use of Plants by the Native People of Alberta, Alberta
    Culture, Circulating Exhibits Program, National Museums of Canada Fund, 1981.
Kershaw, Linda. Edible & Medicinal Plants of the Rockies, Lone Pine, Edmonton 2000.
_____ Alberta Wayside Wildflowers. Lone Pine, Edmonton, 2003.
_____ Saskatchewan Wayside Wildflowers. Lone Pine, Edmonton, 2003.
_____ Manitoba Wayside Wildflowers. Lone Pine, Edmonton, 2003.
Kershaw, L. et al. Rare Vascular Plants of Alberta. U. of Alberta Press, Edmonton, 2001.
Kershaw, MacKinnon & Pojar. Plants of the Rocky Mountains. Lone Pine, Edmonton 1998.
Keys, John. D. Chinese Herbs, Charles E. Tuttle Co. 1976.
Kimmerer,Robin. Gathering Moss. Oregon State University Press, Corvallis, 2003.
Kindscher, Kelly. Medicnal Wild Plants of the Prairies. Univ. Press of Kansas. 1987.
King, Francis X. Rudolf Steiner and Holistic Medicine. Rider & Co. England, 1986.
Klein, Carol. Plant Personalities. Timber Press, Portland, Oregon. 2005.
Klein, Richard. The Green World. 2nd edition. Harper Collins, 1987.
Kloss, Jethro. Back to Eden. Woodbridge Press Pub.Co. Santa Barbara, Ca. 1975.
Knab, Sophie H. Polish Herbs, Flowers and Folk Medicine. Hippocrene Books, N.Y. 1999.

Knowles, Hugh. Woody Ornamentals for the Prairies. U. of Alberta , 1995.

Knudtson,P & Suzuki D. Wisdom of the Elders. Greystone Books. Vancouver BC 2006.

Kraft, K & Hobbs C. Pocket Guide to Herbal Medicine. Thieme, N.Y. 2004.

Kranich, Ernst M. Planetary Influences Upon Plants. Bio-Dynamic Lit. Wyoming RI 1984.

Krymow, V. Healing Plants of the Bible. Wild Goose Pub. Glasgow, UK 2002.

Kuhnlein, Harriet and Turner, Nancy. Traditional Plant Foods of Canadian Indigenous Peoples. Gordon and Breach Science Publishers. 1991.

Kuijt, Job. The Biology of Parasitic Flowering Plants, U. of California Press, 1969

Kunkele, U. & Lohmeyer, T. Herbs for Healthy Living. Parragon Pub. Bath UK 2007.

Lacey, Laurie. Micmac Medicines Remedies and Recollections. Nimbus Pub. Halifax, 1993.

Lahring, Heinjo. Water and Wetland Plants of the Prairie Provinces, Can Plains Research Center, U. of Regina, 2003

Lambert, Grant. Falling Leaf Essences. Healing Arts Press, Rochester Vermont, 2002.

Lamont, SM. The Fisherman Lake Slave and their environment: a story of floral and faunal resources. Master's thesis. U. of Saskatchewan, Saskatoon, 1977.

Langenheim, Jean. Medicinal Plant Resins. Timber Press Portland Oregon 2003.

Larsen,Henning. An Old Icelandic Medical Miscellany, Norske Akademi, Oslo, Norway '31

Lavabre, Marcel. Aromatherapy Workbook. Healing Arts Press, Vermont. 1990.

Lawless, Julia, The Encyclopedia of Essential Oils , Element Books, 1992.

LeClaire,N &Cardinal,G. Alberta Elders' Cree Dictionary, U of Alberta Press, 1998.

Leduc, M.A. The Explorers Guide to Boreal Forest Plants, Hwy Book Shop, Cobalt, Ont. 1997

Leighton, Anna L. Wild Plant Use by the Woods Cree (NIHITHAWAK) of East-Central Saskatchewan . Paper no. 101, National Museums of Canada, Ottawa, 1985

Lepore, Donald. The Ultimate Healing System. Woodland Books, Provo, Utah, 1988.

Le Strange, Richard, A History of Herbal Plants. Arco Pub. New York. 1977.

Leung, Albert. Chinese Herbal Remedies. Universe Books, New York, 1984.

Leung & Foster, Encyclopedia of Common Natural Ingredients, J. Wiley&Sons, N.Y. 1996.

Levey,M. The Medical Formulary or Aqrabadhin of Al-Kindi U of Wisconsin Press, 1966

Leyel, C.F. Elixirs of Life, Faber and Faber, London.1948

Li, Thomas. Medicinal Plants, Culture, Utilization & Phytopharmacology. Technomic Publishing, Lancaster, Pennsylvania, 2000.

Li, Thomas. Chinese and related North American Herbs. CRC Press, Boca Raton, 2002.

Libster, Martha. Delmar's Integrative Herb Guide for Nurses. Delmar, 2002.

Lininger et al. The Natural Pharmacy. Healthnotes, Prima Pub. Rocklin Ca, 1999.

L'Orange Darlena, Herbal Healing Secrets of the Orient. Prentice Hall, New Jersey, 1998.

Lock, Carolyn. Country Colours. Nova Scotia Museum. 1981

Lovejoy, Sharon. Sunflower Houses. Workman Pub Co. New York 2001.

Lu, Henry. Using Foods to Stay Young, Sterling Press, New York, 1996.

_____ Chinese Natural Cures. Black Dog & Leventhal Pub. New York, 1994

Luetjohann, Sylvia. The Healing Power of Black Cumin. Lotus Light, Twin Lakes, WI, 1998

Lyle, Katie Letcher. The Wild Berry Book, NorthWord Press, Minocqua, WI, 1994.

Mabey, Richard. Plantcraft. Universe Books. 1978.

MacKinnon, Pojar, Coupe. Plants of Northern British Columbia. Lone Pine Press, 1992.

Mailhebiau, Philippe. Portraits in Oils. C.W. Daniel Company, Essex, England, 1995.

Malmud, René. The Amazon Problem, trans by M. Stein, Spring Pub. Dallas TX, 1980.

Maloof, Joan. Teaching the Trees, Lessons from the Forest. U Georgia Pr, Athena GA. 2005.

Manandhar, N.P. Plants and People of Nepal. Timber Press, Portland, Oregon, 2002.

Maple, Eric. The Secret Lore of Plants and Flowers. Robert Hale Ltd. London 1980.

March, Kathryn & Andrew. The Wild Plant Companion. Meridian Hill Pub. 1986.

Marles, Robin. The Ethnobotany of the Chipewyan of Northern Saskatchewan, 1984. Thesis.

319

_____ et al. Aboriginal Plant Use in Canada's Northwest Boreal Forest. UBC Press, Vancouver, and Natural Resources Canada, 2000

McBride, L.R. Practical Folk Medicine of Hawaii. Petroglyph Press, Hilo,Hawaii, 1975.

McCune B. & Geiser L. Macrolichens of the Pacific Northwest. Oregon State U. Press, 1997

McFarland, Phoenix. The Complete Book of Magical Names. Llewellyn Pub. St Paul 1996

McGrath, Judy. Dyes from Lichens and Plants. Van Nostrand Rheinhold, 1977.

McGuffin, Nancy. Spectrum: dye plants of Ontario. Burr House Spinner, Richmond Hill '86

McIntyre, Anne. The Complete Woman's Herbal, Henry Holt, New York, 1995.

Mears, R & Hillman,G. Wild Food. Hodder and Stoughton

MELODY. Love is in the Earth, A Kaleidoscope of Crystals. Earth Love Pub. Col. 1995.

Mercatante, A. S. The Facts on File Encyclopedia of World Mythology. New York 1988

Merriam, C. Hart. Dawn of the World, Weird Tales of Mewan Indians. Arthur H. Clark, Cleveland, 1910

Meyer, George et al. Folk Medicine and Herbal Healing, Charles Thomas, Springfield, 1981

Meyerowitz,Steve. Sprout It! The Sprout House, Box 1100,Great Barrington, MA, 1993.

Meyers, Edward C. Basic Bush Survival, Hancock House, Surrey, B.C. 1997.

Miller, L &Murray,W. Herbal Medicinals A Clinician's Guide. Hawthorn Press, N.Y. 1998.

Miller, Sandra. Editor Echinacea- Medicinal and Aromatic Plants. CRC Press, 2004.

Mills S. & Bone,K. Principles and Practice of Phytotherapy. Churchill Livingstone, 2000.

_____ The Essential Guide to Herbal Safety. Churchill Livingstone, 2005.

Mills, Simon. Out of the Earth. Viking Penquin Books, Toronto. 1991.

Millsbaugh, Charles. American Medicinal Plants, Dover Pub. New York, 1974

Milne, Courtney. Visions of the Goddess, Penguin Studio, Toronto, 1998

Minnis & Elisens. Biodiversity and Native America. U. Oklahoma Press, 2000.

Mitchel, Jr. Wm. Plant Medicine in Practice. Churchill Livingstone, St. Louis, 2003.

Moerman, Daniel, Medicinal Plants of Native America. U of Michigan No. 19, 1986

Mohammed, G. Catnip & Kerosene Grass Candlenut Books, Sault Ste. Marie, Ont, 2002.

Montgomery, Pam. Plant Spirit Healing. Bear and Company, Rochester, VT 2008.

Moore, Michael. Los Remedios. Red Crane Books, 1990

_____ Medicinal Plants of the Desert and Canyon West. Museum of New Mexico Press 1989

_____ Medicinal Plants of the Mountain West, Museum of New Mexico Press '79

_____ Med Plants of the Mountain West. Revised, expanded. 2003

_____ Medicinal Plants of the Pacific West, Red Crane Books, 1993

More, Daphne. The Bee Book, Universe Books, New York, 1976.

Morelli, I. et al. Selected Medicinal Plants. University of Pisa. FAO 53/1

Morton, Julia. Major Medicinal Plants . Charles Thomas, Springfield, Illinois 1977

_____ Atlas of Medicinal Plants of Middle America, Bahamas to Yucatan. 1981

Moss, E.H. Flora of Alberta. University of Toronto Press. 1983

Mother, The. Flowers and their Messages. Sri Aurobindo Ashram Trust, India 1979.

Mourning Dove. Coyote Stories. Caxton Press Caldwell Idaho. 1933.

Mowrey, Daniel. The Scientific Validation of Herbal Medicine. Cormorant Books, 1986.

Mucz, Michael. Baba's Kitchen Medicines. U of Alberta Press, Edmonton, 2012.

Mulders, Evelyn. Western Herbs for Eastern Meridian & 5 Element Theory. Self publ. 2006.

Mulligan, G editor The biology of Canadian Weeds, 1-32 Pub. 1693 Ag Canada 1979

_____ 33-61 Pub. 1765 Ag Canada 1984

Murphy, Cristine Editor, Practical Home Care Medicine, Lantern Books, New York, 2001

Murray, Michael. The Pill Book Guide to Natural Medicines. Bantam Books, April, 2002.

_____ & Pizzorno, J. The condensed Encycl of Healing Foods. Pocket Books NY 2005.

Naegele, Thomas A. Edible and Medicinal Plants of the Great Lakes Region, Wilderness Adventure Books, Davisburg, Michigan. 1996.

Naiman, Ingrid. Cancer Salves, A Botanical Approach to Treatment. N. Atlantic Books, 99.
Nesse R & Williams G. Why We Get Sick. Vintage Books/Random House, New York, 1996.
Neuwinger H.D. African Traditional Medicine. Medpharm Sci. Pub. Stuttgart 2000.
_____ African Ethnobotany, Poisons and Drugs. Chapman & Hall, London 1996.
Newcombe C.F. unpub notes on Haida plants. Dept of Anthro. Am Mus Nat Hist. NY 1897
_____ unpublished papers. Prov Archives B.C. Victoria. 1898-1913.
Nicander. The Poems and Poetical Fragments. Cambridge U. Press, New York, 1953.
Norman,Howard. Northern Tales. Pantheon Books, New York, 1990.
Northcote, Rosalind. The Book of Herbs. John Lane: The Bodley Head, London, 1912.
Null, Gary. The Clinician's Handbook of Natural Healing. Kensington Books, N.Y. 1997.
Olive, Barbara. The Flower Healer. Cico Books, London and New York. 2007.
Ollsin, Don. Herbal Healing Journey-Playful Workbook. Aquiline Comm, Victoria,BC 1998.
Ootoova I. et al. Interviewing Inuit Elders, Perspectives on Traditional Health. Vol 5,
Nunavut Arctic College, Box 600, Iqaluit, Nunavut X0Z 0H0.
Page, George. Inside the Animal Mind. Doubleday, New York, 1999.
Pallasdowney, Rhonda. The Complete Book of Flower Essences. New World Library, 2002.
Pappalardo, Joe. Sunflowers (the secret history). The Overlook Press. Woodstock NY 2008.
Parish, Coupé & Lloyd. Plants of S. Interior British Columbia. Lone Pine Edmonton 1996
Park, Willard Z. Ethnographic Notes on the Norhern Paiute of Western Nevada, 1933-40
compiled by Catherine Fowler, U. of Utah, Salt Lake City, 1989.
Parvati, J. Hygieia, A Woman's Herbal. Freestone Collective. 1978
Paturi, Felix Nature, Mother of Invention. Harper and Row Pub. New York. 1976.
Peirce,Andrea. Practical Guide to Natural Medicines. Stonesong Press. 1999.
Pelikan, W. Healing Plants. Mercury Press, Spring Valley NY 1997.
Pellowski, Anne. Hidden Stories in Plants. MacMillan Pub. New York. 1990.
Penoel,Daniel & Franchomme, P. L'Aromatherapie Exactement , Roger Jollois, France, 1990
Peneol, Daniel. Medecine Aromatique, Medecine Planetaire. Roger Jollois France 1991.
_____ & Peneol, Rose-Marie. Natural Home Health Care Using Essential Oils. Osmobiose
Pub. 1998.
People of 'Ksan, The. Gathering What the Great Nature Provided. Douglas & McIntyre.
Vancouver, B.C. 1980.
Peters, Josephine & Ortiz B. After the First Full Moon in April. Left Coast Press. Walnut
Creek CA, 2010.
Pettitt,Sabina. Energy Medicine, Healing from the Kingdoms of Nature, Pacific Essences, Box
8317, Victoria, B.C. V8W 3R9 Canada, 1999
Phaneuf, Holly. Herbs Demystified. Marlowe and Company, New York. 2005
Pielou, E.C. The Naturalist's Guide to the Arctic. U. of Chicago Press. 1994.
Pieroni, A & Price L. Eating and Healing, Trad Food as Medicine. Haworth Press. N.Y. 2006.
Pfeiffer E. The Earth's Face and Human Destiny, Rodale Press, Emmaus, Pa. 1947.
Plotkin, Mark. Medicine Quest. Viking Penguin Books, New York, 2000.
Pojar, J & MacKinnon, A. Plants of Coastal British Columbia Lone Pine Edmonton 1994.
Pollock, L. With Faith and Physic: the life of a tudor gentlewoman. Collins & Brown,1993.
Polya, Gideon. Biochemical Targets of Plant Bioactive Comp. CRC Press, Boca Raton 2003
Pond, Barbara, A Sampler of Wayside Herbs, Chatham Press, Riverside, Conn.
Pressor, Arthur, Pharmacist's Guide to Medicinal Herbs, Smart Pub. Petaluma, CA,2000
Price, Len & Shirley. Understanding Hydrolats. Churchill Livingstone, Toronto, 2004.
_____ Aromatherapy for Health Professionals. Churchill Livingstone 1995.
Purvis, William. Lichens. Smithsonian Institution Press. Washington D.C. 2000
Quin, Frederick F. The Flora Homoeopathica. B. Jain Pub. New Delhi, India. 1997.
Radin, Paul. The Winnebago Tribe, Bur of Am Ethnology, Smithsonian Inst. 37th. 1923.

Rätsch, C. Plants of Love, The History of Aphrodisiacs. Ten Speed Press, Berkeley,1997.
_____ The Dictionary of Sacred & Magical Plants. ABC-CLIO St Barbara 1992.
_____ The Encyclopedia of Psychoactive Plants. Park St Press. 2005.
Reaume, Tom. 620 Wild Plants of North America. Nature Manitoba. Canadian Plains Research Center, U of Regina, U of Toronto Press. 2009.
Reckeweg, Hans-Heinrich, Materia Medica, Vol 1. Aurelia-Verlag GmbH, Baden Baden 1996.
Reich, Lee. Uncommon Fruits Worthy of Attention, Addison-Wesley Pub. 1991.
Reid, Daniel, A handbook of Chinese Healing Herbs, Shambala, Boston, 1995
Rhode, David. Native Plants of Southern Nevada. U of Utah Press. 2002.
Richards B & Kanecko A. Japanese Plants- Know Them &Use Them. Shufunotomo, Tokyo 1995
Richardson, David. The Vanishing Lichens. David and Charles, Vancouver, BC, 1975
Riddle, John M. Eve's Herbs. Harvard U Press. Cambridge Mass. 1997.
_____ Goddesses, Elixirs and Witches. Palgrave MacMillan. England 2010.
Rister, Robert. Healing Without Medication. Basic Health Pub. N. Bergen, N.J. 2003.
Roberts, Jonathan. The Origins of Fruit and Vegetables. Universe Pub. New York. 2001.
Robicsek, F. The Smoking God: Tobacco....Norman: U. of Oklahoma Press, 1978.
Robinson, Peggy. Profiles of Northwest Plants. Far West Book Service. Portland, OR 1979
Rogers, Dilwyn. Edible, Medicinal, Useful & Poisonous Wild Plants of the Northern Great Plains —South Dakota Region. Buechel Memorial Lakota Museum, St. Francis,SD, 1980.
Rogers, Pattiann. Firekeeper:New & Selected Poems. Milkweed Editions, 1994.
Rogers, Robert Dale. Sundew Moonwort Vols-1-7, self-published. Edmonton 1995-present.
_____ Rogers' Herbal Manual. Karamat Wilderness Ways, Edmonton, 2000.
_____ & Capital Health, Herbal Drug Interactions. Mediscript Comm. 2003.
_____ The Fungal Pharmacy, The Complete Guide to Medicinal Mushrooms and Lichens of North America, North Atlantic Books 2011.
Rombi, Max. Phytotherapy. Herbal Health Publishers. U.K. 1990.
Rosengarten,Jr. F. The Book of Edible Nuts. Walker and Co. New York. 1984.
Ross, Gary. Nature's Guide to Healing. Freedom Press, Topanga, Ca. 2000.
Ross, Ivan. Medicinal Plants of the World. Vol 1 Humana Press, Totowa, New Jersey. 1999.
_____ Vol 2 Humana Press, Totowa, N. J. 2002.
Rotella, Rev. Alexis. The Essence of Flowers, Jade Mountain Press, N.J. 1991.
Royer F. & Dickinson R. Plants of Alberta. Lone Pine Pub. Edmonton, AB. 2007.
Rudginsky, Marlene The Flower Speaks. U.S. Games Systems, Stamford, Conn. 1999.
Rupp, Rebecca. Red Oaks and Black Birches , Storey Comm. Garden Way Publishing. 1990
Russell, Sharman Apt. Anatomy of a Rose. Perseus Pub. Cambridge, Mass. 2001.
_____ An Obsession with Butterflies. Perseus Publishing 2003.
Ryan, J et al, Traditional Dene Medicine. Lac La Martre NWT, 1993.
Ryden, Hope. Wildflowers around the year. Clarion Books, New York. 2001.
Ryrie, Charlie. Garden Folklore That Works. Reader's Digest. Pleasantville, NY 2001.
Sagadic O. & Ozcan M. Food Control 2003 14.
Salmon, Wm. Botanologia: The English Herbal. London: I. Dawkes, 1710.
Sandberg & Corrigan. Natural Remedies, their origins and uses. Taylor & Francis 2001.
Sanders, Jack. The Secrets of Wildflowers. The Lyons Press, Guilford, CT, 2003.
Sapolsky, Robert. The Trouble with Testosterone. Scribner, New York. 1997.
Sauer, Johann Christopher, Compendious Herbal-see Weaver below.
Savage, Candace. Bees, Nature's Little Wonders. Greystone Books. Vancouver 2008.
Schalkwijk-Barendsen, Helene. Mushrooms of Western Canada . Lone Pine Pub. 1991.
Schar, Douglas. The Backyard Medicine Chest. Elliott&Clark Pub. Washington, DC. 1995.

Scheffer, Mechthild, Bach Flower Therapy, Theory and Practice, Healing Arts Press, 1988
Schenk, George. Moss Gardening. Timber Press, Portland Oregon. 1997.
Schnaubelt, Kurt. Medical Aromatherapy. Frog Ltd. Berkeley CA. 1999.
Schneider, Anny. Wild Medicinal Plants. Key Porter Books, Toronto. 2002.
Schnell, Donald. Carnivorous Plants. 2nd Ed. Timber Press, Portland, Oregon, 2002.
Schofield, Janice. Discovering Wild Plants. Alaska Northwest Books. 1989.
_____ Nettles. Keats Publishing, New Canaan, Conneticut, 1998.
Schulman, Robert. Solve It With Supplements. Rodale Press. New York. 2007.
Shapiro, R & Rapkins J. Awakening to the Plant Kingdom, Cassandra Press 1991.
Shauenberg, Paul and Paris. Guide to Medicinal Plants. Keats Publishing, 1977.
Shook, Edward Dr. Advanced Treatise on Herbology . Reprint Health Research.
Shosteck,Robert. Flowers and Plants. Quadrangle/The New York Times Book Co. 1974.
Siegfried, EV. Masters Thesis, Ethnobotany of the Northern Cree of Wabasca/Desmarais. U of
    Calgary, Alberta. 1994.
Silverman, Maida. A City Herbal. David R. Godine , 1990.
Silvertown, Jonathan. An Orchard Invisible. U of Chicago Press. 2009.
Simonot, Danielle. Bio-Manufacturing in Saskatchewan- Assessment of the Manufacturing
    Potential of Select Saskatchewan Plants, Sask. Nutraceutical Network, Saskatoon, 2000
Simpson, Brenan, M. Flowers At My Feet, Hancock House, Surrey, B.C. 1996.
Sionneau, P. An Introduction to the Use of Processed Chinese Medicinals. Blue Poppy Press,
Second Printing 2003, Translated by Bob Flaws.
Smagghe, Guy Ed. Ecdysone: Structures and Functions. Springer Sci 2009.
Small, E & Catling, P. Canadian Medicinal Crops, NRC Research Press, Ottawa 1999.
Small, Ernest. Culinary Herbs, Second Ed. NRC Research Press, Ottawa, 2006.
_____ Medicinal Herbs, NRC Research Press, Ottawa, 2000.
_____ Top 100 Food Plants. NRC Press, Ottawa. 2009.
Smith, Andrew. Strangers in the Garden, the Secret Lives of Our Favorite Flowers.McClelland
    & Stewart 2004.
Smith, Annie Lorrain. Lichens, Cambridge at the University Press, 1921.
Smith, Harlan, Ethnobotany of the Gitksan Indians of B.C. Edited by B. Compton, B. Rigsby,
    and M.L. Tarpent, Mercury Series, Can Ethno Service, Paper 132, Can Mus of Civil.
    1997.
Smith, Huron H. Manataka American Indian Council. www.manataka.org.
Snell, Alma Hogan. A Taste of Heritage. Crow Indian Recipes and Herbal Medicines.
    University of Nebraska Press 2006.
Soule, Deb. The Roots of Healing, A Woman's Book of Herbs. Citadel Press, 1995.
Spencer, Kate. The Magic of Green Buckwheat ,Richard Clay, England, 1987.
Spinella, Marcello. The Psychopharmacology of Herbal Medicine. MIT Press, 2001.
Steedman, E.V. The Ethnobotany of the Thompson Indians of British Columbia. 1930.
Stein, Sara. My Weeds, A Gardener's Botany. Harper and Row, 1988.
Stern, Gai. Australian Weeds. Harper and Row, Australia 1986
Stern Wm. Stern's Dictionary of Plant Names for Gardeners. Cassell Pub, London, 1972
Stewart, Hilary. CEDAR. Douglas & McIntyre. Vancouver/Toronto, 1984.
Storl, Wolf D. Healing Lyme Disease Naturally. NorthAtlantic Books, Berkeley, CA 2010.
Strehlow,W & Hertzka,G. Hildegard of Bingen's Medicine Bear & Co. Santa Fe 1988
Stuart, David. Dangerous Garden. Harvard University Press, Cambridge, Mass. 2004
Sturdivant L.&Blakley,T. Medicinal Herbs in the Garden, Field and Marketplace Bootstrap
    Guide, San Juan Naturals, Friday Harbor,WA, 1999.
Sumner, Judith. The Natural History of Medicinal Plants. Timber Press, Oregon, 2000.

Swanton, J.R. Haida Texts and Myths. Bureau Am Ethnol, Bull #29. Smithsonian Inst. Washington, D.C. 1905.
_____ Bureau of Am Ethno 26th Ann Report. Smithsonian Inst. Washington, 1908.
Szczeklik, Andrzej. Kore: On Sickness, the Sick and the Search for the Soul of Medicine. Counterpoint Berkeley 2012.
Tainter, D& Grenis A, Spices and Seasonings , VCH Pubishers, New York, 1993.
Talalaj,S.& Czechowicz,A S. Herbal Remedies, Hill of Content Press, Melbourne, 1989
Taylor, Wm &Farnsworth,N. The Vinca Alkaloids, Marcel Dekker, New York, 1973.
Teeguarden, Ron. The Ancient Wisdom of the Chinese Tonic Herbs. Warner Bros. 1998.
Telesco, Patricia. The Victorian Flower Oracle, Llewellyn Pub. St. Paul 1994
Temple, Robert. The Genius of China. Simon and Schuster. New York. 1986.
Thompson, Gerry, Astral Sex to Zen Teabags. Findhorn Press, 1994.
Thoreau, Henry David. Wild Fruits. W. W. Norton & Co. New York, 2000.
Throop, Priscilla. Hildegard von Bingen's Physica. Healing Arts Press, Vt. 1998.
Tick, Edward. The Practice of Dream Healing. Quest Books Wheaton, Illinois, 2001.
Tierra, Michael. The Way of Herbs- revised Pocket Rooks, New York, 1998.
Tigner, Daniel. Canadian Forest Tree Essences, self published,1998. ISBN 0968365809
Tilford, Gregory. Edible and Medicinal Plants of the West. Mountain Press, Missoula 1997.
Timbrook, Jan. Chumash Ethnobotany. St. Barbara Mus, Heyday Books, Berkeley Ca 2007.
Traill, E.C. Studies of Plant Life in Canada. A. S. Woodburn, Ottawa, 1885.
Traill, C. P. The Backwoods of Canada. McClelland and Stewart. Toronto. 1846.
Tobyn, G., Denham, A., Whitelegg, M. The Western Herbal Tradition. 2000 years of medicinal herbal knowledge. Churchill Livingstone Toronto 2011.
Toop, Edgar W & Williams, Sara. Perennials for the Prairies. U of A&Saskatchewan. 1991.
Treben, Maria. Health Through God's Pharmacy. Wilhelm Ennsthaler. 1982.
Tresidder, Jack. Symbols and Their Meaning. Friedman/Fairfax Pub. 2007.
Tucker A. & DeBaggio,T. The Big Book of Herbs. Interweave Press. Loveland CO. 2000.
_____ The Encylcopedia of Herbs. Timber Press, Portland. 2009.
Turkington, Carol. The Home Health Guide to Poisons and Antidotes, Facts on File 1994
Turner, Nancy J. Food Plants of Interior First Peoples. UBC Press, Vancouver, 1997.
_____ Food Plants of Coastal First Peoples. UBC Press, Vancouver, 1995.
_____ Plant Technology of First Peoples in B.C. UBC Press, Vancouver, 1998.
_____ et al. Thompson Ethnobotany. Memoir #3, Royal B.C. Museum, 1996.
_____ Plants of Haida Gwaii. Sononis Press, Winlaw, B.C. 2004.
_____ The Earth's Blanket. Douglas & McIntyre. Vancouver. 2005.
Turner, N & von Aderkas, P. Common Poisonous Plants and Mushrooms. Timber Press 2009
Turner, W.B. Fungal Metabolites, Academic Press, London and New York, 1971.
Twitchell, Paul. Herbs The Magic Healers. Eckankar, Box 3100 Menlo Park, CA, 1986.
Vermeulen, Nico. Encyclopedia of Herbs. Whitecap Books, Vancouver B.C. 1998.
Viereck, Eleanor, G. Alaska's Wilderness Medicines. Alaska Northwest Pub. 1987
Vitt, Marsh and Bovey, Mosses, Lichens, and Ferns, Lone Pine Press, 1988.
Vogel, A. Swiss Nature Doctor. A. Vogel, Switzerland. 1952
_____ Nature-Your Guide to Healthy Living. Verlag A. Vogel, Teufen, Switzerland 1986.
Vogel, Virgil. American Indian Medicine, U. of Oklahoma Press, Norman, 1970
Walker, Barbara. The Woman's Dictionary of Symbols&Sacred Objects. Csstle Books, 1988.
Walker, Marilyn. Wild Plants of Eastern Canada. Nimbus Pub. Halifax NS. 2008.
Ward, Bobby J. The Plant Hunter's Garden. Timber Press, Portland. 2004.
Ward-Harris, Joan.More Than Meets the Eye, The Life and Lore of Western Wildflowers Oxford University Press, Toronto, 1983

Watanabe & Shibuya. Pharmacological Research on Traditional Herbal Medicines. Harwood Academic Publishers, 1999.

Watt, John, and Breyer-Brandwijk, Maria The Medicinal and Poisonous Plants of Southern and Eastern Africa . E and S. Livingstone. Edinburgh and London. 1962.

Watts, Donald. Elsevier's Dictionary of Plant Lore. Elsevier. 2007.

Waugh, F.W. Iroquois Foods and Food Preparation #12 Anthropological Series, Ottawa. 1916. Reprinted by Iroqrafts, RR #2, Ohsweken, Ontario N0A 1M0, 1991.

Weaver, Wm. 100 Vegetables & Where They Came From. Workman Pub. New York, 2000.

_____ Sauer's Herbal Cures America's First Book of Botanic Healing 1762-1778, Routledge, New York, 2001.

Weed, Susan. Menopausal Years, The Wise Woman Way. Ash Tree Pub. Woodstock NY, 1992

Weigle, Marta. Spiders and Spinsters. U. of New Mexico Press, Albuquerque, 1982.

Weiner, M. The People's Herbal, A family guide. Putnam Publishing, New York, 1984.

Weiss, Rudolf. Herbal Medicine. Beaconsfield Publishers, 1988.

_____ Herbal Medicine 2nd Edition. Thieme, Stuttgart, New York, 2000.

Wells, Diana.100 Flowers and How They Got Their Names, Algonquin Books, Chapel Hill,97

Westcott, Frank. The Beaver Nature's Master Builder. Hounslow Press, Willowdale, ON '89.

Westrich, LoLo, California Herbal Remedies, Gulf Pub Co. Houston, TX, 1989.

Wetzel, Suzanne et al. Bioproducts from Canada's Forests. Springer Netherlands 2006.

WHO monographs on selected medicinal plants, vol 1, 1999; vol 2, 2002.

White, Ian. Australian Bush Flower Essences. Bantam Books, 1991

White, Florence. Flowers as Food . Jonathan Cape. 1934

Whitmont, Edward. Psyche and Substance. North Atlantic Books. 1980

Wilkinson, Kathleen. Trees and Shrubs of Alberta. Lone Pine Books, Edmonton 1990.

_____ Wildflowers of Alberta. U of A/Lone Pine Books, Edmonton 1999.

Williams, Jude. Nature's Gentle Cures. Sterling Publishing. New York. 1997.

Williamson, Darcy. 130 Medicinal Plant Monographs of the NW. self pub. E-book. 2011.

Williamson, E. Major Herbs of Ayurveda. Churchill Livingstone, Elsevier Science, 2002.

Winston, David. Herbal Therapeutics. HT Research Library Broadway NJ 8th Ed 2003.

_____ & Maimes, S. Adaptogens: Herbs for Strength, Stamina and Stress Relief. Healing Arts Press, Rochester, Vermont 2007

Wolf, Adolf Hungry, Teachings of Nature/Good Med Book,#14 Box 844 Invermere 1975.

Wolfson, Evelyn. From the Earth to Beyond the Sky. Houghton Mifflin Co. Boston, 1993.

Wood, Matthew. The Book of Herbal Wisdom. North Atlantic Books, Berkeley, 1997.

_____ Seven Herbs: Plants as Teachers, North Atlantic, Berkeley, 1986.

_____ Vitalism, the history of Herbalism, etc. N. Atlantic, Berkeley 1992.

_____ The Practice of Traditional Western Herbalism. N. Atlantic, Berkeley 2004.

_____ The Earthwise Herbal. Two vols. North Atlantic, Berkeley, 2008 and 2009.

Wood, Rebecca. The New Whole Foods Encyclopedia, Penguin Arkana, New York, 1999.

Worwood, Valerie. The Fragrant Heavens. New World Library. Novato CA, 1999.

Wren, R.C. Potter's New Cyclopaedia of Botanical Drugs and Prep. C.W. Daniel, 1988.

Wright, Clarrisa D. Food What We Eat and How We Eat . Ebury Press, London, 2000.

Wu, Jing-Nuan. An Illustrated Chinese Materia Medica. Oxford U Press. New York 2005.

Wulf-Tilford M. & G. All You Ever Wanted to Know About Herbs for Pets. BowTie Press, 1999

Yance Jr, D. Herbal Medicine, Healing and Cancer. Keats Publishing, Chicago, 1999.

Yang Shou-zhong. The Divine Farmer's Materia Medica. Blue Poppy Pr, Boulder, Co 1998.

Yang Xinrong. Encyclo Reference of Traditional Chinese Medicine. Springer Berlin 2003.

Yarnell, Eric et al. Clinical Botanical Medicine. Mary Ann Liebart Pub. NY 2002.

Yeager, S et al. New Foods for Healing. Prevention Health Books, Rodale Press, 1998.

Ying, Jianzhe, et al. Icones of Medicinal Fungi from China. Science Press, Beijing 1987

Young David et al. Cry of the Eagle, Encounters with a Cree Healer, U of Toronto Press, '89

Young, Jane & Hawley, Alex. Plants and Medicines of Sophie Thomas. 2nd Ed. 2004.

Yun, Henry. Herbal Holistic Approach to Arthritis. Dominion College. 1988.

Zevin, Igor V. A Russian Herbal. Healing Arts Press, Rochester, Vermont. 1997

Zheleznova, Irina. Northern Lights, Fairy Tales of the Peoples of the North, Progress Publishers, 1976.

Zinmeister & Mues. Bryophytes-Their Chemistry... Clarendon Press, Oxford, 1990.

FLOWER ESSENCE RESOURCES

Aditi Himalaya Flower Essences, 15,Jaybharat Society, 3rd Road, Khar (W), Bombay 400 052, India.

Alaskan Flower Essence Project, P.O. Box. 1369, Homer, Alaska USA 99603-1369. www.alaskanessences.com.

Australian Bush Flower Essences. Australia. www.ausflowers.com.au.

Bach- Healing Herbs English Flower Essences- in Canada by Self Heal Distributing, Box 95008, Whyte Postal Outlet, Edmonton, AB T6E 0E5, 1800-593-5956 or www.selfhealdistributing.com Also www.healingherbs.co.uk or www.fesflowers.com

Bailey Flower Essences, 8 Neslon Road, Ilkley, West Yorkshire England, LS298HN. www.flowervr.com

Bloesem Remedies. Netherlands. www.bloesem-remedies.com

BrynaHerb Essences. www.brynaherbessences.uk

Canadian Forest Essences, PO Box 29128,1996 W. Broadway, Vancouver, BC V6J 1Z0

Canadian Forest Tree Essences. Ottawa. www.essences.ca. 613-725-9764.

Choming Flower Essences. www.mkprojects.com

Clear Path Essences. www.clearpathessences.com

Dancing Light Orchid Essences. Fairbanks, Alaska. www.orchidessences.com

Desert Alchemy, PO Box 44189, Tucson, Arizona, USA 85733. www.desert-alchemy.com.

Deva Flower Essences BP3 38880, Autrans, France. www.lab-deva.com

Eastern Flower Herbal Essences. julied@hfx.eastlink.ca.

Falling Leaf Essences. Box 78, Kallista, Victoria 3791, Australia. www.advancedalchemy.com.au.

Findhorn Flower Essences, Morayshire, Scotland IV36 0TY. www.findhornessences.com

Florais des Minas, Rua Albita, 194-Sala 408, Cruziero, CEP 30310-160,BH, MG, BRAZIL

FlorAlive®, Brent Davis. Contact info@floralive.com

FES Flower Essence Society, PO Box 1769, Nevada City, California, USA, 95959. www.fesflowers.com

Canadian Distributor- Self Heal Distributing, Box 95008, Whyte Postal Outlet, Edmonton, AB T6E 0E5 – www.selfhealdistributing.com

Green Hope Farm Flower Essences, PO Box 125, Meriden, New Hampshire USA 03770

Green Man Tree Essences. www.greenmantrees.demon.co.uk.

Habundia Flower Essences. c/o Peter Aziz. PO Box 90, Totnes, Devon, England TQ11 0YG.

Harebell Remedies. Scotland. ellie@harebellremedies.co.uk.

Hawaiian Gaia Flower Essences. www.gaiaessences.com

High Sierra Flower Essences. PO. Box 4275 Truclee, CA 96160.

holly.hsb@highoctavehealing.com

Horus Flower Essences- horus@floweressences.de.

Hummingbird Remedies, PO Box 50161, Eugene, Oregon, USA 97405

Icelandic Flower Essences. www.kristbjorb.is.

Jade Mountain Flower Essences, Box 125, Mountain Lakes, New Jersey USA 07046-0125

Korte Phi. www.PHIessences.com

Light Heart Essences. England. www.lightheartessences.co.uk.

Light Mountain Flower Essences, Michael A. Vertolli, 1-800-667-HERB.

Living Essences of Australia, Box 355, Scarborough, 6019, Perth, Australia. www.livingessences.com.au

Living Flower Essences, www.livingfloweressences.com . Rhonda Pallasdowney.

Master's Flower Essences, 14618 Tyler Foote Rd Nevada City, California, USA, 95959.
    www.masteressences.com
Miriana fortem Flower Essences. www.mirianaflowers.com and info@miraflowers.com.
naturaSacredplay, PO Box 32, Buckhorn, New Mexico, 88025, (505-535-2255).
New Millenium Flower Essences of New Zealand. info@nmessences.com.
New Zealand New Perception Flower Essences, PO Box 60-127,Titirangi, Auckland 7, NZ
Pacific Essences, Box 8317, Victoria, B.C. V8W 3R9. www.pacificessences.com.
Pegasus Products, PO Box 228, Boulder, Colorado, USA 80306-0228. 1-800- 527-6104.
Perelandra, Box 3603, Warrenton, VA. 22186. www.perelandra-ltd.com
Petite Fleur Essence, 8524 Whispering Creek Trail, Fort Worth, Texas, USA 76134.
    www.aromahealthtexas.com
Prairie Deva Flower Essences, Box 95008, Whyte Postal Outlet, Edmonton, AB T6E 0E5
    1-(780) 433-7882. www.selfhealdistributing.com
Ravenworks- joni@ravenworksministries.org
Running Fox Farm PO Box 381,Worthington, Maryland USA 01098
Star Peruvian Flower Essences. Santa Barbara. www.starfloweressences.com
Stars of the Meadow, David Dalton, Lindisfarne Books, Mass. 2006.
Sun Essences. Norfolk, England. www.sunessence.co.uk
Sweetwater Sanctuary Essences. www.plantspirithealing.com
Tree Frog Farm Flower Essences. www.treefrogfarm.com
Whole Energy Essences, PO Box 285, Concord, Mass. 01742
Wild Rose Essences. www.wildrose.com
Woodland Essence, PO Box 206, Cold Brook, New York, USA 13324.

7232178R10188

Printed in Great Britain
by Amazon.co.uk, Ltd.,
Marston Gate.